Gastroenterology

CLINICAL CASES UNCOVERED

Satish Keshav

MBBCh (Wits), DPhil (Oxon), FRCP (London)

Consultant Gastroenterologist and Honorary
Senior Lecturer
Translational Gastroenterology Unit
Nuffield Department of Medicine
John Radcliffe Hospital
Oxford

Emma Culver

MBChB, BSc (Hons), MRCP

Gastroenterology Registrar and Academic
Research Fellow
Gastroenterology Department
Nuffield Department of Medicine
John Radcliffe Hospital
Oxford

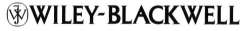
WILEY-BLACKWELL

A John Wiley & Sons, Ltd., Publication

Library of Congress Cataloging-in-Publication Data

Keshav, Satish.
   Gastroenterology / Satish Keshav, Emma Culver.
     p. ; cm. – (Clinical cases uncovered)
   Includes bibliographical references and indexes.
   ISBN 978-1-4051-6975-2 (pbk. : alk. paper)
  1.   Gastroenterology–Case studies. 2.   Digestive organs–Diseases–Case studies. I. Culver, Emma. II. Title. III. Series: Clinical cases uncovered.
   [DNLM: 1.   Digestive System Diseases–diagnosis–Case Reports. 2.   Digestive System Diseases–diagnosis–Problems and Exercises. WI 18.2]
   RC808.K47 2011
   616.3′3–dc22
                    2010039153

Set in 9/12 pt Minion by Toppan Best-set Premedia Limited
Printed and bound in Singapore by Markono Print Media Pte Ltd

1 2011

Contents

Preface, vii

How to use this book, viii

List of abbreviations, ix

(**Part 1**) **Basics, 1**

Basic science, 1

Approach to the patient, 14

(**Part 2**) **Cases, 29**

Upper gastrointestinal

Case 1 A 61-year-old woman with progressive dysphagia, 29

Case 2 A 52-year-old man with atypical chest pain, 34

Case 3 A 57-year-old woman with upper abdominal discomfort, 40

Case 4 A 36-year-old man with upper abdominal discomfort and heartburn, 45

Case 5 A 27-year-old woman with nausea and vomiting, 51

Case 6 A 73-year-old man with haematemesis and melaena, 56

Case 7 A 68-year-old woman with fatigue, weight loss and altered bowel habit, 63

Lower gastrointestinal

Case 8 A 23-year-old woman with constipation, 69

Case 9 A 24-year-old woman with chronic diarrhoea, 74

Case 10 A 51-year-old woman with acute nausea, vomiting and diarrhoea, 80

Case 11 A 79-year-old woman with altered bowel habit and weight loss, 85

Case 12 A 54-year-old man with rectal bleeding, 90

Case 13 A 66-year-old woman with anaemia, 95

Liver disease

Case 14 A 64-year-old man with abnormal liver function tests, 100

Case 15 A 45-year-old man with acute jaundice, 109

Case 16 A 53-year-old woman with jaundice and abnormal liver tests, 115

Case 17 A 53-year-old man with abdominal swelling, 120

Case 18 A 36-year-old man who drinks alcohol, 125

Biliary and pancreatic disease

Case 19 A 79-year-old man with right upper quadrant colicky abdominal discomfort, 131

Case 20 A 19-year-old man with acute abdominal pain, 136

Nutrition

Case 21 A 35-year-old woman with anorexia, 143

Case 22 A 48-year-old man with an increased body mass index, 148

Functional disorders

Case 23 A 21-year-old student with chronic abdominal pain, 153

(**Part 3**) **Self-assessment, 159**

MCQs, 159

EMQs, 162

SAQs, 166

Answers, 167

Further reading, 173

Index of cases by diagnosis, 175

Index, 177

The colour plate section can be found facing p.54.

Preface

Clinical gastroenterology is both simple and complex. The simplicity comes from the finite number of diagnoses that are commonly encountered, and the relatively limited number of symptoms that typically indicate disease of the gastrointestinal system. However, there are hidden depths to the practice of the speciality. Gastroenterologists deal with disease affecting many separate organs that all form part of the same system – the liver, pancreas, stomach, etc. The clinical consequences of some diseases can be dramatic and complex, particularly, for instance, dysfunction of the liver. Symptoms such as abdominal pain, altered bowel function and changes in weight can be combined in myriad ways to pose true clinical puzzles. This book aims to guide the reader through this complexity by offering real case studies and showing how, in practice, clinicians can achieve some degree of clarity, and offer to patients a reasonable diagnostic and therapeutic plan.

In the first section, the book offers a basic and brief overview of anatomical, physiological and pharmacological facts that inform our thinking about gastroenterological problems, and suggests how best to approach the patient in the second chapter. Thereafter, in the second section, each chapter deals with presenting symptoms and signs and the subsequent chapters are arranged in six sections to cover disease processes affecting the upper gastrointestinal tract, lower gastrointestinal tract, liver, pancreas and biliary tract, nutrition, and so-called functional bowel disorders. These are important and often overlooked because there is a profound lack of understanding about their pathogenesis. However, there are many patients with irritable bowel syndrome and the like, and a robust and reliable clinical approach to treating them is essential.

In each of the symptom- or sign-based chapters, the emphasis is on clinical reasoning and strategy, and the reader will have an opportunity to examine how the many possible paths are in practice negotiated to reach a diagnosis and formulate a plan for managing the situation. Exact doses and tests are de-emphasised, while strategies, categories and context are highlighted, all within the framework of dealing with the particular human patient whose predicament is being examined.

Boxes and lists are strategically placed to aid memory and recall, and to emphasise key facts. The last section, which comprises a set of questions to test understanding, is based on the contents of each chapter, and the emphasis in these is on core knowledge rather than the esoteric or arcane.

Writing this book has proved to be an education as well being hugely enjoyable, and our hope is that the reader too will gain knowledge and understanding of the complexity of gastroenterological medicine, whilst acquiring some practical understanding of how to approach the patient with gastrointestinal problems, and some sense of satisfaction and fun. The typical reader might be a medical or nursing student in their clinical years, or a doctor in training, either in their foundation years or in early speciality training. The book will be useful as preparatory reading before joining the gastroenterology firm in a clinical rotation, or as an aid to revision before written and clinical examinations.

Satish Keshav
Emma Culver

How to use this book

Clinical Cases Uncovered (CCU) books are carefully designed to help supplement your clinical experience and assist with refreshing your memory when revising. Each book is divided into three sections: Part 1, Basics; Part 2, Cases; and Part 3, Self-assessment.

Part 1 gives you a quick reminder of the basic science, history and examination, and key diagnoses in the area. Part 2 contains many of the clinical presentations you would expect to see on the wards or to crop up in exams, with questions and answers leading you through each case. New information, such as test results, is revealed as events unfold and each case concludes with a handy case summary explaining the key points. Part 3 allows you to test your learning with several question styles (MCQs, EMQs and SAQs), each with a strong clinical focus.

Whether reading individually or working as part of a group, we hope you will enjoy using your CCU book. If you have any recommendations on how we could improve the series, please do let us know by contacting us at: medicalstudent@wiley.co.uk.

Disclaimer

CCU patients are designed to reflect real life, with their own reports of symptoms and concerns. Please note that all names used are entirely fictitious and any similarity to patients, alive or dead, is coincidental.

List of abbreviations

ACE	angiotensin-converting enzyme		G6PD	glucose-6 phosphate dehydrogenase
ADH	antidiuretic hormone		GTN	glyceral trinitrate
AFP	α-fetoprotein		HBcAb	hepatitis B core antibody
AIDS	acquired immune deficiency syndrome		HBeAb	hepatitis B 'e' antibody
AIH	autoimmune hepatitis		HBeAg	hepatitis B 'e' antigen
ALP	alkaline phosphatase		HBsAb	hepatitis B surface antibody
ALT	alanine aminotransferase		HBsAg	hepatitis B surface antigen
AMA	antimitochondrial antibody		HBV	hepatitis B virus
ANAs	antinuclear antibodies		HCC	hepatocellular carcinoma
anti-SMAs	anti-smooth muscle antibodies		HCV	hepatitis C virus
ARDS	acute respiratory distress syndrome		HCVAb	hepatitis C antibody
5-ASA	5-aminosalicylates		HHC	hereditary haemochromatosis
ASCA	anti-*Saccharomyces cerevisiae* antibody		HIV	human immunodeficiency virus
AST	aspartate aminotransferase		HLA	human leukocyte antigen
β-HCG	beta-human chorionic gonadotrophin		H_2RA	H_2-receptor antagonist
BCG	bacille Calmette–Guérin (vaccine)		HUS	haemolytic uraemic syndrome
BMI	body mass index		IBD	inflammatory bowel disease
BSG	British Society of Gastroenterology		IBS	irritable bowel syndrome
CBD	common bile duct		IgA	immunoglobulin A
CMV	cytomegalovirus		INR	international normalised ratio
COPD	chronic obstructive airways disease		JVP	jugular venous pressure
CRP	C-reactive protein		LDH	lactate dehydrogenase
CT	computed tomography		LDL	low density lipoprotein
CXR	chest X-ray		LFTs	liver function tests
DEXA	dual energy X-ray absorptiometric scan		LKMAs	liver–kidney microsomal antibodies
DIC	disseminated intravascular coagulation		MALT	mucosal-associated lymphoid tissue
DRE	digital rectal exam		MCV	mean corpuscular volume
EBV	Epstein–Barr virus		mDF	Maddrey's discriminant function
ECG	electrocardiogram		MDT	multidisciplinary team
ERCP	endoscopic retrograde cholangiopancreatography		MHC	major histocompatibility complex
			MRCP	magnetic resonance cholangiopancreatography
EUS	endoscopic ultrasound			
FDA	Food and Drug Agency of the USA		MRI	magnetic resonance imaging
FDG	fluorodeoxyglucose		NAFLD	non-alcoholic fatty liver disease
FOB	faecal occult blood		NASH	non-alcoholic steatohepatitis
γ-GT	gamma glutamyl transferase		NSAIDs	non-steroidal anti-inflammatory drugs
GAHS	Glasgow alcoholic hepatitis score		PBC	primary biliary cirrhosis
GI	gastrointestinal		PCR	polymerase chain reaction
GORD	gastro-oesophageal reflux disease		PDH	pyruvate dehydrogenase

PET	positron emission tomography	TNF-α	tumour necrosis factor α
PPI	protein pump inhibitor	TSH	thyroid-stimulating hormone
PT	prothrombin time	tTG	tissue transglutaminase
SA-AG	serum ascites–albumin gradient	TTP	thrombotic thrombocytopenic purpura
SIRS	systemic inflammatory response syndrome	VIP	vasoactive intestinal peptide
T_3	tri-iodothyronine	vWF	von Willebrand factor
T_4	thyroxine	WBC	white blood cell count
TIBC	total iron-binding capacity		
TIPSS	transjugular intrahepatic portal-systemic shunt		

Basic science

Introduction

The intestinal tract is essential for maintaining nutrition by appropriate intake of macronutrients, micronutrients, fluid and electrolytes. Intestinal failure can lead to nutritional catastrophe and imbalances in fluid and electrolytes.

The pancreas is the main producer of digestive enzymes that facilitate the extraction of nutrients from food. Pancreatic dysfunction can cause malabsorption of food.

The liver has an essential and central role in metabolism, critical functions in detoxifying and excreting endogenous and exogenous molecules in bile, and in synthesising essential serum proteins such as albumin and clotting factors. Liver failure is rapidly fatal.

Embryology

The entire intestinal tract is derived embryologically from the endoderm, and can be conceptualized as a hollow tube stretching from the mouth to the anus, with the liver and pancreas as gland-like specialised appendages, connected to the main tract by ducts.

Structure

The main intestinal tract has a basic structure that is preserved throughout:
• The innermost layer, facing the hollow lumen, is lined by a specialised layer of epithelial cells that vary from region to region.
• The epithelium is supported by a layer of connective tissue, the lamina propria.
• The lamina propria is surrounded by a layer of smooth muscle, the muscularis mucosae.
• The muscularis is surrounded by the submucosal connective tissue.

Gastroenterology: Clinical Cases Uncovered, 1st edition.
© S. Keshav and E. Culver. Published 2011 by
Blackwell Publishing Ltd.

• Outside of this are strong layers of muscle, the muscularis propria. This is generally organised in an inner circular layer with fibres running at right angles to the long axis of the tube, and an outer longitudinal layer with fibres running along the long axis.
• The outermost layer of much of the intestinal tract is the visceral peritoneum, which is an epithelial layer.

Most lengths of the small and large intestine are attached to the posterior wall of the abdominal cavity by a length of mesentery, which is comprised of connective tissue covered by a continuation of the visceral peritoneal layer, and through which blood and lymphatic vessels and nerves run.

Blood supply

The arterial blood supply to the intra-abdominal intestinal organs, from stomach to rectum, and including the liver and pancreas, is derived from the coeliac, superior mesenteric and inferior mesenteric arteries, which are direct branches of the abdominal aorta.

The venous drainage of most of the intra-abdominal organs is via the hepatic portal vein, which enters the liver, and provides 75% of the hepatic blood supply. This hepatic portal flow system means that absorbed nutrients first enter the liver, before reaching the systemic circulation.

Nerve supply

Most of the gastrointestinal tract is innervated by the autonomic nervous system with parasympathetic and sympathetic branches. The intestine also contains an intrinsic nervous system organised into interconnected plexuses in the submucosa and the muscularis propria, which is termed the enteric nervous system. This provides isolated segments of intestine with the ability to coordinate secretion and motility without external innervation.

Immune system

The intestinal tract encounters food particles, antigens and potentially harmful microorganisms constantly.

Arguably, it must contend with the greatest challenge in defending the organism against infection and other danger, as unlike other areas exposed to the external world, such as the skin and lungs, it also has to make fine distinctions between substances that could be either essential food or lethal foe – 'salmon or *Salmonella*?'.

As a consequence, the immune system of the gastrointestinal tract is highly developed and specialised, and contains approximately 70% of all the immune cells in the body.

Anatomy and function
The intestinal tract
Mouth, pharynx and oesophagus

The mouth with teeth, tongue and salivary glands is essential for ingestion of food and nutrition. The senses of taste and smell serve to identify healthy food, and coordinated activity of the muscles of mastication, the tongue and pharynx allow food to be processed and swallowed safely.

The mouth, pharynx and oesophagus are all lined by a stratified squamous epithelium. The muscle layers of the

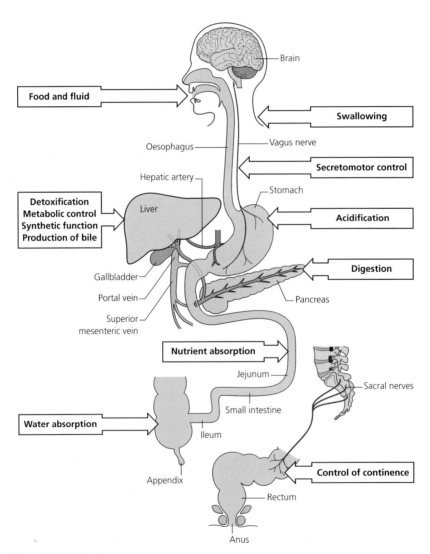

Fig. A Overview of gastrointestinal function.

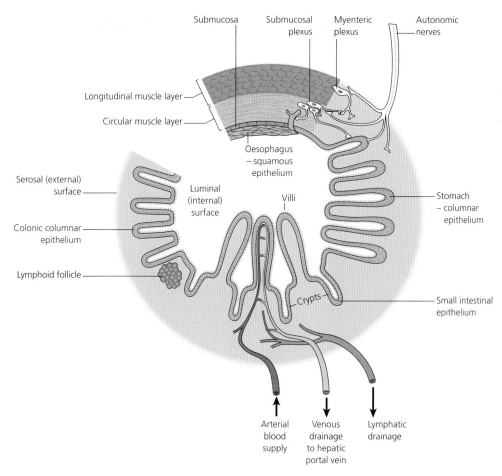

Fig. B Organisation of the hollow organs.

upper oesophagus are striated skeletal-type muscle, while the muscle layers of the distal oesophagus, like the rest of the intestinal tract, comprise smooth, non-striated fibres.

Stomach

The stomach is J-shaped, wider at the proximal, upper end, known as the body, and narrowing distally to form the antrum, from which the pylorus leads to the duodenum. This shape means that the stomach can act as a reservoir for food after a meal. Strong churning movements of the stomach convert solid food boluses from the oesophagus into slurry called chyme, which passes easily into the duodenum.

The gastric epithelial lining is comprised of a single layer of columnar cells, which is also the case for the rest of the intestinal tract distal to the stomach. In the stomach this epithelial layer is specialised to produce hydrochloric acid from parietal cells, via a specialized K^+/H^+ transporter, popularly known as the proton pump. This initiates the process of digestion by activating the enzyme pepsinogen, produced by oxyntic cells in the gastric epithelim.

Duodenum

Anatomy

The epithelium of the duodenum is specialised for absorption, comprising a single layer of columnar cells that are lined with microscopic microvilli to increase the surface area for absorption. Furthermore, specialised molecules on the cell surface, including transporters and enzymes, are critically important for this digestive and absorptive function.

The lining of the duodenum, like the rest of the small intestine, is arranged into finger-like projections into the lumen, called villi, which serve to increase the surface area, and indentations into the wall of the intestine, called crypts. The stem cells, from which the entire epithelial lining is renewed, approximately every 7 days, are located in the crypts. The stem cells provide, by division and differentiation, all the major cells of the intestinal lining; these include:

- Absorptive enterocytes.
- Goblet cells, which produce mucus.
- Paneth cells, which have a role in antibacterial defence.
- Neuroendocrine cells, which produce a variety of enteric hormones such as somatostatin, cholecystokinin, gastrin, vasoactive intestinal peptide (VIP) and glucacon-like peptides.

Function

Bile from the gallbladder, and pancreatic secretions enter the duodenum through the ampulla of Vater, providing bicarbonate-rich alkaline secretions, bile salts to emulsify fats, and carbohydrate, protein and fat-digesting enzymes, which neutralise acid chyme from the stomach, and begin the major work of digestion. Thus the duodenum is a crucial region for digestion and absorption.

Jejunum and ileum
Anatomy

The basic structure of the distal small intestine is identical to the duodenum, with villi, crypts, submucosa and circular and longitudinal muscle layers.

Blood and lymphatic supply

The blood supply is from the superior mesenteric artery. The venous drainage is via the superior mesenteric vein, joining the splenic vein to form the hepatic portal vein, which enters the liver carrying nutrients from the small intestine.

The lymphatic drainage of the small intestine, which carries fat-rich particles absorbed from food, enters the thoracic duct, emptying into the systemic venous circulation. The smallest lymph channels, called lacteals, are found in the central core of each villus, strategically placed to absorb triglyceride-rich chylomicrons.

Function

These segments of the small intestine are essential for absorbing food. The minimum length of small intestine necessary to sustain life is approximately 100 cm, and the function of this minimum length is enhanced if the ileocaecal valve is intact.

There is some regional specialisation – the jejunum is the main site of absorption of folic acid, and the ileum is essential for the absorption of vitamin B_{12} and of bile salts, which are recycled via an enterohepatic circulation.

> **Box A Specialisation in the small bowel**
>
> - Ileum: absorption of vitamin B_{12} and bile salts
> - Jejunum: absorption of folic acid

Constant peristaltic activity of the small intestine, including a daily migrating motor complex wave that clears the intestine, together with many antibacterial substances secreted into the intestine, keep the number of bacteria in the small intestine relatively low, certainly compared to the large intestine. This may be important for optimum absorption of nutrients, and, in certain pathological conditions, bacterial overgrowth in the small intestine can cause diarrhoea and malabsorption.

The large intestine
Anatomy

The basic structure of the large intestine is similar to the small intestine. The differences are:

- The external longitudinal layer of smooth muscle in the large intestine is collected into bands called taenia.
- There are no villi in the large intestine.

The ileum enters the caecum, which is the most proximal part of the large intestine, via the ileocaecal valve, which partially prevents the reflux of bacteria into the small intestine. Distal to the caecum is the ascending colon, situated along the right flank, the transverse colon extending from just below the liver to just below the spleen, the descending colon situated along the left flank, the sigmoid colon curving over the pelvic brim, and the rectum which is situated in front of the sacrum and ends at the junction of rectum and anus.

The anus is the muscular sphincter that maintains the continence of faeces and flatus in the rectum, and is comprised of an inner layer of smooth muscle, the internal sphincter, and an outer layer of voluntary muscle, the external sphincter. The lining of the anus is a stratified squamous epithelium that blends into the skin at the anal verge.

Box B Structural components of the large intestine (proximal to distal)

- Ileocaecal valve
- Caecum
- Ascending colon
- Hepatic flexure
- Transverse colon
- Splenic flexure
- Descending colon
- Sigmoid colon
- Rectum
- Anus

Blood supply

The vascular supply of the colon is derived from the superior and inferior mesenteric arteries, and the venous drainage is via the superior and inferior mesenteric veins. The venous return from the rectum is into the systemic circulation so that portosystemic shunts can form in this region, as they can in the distal oesophagus.

Nerve supply

Defecation is controlled by both autonomic and somatic nerves, and the nerve supply of the rectum is from the sacral plexus.

Function

The main function of the large intestine is to reabsorb water from the small intestinal effluent. When patients undergo a colectomy and are left with an ileostomy, fluid losses from the stoma can be of the order of litres per day; this is in contrast to the normal volume of faecal output, which is approximately 200 mL.

Specialised cells

The main epithelial cells, colonocytes, are specialised for the absorption of electrolytes and water, and there are many goblet cells and few or no Paneth cells in the crypts of the colon.

Hepatobiliary system and pancreas
Liver
Anatomy

The liver is the largest single organ in the body at approximately 1.5 kg in weight. It is located in the right upper quadrant of the abdomen, directly under the right hemidiaphragm. The arterial supply is via the hepatic branch of the celiac artery, and the portal vein. The venous drainage via the hepatic veins is into the inferior vena cava.

The secretory product of the liver, bile, is excreted via biliary canaliculi that coalesce to form bile ducts. The bile ducts in turn form the main intrahepatic bile ducts, which form the hepatic duct. This is joined by the cystic duct from the gallbladder, which has the capacity to store and concentrate bile, to form the common bile duct. This exits the liver, and is joined by the main pancreatic duct before entering the duodenum at the ampulla of Vater.

Box C Functions of the liver

- Amino acid synthesis
- Carbohydrate metabolism (gluconeogenesis, glycogenolysis, glycogenesis)
- Protein metabolism, synthesis and degradation
- Lipid metabolism, cholesterol synthesis and lipogenesis
- Coagulation factor production (fibrinogen, prothrombin) and protein C, protein S and antithrombin
- Albumin production
- Angiotensinogen synthesis (hormone raising blood pressure if activated by renin)
- Bile production and excretion
- Immunological effects via the reticuloendothelial system
- Storage of glucose (as glycogen) and vitamins
- Detoxification, converting ammonia to urea
- Breakdown of toxic substances
- Breakdown of haemoglobin, insulin and other hormones
- Excretion of waste products

Function

The liver is the main organ of metabolic control, maintaining circulating levels of glucose and fats, and providing essential circulating proteins such as albumin, carrier proteins and a number of clotting factors and complement components. The liver also receives almost the entire venous drainage of the intestinal tract, performing an essential regulatory and detoxifying role. When this circulation is disrupted, patients suffer consequences such as severe neurological dysfunction, which can lead to coma and death, known as hepatic encephalopathy. In addition, the liver metabolises and is essential for the excretion of endogenous and exogenous waste products such as bilirubin derived from the breakdown of haem, and of ammonia from the breakdown of amino acids, which is excreted in the form of urea.

Without the liver, life cannot be sustained for more than a few hours, and there is as yet no adequate artificial liver substitute.

Specialised cells

The liver is composed of a huge number of hepatocytes, which are arranged in columns and sheets with intervening channels through which blood courses, known as sinusoids; between adjacent hepatocytes are the microscopic biliary canaliculi into which bile is secreted. The sinusoids are lined by an endothelial cell layer that, unlike vascular endothelia in other organs, is relatively loosely organised, with many gaps in the lining.

Between the vascular endothelium and the hepatocytes is the space of Disse in which specialised stellate cells of the liver are located. These cells store retinoic acid and have a critical function in repairing liver injury and forming scar tissue that can lead to hepatic cirrhosis. Immune cells including lymphocytes and resident hepatic macrophages known as Kupffer cells reside in the sinusoidal and peri-sinusoidal spaces.

Hepatocytes are specialised to process, store and export sugars, fats and proteins, and to metabolise and detoxify endogenous and exogenous organic compounds. Typical ultrastructural features of hepatocytes include numerous mitochondria, extensive rough and smooth endoplasmic reticulum, Golgi apparatus, fat-filled vacuoles and glycogen-storage granules.

Pancreas

Anatomy

The pancreas is a large exocrine secretory organ located in the epigastrium, inferior to the stomach and to the left of the duodenum. The pancreas also contains endocrine islets that produce the essential hormones insulin and glucagon, which maintain glucose homeostasis.

The exocrine pancreas comprises secretory epithelial cells organised into acini, with the secretions draining into ducts. These ducts coalesce to form the main pancreatic duct; this drains into the duodenum at the ampulla of Vater.

Function

Pancreatic secretions provide the great bulk of digestive enzymes, including proteases, lipases and amylases. The pancreas also produces HCO_3^- to neutralise stomach acid and create the optimal pH for digestive action.

Pancreatic enzymes have the capacity to cause autodigestion of the gland itself, and of intestinal tissues. Enzymes are therefore produced as larger proteins, known as pro-enzymes that are inactive; they are activated by cleavage after they have been secreted into ducts and the intestine.

Damage to the pancreas, which may release enzymes into the gland itself, can cause severe damage and a life threatening condition – acute pancreatitis. Diseases that damage the pancreatic capacity to produce enzymes, such as chronic pancreatitis, reduce the digestive capacity and cause malabsorption of fats, carbohydrates and proteins.

Digestion and absorption

The intestine is essential for processing and obtaining nutrition from food, regulating metabolism, and maintaining aspects of fluid and electrolyte balance. This is mediated by integrated action of all parts of the gastrointestinal tract, including the luminal organs from oesophagus to colon, and the pancreas and liver.

Digestion

Mechanical dissolution of food after chewing and swallowing is continued by the stomach, producing slurry known as chyme. The smaller the particles of food, the greater the surface area to volume ratio, providing a more tractable target for digestive enzymes including those produced by the pancreas and secreted into the duodenum. Fat is poorly soluble in the aqueous chyme, and bile salts secreted in bile help to disseminate fat from the diet into micelles, allowing greater access for fat-digesting enzymes. Thus obstruction to bile flow compromises the digestion and absorption of fats and fat-soluble vitamins such as D and K.

Digestion is the process of enzyme-mediated hydrolysis of macromolecules such as starch, triglycerides and proteins in food. The products of digestion are the constitutive components of these macromolecules – monosaccharides, free fatty acids, amino acids and short peptides – which are absorbed through the intestinal epithelium into the vascular and lymphatic circulation via specific transporter proteins. These transporters typically have exquisite specificity, for example for glucose coupled with Na^+ ions, or fructose, or acidic, basic and neutral amino acids.

Fatty acids absorbed from the diet are reconstituted in the epithelial cells into triglycerides and are secreted into lacteals as chylomicrons, for transport into the circulation. Other transport systems are responsible for the transport of micronutrients, that is, mineral

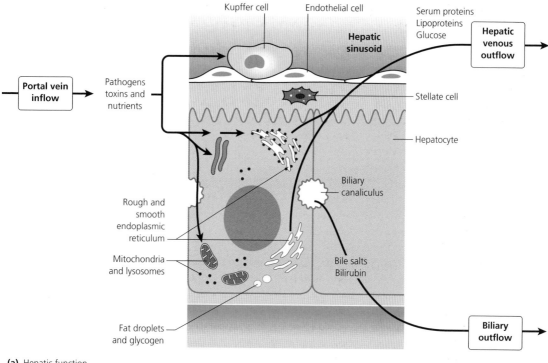

(a) Hepatic function

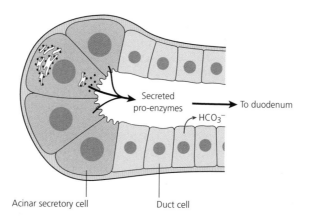

(b) Pancreatic exocrine acinus

Fig. C Hepatobiliary and pancreatic function.

elements and vitamins. These systems are regionally distributed, so that, for example, most absorption of iron occurs in the duodenum, while absorption of vitamin B_{12} occurs in the terminal ileum. Damage to the intestinal epithelium in different regions may therefore produce distinct patterns of malabsorption and deficiency.

Reabsorption

Digestive enzymes are secreted in large quantities of fluid and electrolytes, and if all of the secreted electrolytes and fluids were not reabsorbed the body would be depleted. Some reabsorption takes place in the distal small intestine; however the greatest capacity is in the colon, and the ileal effluent of over 1 L of fluid per day is reduced to

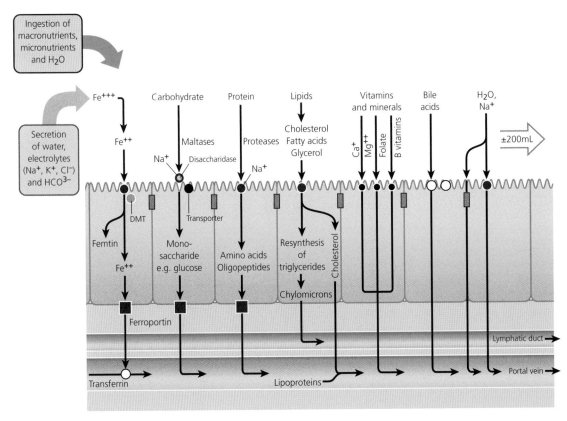

Fig. D Digestion and absorption.

approximately 200 mL. Reabsorption of water is accompanied by the reabsorption of salts, particularly Na^+, Cl^- and HCO_3^-.

Diarrhoeal illness

In diarrhoeal illnesses, the overall volume of stool is increased. It is possible to distinguish if this is due to one of the following processes:
- Hypersecretion, for example caused by cholera toxin, which activates secretion from intestinal epithelial cells.
- Inflammation, where secretion may be stimulated and the reabsorptive capacity of the intestine is compromised.
- Osmotic diarrhoea, whereby osmotically active substances in the intestinal content prevent reabsorption of water by creating a steep osmotic pressure gradient.
- Hypermotility, where increased peristalsis results in a rapid transit of intestinal contents through the intestine, exceeding the rate at which fluid can be reabsorbed.

Because absorption of water from the intestine follows electrolytes and osmotically active molecules such as sugars, diarrhoeal losses can be counteracted by providing luminal salt and sugar in the correct proportions. This is the basis of oral rehydration solutions to combat diarrhoea, which typically provide Na^+ and glucose to exploit the Na^+/glucose transporter. Hypotonic fluids such as plain water dilute the luminal Na^+ and reduce the capacity for absorption of water.

Gastrointestinal pathology
Infection

Gastrointestinal infection accounts for a major part of morbidity and mortality worldwide. Simple enteric infections, food poisoning and gastroenteritis, and specific infections such as cholera, which occur in outbreaks following the ingestion of contaminated food and water, can cause severe illness and death, particularly in the very young and the elderly and frail. Lack of sanitation and

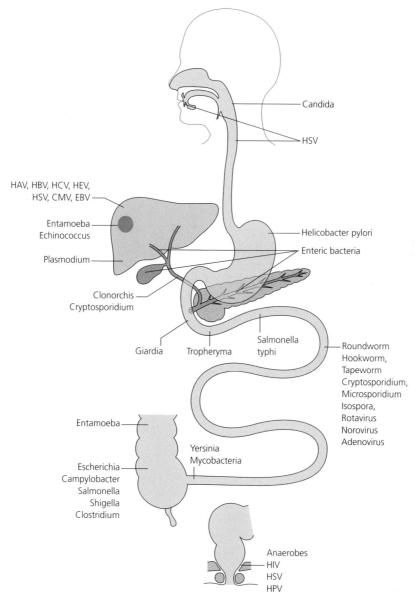

Candida

HSV

HAV, HBV, HCV, HEV, HSV, CMV, EBV

Entamoeba
Echinococcus

Plasmodium

Helicobacter pylori

Enteric bacteria

Clonorchis
Cryptosporidium

Giardia   Tropheryma   Salmonella typhi

Roundworm
Hookworm,
Tapeworm
Cryptosporidium,
Microsporidium
Isospora,
Rotavirus
Norovirus
Adenovirus

Entamoeba

Escherichia
Campylobacter
Salmonella
Shigella
Clostridium

Yersinia
Mycobacteria

Anaerobes
HIV
HSV
HPV

Fig. E Infections of the gastrointestinal tract.

reliable, safe drinking water, coupled with inadequate basic health care in poor regions of the world mean that gastroenteritis and diarrhoeal illness causes over 1 million excess deaths in childhood worldwide.

Gastroenteritis

Gastroenteritis is usually self-limiting. However, gastroenteritis can lead to dehydration that may cause death; and malnutrition and enfeeblement, where social circumstances and health care are inadequate, predispose to illnesses such as pneumonia. Agents that cause gastroenteritis include the following:

• Viruses such as rotavirus, adenovirus and norovirus.
• Bacteria such as *Escherichia coli*, *Campylobacter*, *Shigella* and *Vibrio cholerae*.
• Parasites such as amoeba can cause dysentery, while others such as round worms, tapeworms and hookworms infest the intestine and cause chronic intestinal disease,

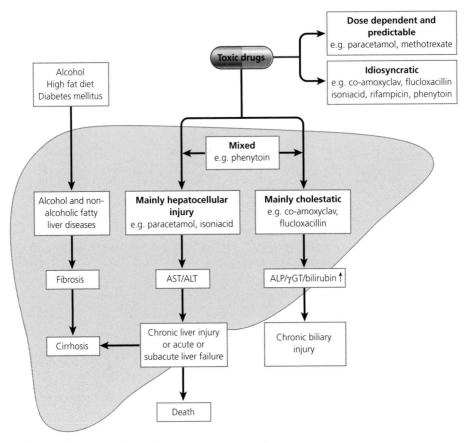

Fig. F Drugs and toxins in the gastrointestinal tract.

malnutrition and iron deficiency by chronic low-volume bleeding.

Helicobacter pylori infection

Helicobacter pylori is a bacteria that is specialised for colonising the gastric mucosa, where it secretes a urease enzyme that locally neutralises gastric hydrochloric acid by hydrolysing urea to CO_2 and NH_4. Approximately 80% of the world's population is chronically infected with *H. pylori*, although the proportion is lower in rich countries with high standards of hygiene. Infection with *H. pylori* predisposes individuals to gastritis, peptic ulceration and stomach cancer – links that were discovered by Drs Warren and Marshall, leading to their winning the Nobel Prize for Medicine in 2005.

H. pylori infection can now be detected and is readily eradicated by a combination of acid suppression and antibiotics.

Viral infections

Viral infections, particularly by the hepatitis viruses A, B, C and E, are a major cause of liver disease. Hepatitis A and E cause acute hepatitis that is usually self-limiting, although patients may be quite ill with malaise and jaundice. Hepatitis viruses C and B cause chronic hepatitis that can progress to cirrhosis and liver cancer. Both forms of chronic viral hepatitis can now be treated with antiviral drugs.

Toxic damage
Alcohol

Alcohol is a major cause of liver disease as well as other illness. Chronic excessive use of alcohol causes chronic liver damage; the healing process, which includes regeneration of liver cells in the form of nodules rather than well-ordered plates and sheets, and fibrotic scarring, can lead to cirrhosis.

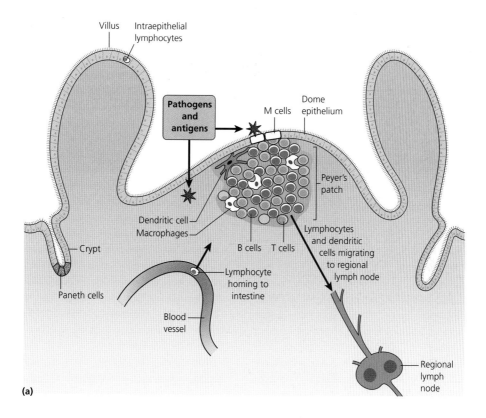

(a)

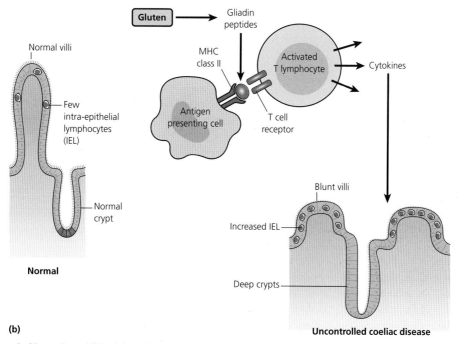

(b)

Fig. G (a) Intestinal immunity and (b) autoimmunity.

Medications

The liver is also readily damaged by a whole range of medical drugs, many of which have a tendency to cause a typical pattern of injury:

• Cholestasis may be due to flucloxacillin, co-amoxiclav and chlorpromazine, which damage the biliary epithelium.
• Acute liver damage may be due to antituberculosis drugs and anticonvulsants, which can mimic viral hepatitis.
• Massive necrosis of the liver may be caused by an overdose of the widely used analgesic paracetamol (acetaminophen). This can lead to acute liver failure, and is a medical emergency.

Autoimmune damage

Immune-mediated damage to the gastrointestinal system is a major cause of luminal disease, liver disease and in some cases pancreatic disease. The aetiology of the major immune-mediated diseases of the intestine remain unknown, although recent advances, particularly in genetic and immunological research, suggest a critical role for the innate immune system and the relation of the host to microorganisms that reside in the intestinal lumen.

Coeliac disease

One of the major immune-mediated diseases of the intestine is coeliac disease, which is caused by an inherited predisposition to react adversely to peptides derived from the digestion of gluten in cereals such as wheat, barley and rye. This affects as many as 1:100 people in parts of Europe and is associated with inheritance of the HLA-DQ2 allele in the MHC (major histocompatibility complex) class II locus.

In people with coeliac disease, gliadin peptides interact with the MHC to stimulate the aberrant proliferation of T lymphocytes, which causes damage to the intestinal mucosa, particularly in the duodenum. This can lead to malabsorption and weight loss, and because iron is mainly absorbed in the duodenum, to anaemia. The only successful treatment for coeliac disease is to avoid gluten in the diet.

Inflammatory bowel disease

Other major immune-mediated disease of the intestine includes inflammatory bowel disease (IBD), which is mainly subdivided into Crohn's disease and ulcerative colitis. Both can cause diarrhoea, abdominal pain, rectal bleeding from the inflamed and ulcerated colonic mucosa, and weight loss. Inflammation is localized to the colonic mucosa in ulcerative colitis, and may affect almost any part of the intestine, extending into the submucosa and deeper layers in Crohn's disease. The treatment remains empirical, and involves immunosuppression in many cases.

Primary biliary cirrhosis

Primary biliary cirrhosis (PBC) is a major cause of chronic liver disease, and is considered an autoimmune disease with damage limited to the biliary epithelium. It tends to affect women more than men, and progresses insidiously.

A simple diagnostic test for PBC is the presence of a circulating autoantibody to the mitochondrial enzyme pyruvate dehydrogenase (PDH). It is unknown why the presence of this autoantibody, which is the basis of the antimitochondrial antibody (AMA) test should be so strongly and specifically associated with PBC. AMA has no pathogenic effect, and the antigen is found in all cells that contain mitochondria.

There is no proven treatment for PBC, and in cases that have progressed to cirrhosis and liver failure, liver transplantation is the only therapeutic option.

Neoplasia

Cancer in the gastrointestinal system is a major cause of disease and death worldwide. For example, colon cancer is now the leading cause of death from cancer in the Western world, after lung and breast cancer in men and women, respectively. All parts of the intestinal tract can develop malignant tumours, although the colon, pancreas, oesophagus, stomach and liver are most frequently affected.

Genetic and environmental factors

Cancer typically develops as a stepwise process in which previously normal cells develop mutations in genes that alter their function and gradually release them from the normal restraints on growth and differentiation. Genetic and environmental factors play a strong role in the pathogenesis of cancer.

There is marked geographic variation in the incidence of various forms of cancer:

• Liver cancer associated with chronic infection with hepatitis B virus is highly prevalent in the Far East.
• Colon cancer is especially prevalent in the West and is associated with a diet rich in red meat.
• Gastric cancer is rare in the West and frequent in Japan.

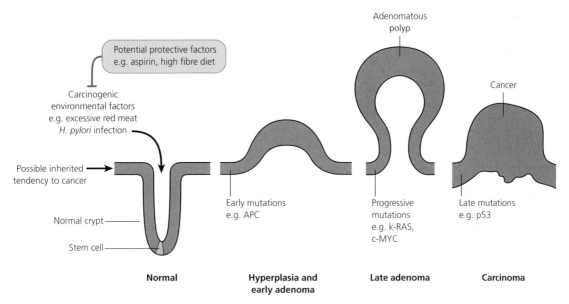

Potential protective factors
e.g. aspirin, high fibre diet

Carcinogenic
environmental factors
e.g. excessive red meat
H. pylori infection

Adenomatous
polyp

Cancer

Possible inherited
tendency to cancer

Early mutations
e.g. APC

Progressive
mutations
e.g. k-RAS,
c-MYC

Late mutations
e.g. p53

Normal crypt

Stem cell

Normal

**Hyperplasia and
early adenoma**

Late adenoma

Carcinoma

Fig. H Neoplasia of the gastrointestinal tract.

• Oesophageal squamous carcinoma is highly prevalent in parts of sub-Saharan Africa.

• Oesophageal adenocarcinoma is increasingly in incidence in the West.

Familial syndromes may increase the risk of certain types of cancer, for example colorectal cancer. It is also known that chronic inflammation, caused for example by *H. pylori* in the stomach, or hepatitis B virus in the liver, predisposes to the development of cancer.

Box D Colorectal cancer hereditary syndromes

• Hereditary non-polyposis colorectal cancer (HNPCC)
• Familial adenomatous polyposis (FAP)
• *MUTYH*-associated polyposis (*MUTYH* is a human gene encoding a DNA glycosylase)
• Peutz–Jeghers syndrome (PJS)
• Juvenille polyposis

Colon cancer

In colon cancer, for example, this progressive change can be detected in pre-malignant lesions that are dysplastic rather than neoplastic. Typically dysplastic colonic epithelial cells form protuberances into the lumen of the colon called polyps which can be removed and examined in the laboratory. The removal of dysplastic polyps also arrests the development of cancer in that particular site.

Partly as a consequence of this reproducible adenoma to carcinoma sequence of development, the sequential genetic changes that lead to cancer are particularly well elucidated in colon cancer. We know, for example, that the earliest genetic change that occurs is a mutation in the APC tumour suppressor gene, and that one of the final changes that occurs before an adenoma becomes malignant is a mutation in the p53 gene.

Prevention

Strategies to prevent cancer in the gastrointestinal tract include measures to arrest chronic inflammation. These include:

• Eradication of *H. pylori* infection.
• Treating oesophagitis caused by the reflux of gastric acid.
• Treating and preventing hepatitis B virus infection.
• Colonoscopy to detect and remove adenomatous polyps before they become malignant also prevents colon cancer. It is increasingly advocated in those regions where there is a high prevalence of this disease, such the USA and UK.

Approach to the patient

Gastrointestinal diagnosis relies heavily on a careful and thorough history. A detailed description of the symptoms and ancillary data, such as exposure to contaminated food or water, previous episodes of illness, consumption of potentially toxic drugs, heritable illness, etc., is critically important.

> **KEY POINT**
>
> - Always introduce yourself and obtain verbal consent from the patient before proceeding with a detailed history and examination.

Presenting complaint

History taking should always start with an open question; asking the patient to 'describe in their own words what the trouble is' is helpful. If the answer is vague or non-specific, more structured questions can then be asked. This is important for two reasons:

1 First, some symptoms, such as heartburn or dysphagia are so characteristically associated with certain conditions that the symptom naturally leads to the appropriate diagnostic hypothesis.

2 Second, where there may be a constellation of symptoms that need to be managed, knowing the patient's priorities guides the appropriate treatment strategy.

Gastrointestinal symptoms are often non-specific. For example, abdominal pain may indicate life-threatening acute pancreatitis or may be a feature of irritable bowel syndrome, which usually runs a benign course. Many serious diseases are asymptomatic until the late stages,

Gastroenterology: Clinical Cases Uncovered, 1st edition.
© S. Keshav and E. Culver. Published 2011 by
Blackwell Publishing Ltd.

and may only manifest with mild, vague symptoms such as malaise and fatigue. Be vigilant for changes – for example a change in bowel habit, change in food tolerance, change in energy levels, etc.

Where patients use terms that are subject to interpretation, clarify the meaning. Words like diarrhoea, constipation, nausea, heartburn, etc., mean different things to different people. People are also frequently embarrassed about bodily functions such as defecation, and will use euphemisms that are even more idiosyncratic.

Use the interview to show that as a professional you are knowledgeable, interested and non-judgemental, and give the patient the opportunity to talk freely, possibly for the first time, about their symptoms.

> **KEY POINT**
>
> - Always clarify the meaning of symptoms, as certain terms are subject to interpretation.

Gastrointestinal symptoms

Disorders of the gastrointestinal system may present with a wide range of symptoms. When enquiring about gastrointestinal illness it is worth asking specifically about certain symptoms, even if only to have a confirmed negative. The following list could guide the consultation:

- Dry mouth (xerostomia) or painful mouth.
- Excess salivation (waterbrash).
- Altered taste sensation (dysgeusia) or smell.
- Bad breath (halitosis).
- Lump in the throat (globus).
- Difficulty with swallowing (dysphagia).
- Pain on swallowing (odynophagia).
- Nausea and vomiting.
- Heartburn and reflux: epigastric or retrosternal burning or acid indigestion.
- Abdominal pain or discomfort.

- Dyspepsia: epigastric discomfort particularly related to eating.
- Bloating or abdominal distension.
- Hiccups.
- Excessive belching or flatulence.
- Diarrhoea: increased frequency or volume of stool, or looser motions.
- Urgency of defecation.
- Incontinence of faeces or flatus.
- Constipation: reduced frequency or volume of stool, difficulty passing stool.
- Incomplete evacuation (tenesmus).
- Defecation difficulty.
- Any altered bowel habit.
- Any altered stool character.
- Rectal bleeding: fresh or altered blood or melaena stool.
- Loss of weight.
- Change in appetite: loss of appetite, increased appetite.
- Jaundice.
- Itch (pruritis).

Painful mouth

Causes of a painful mouth include infections, trauma, vitamin deficiency, medications, systemic disorders and dermatological conditions. Gastrointestinal disorders causing painful mouth ulceration include coeliac disease and inflammatory bowel disease. Idiopathic apthous ulcers may run in families and be exacerbated by menstruation.

> **Box E Causes of a painful mouth**
>
> - Infection: candidiasis, herpes simplex, ulcerative gingivitis, infectious mononucleosis
> - Trauma: dentures or teeth
> - Medication: cytotoxic drugs, sulphonamides
> - Vitamin deficiency: vitamin B_{12}, folate, iron
> - Ulceration from systemic disease: inflammatory bowel disease, coeliac disease, Behçet's disease
> - Dermatological condition: lichen planus, erythema multiforme, pemphigoid and pemphigus
> - Malignant: leukoplakia, carcinoma
> - Idiopathic: apthous mouth ulcers

Dysphagia and odynophagia

Key factors to define are:

1 *Level of swallowing difficulty*: oropharangeal dysphagia causes difficulty in initiating a swallow, problems within

a second of initiating a swallow or repeated attempts at swallowing. Oesophageal dysphagia causes difficulty in swallowing seconds after initiating a swallow.

2 *Type of swallowing difficulty*: this may be for solids, liquids or both. Swallowing solids with 'sticking' and impact pain suggests a mechanical cause such as a stricture. Difficulty with liquids with spluttering and repeated swallows may represent a high pharyngeal cause. Nasal regurgitation, spluttering and aspiration may be due to achalasia or a pharyngeal pouch. A pouch may also cause bulging of the neck, gurgling or a nocturnal cough. The inability to swallow both solids and liquids may be a feature of oesophageal dysmotility or a more worrisome oesophageal carcinoma; the order of symptoms, speed of onset and associated alarm features are important to differentiate this.

3 *Duration and pattern of swallowing difficulty*: the duration and progression of dysphagia will determine if this is a benign or malignant process. A short progressive history is more suggestive of malignancy. A longer history intermittently over years suggests a more benign cause such as oesophageal dysmotility or an oesophageal web.

4 *Pain on swallowing (odynophagia)*: retrosternal chest pain on swallowing is characteristic of inflammatory disorders of the oesophagus. This may be the result of oesophageal candidaisis, herpes simplex oesophagitis, severe ulcerated reflux oesophagitis, oesophageal spasm or achalasia.

5 *Previous history of reflux disease or swallowing disorder*.

> **!RED FLAG**
>
> The following symptoms should act as an alarm:
>
> - Unintentional weight loss.
> - Short history of progressive dysphagia.

Predisposing factors for dysphagia

- Foreign body (fibrous or dry foods, tablets, solid objects).
- Corrosive material.
- Prolonged acid reflux and heartburn.
- Medication: bisphosphonates, non-steroidal anti-inflammatory drugs (NSAIDs), steroid inhalers.
- Smoking.
- Alcohol consumption.
- Previous history of Barrett's or peptic stricture.

- Neck surgery or radiotherapy.
- Connective tissue disease such as scleroderma.
- Neurological disorder with a bulbar palsy.
- Family history of gastrointestinal malignancy or familial tylosis.

Complications of dysphagia

- Aspiration of oesophageal contents into the bronchial tree.
- Oesophageal rupture or tear.

Nausea and vomiting

Nausea and vomiting may be caused by gastrointestinal disorders or conditions affecting other organ systems. In most cases, vomiting is preceded by nausea, but in the case of intracranial tumour or hyperemesis of pregnancy, there may be no warning. Vomiting may also be self-induced in cases of bulimia or to relieve symptomatic pain or satiety. A careful description of what is meant by each of these terms is required.

Features of history

- Duration of symptoms.
- Timing and frequency of vomiting, such as early morning.
- Contents of vomit, taste, colour, quantity and smell. Bile is yellow-green and bitter and from the distal duodenum. Faeculant vomit is brown and malodorous suggesting small bowel of colonic obstruction or a fistula.
- Presence of blood: fresh red blood may arise from an oesophageal lesion, dark blood with clots suggests profuse bleeding from a peptic ulcer or varicies, coffee ground vomit is altered blood due to gastric acid exposure. Also ask if there was intense retching prior to this, suggesting a Mallory–Weiss tear.
- Exacerbating factors, such as certain foods or smells.
- Relieving factors.

Associated gastrointestinal symptoms that may give a clue about aetiology

- Swallowing difficulties: perhaps a pouch or stricture is present.
- Abdominal pain or discomfort, such as in peptic ulceration, pancreatitis and gallstones.
- Reflux of acid or heartburn in ulcer disease.
- Loss of appetite or weight: think malignancy and malabsorption.
- Jaundice with or without pruritis in hepatobiliary disease.

- Fever or rigors.
- Change in colour of the stools or urine.
- Change in bowel habit.

Associated non-gastrointestinal symptoms that may give a clue about aetiology

- Menstrual disturbance: could patient be pregnant?
- Neurological symptoms: headaches, visual disturbance, neck stiffness, weakness or paraethesia, vertigo.
- Disorder of hearing or balance in labyrnthitis or Menière's disease.
- Excessive thirst or urination, indicating diabetes.
- Rash (hyperpigmentation) of Addison's disease.

Predisposing factors

- Medical conditions: neurological disorder, diabetes, thyroid disease, cardiovascular disease, arrhythmia.
- Psychiatric history, asking specifically about bulimia.
- Medications, such as chemotherapy agents, analgesics, antiarrthymics, diuretics, hormonal drugs, antibiotics and antivirals, anticonvulsants, anti-parkinsonian drugs.
- Infection exposure.
- Travel history.
- Smoking and amount.
- Alcohol consumption.
- Recreational drug use.

Box F Causes of nausea and vomiting

Gastrointestinal
- Achalasia
- Pyloric stenosis
- Intestinal strictures
- Gastroparesis
- Peptic ulcer disease
- Non-ulcer dyspepsia
- Pseudo-obstruction
- Gastrointestinal infections and food poisoning
- Pancreatitis
- Cholecystitis and cholangitis
- Acute hepatitis
- Mesenteric ischaemia
- Gastric cancer

Other causes
- Pregnancy
- Intracranial pathology: raised ICP, meningitis, migraine, seizures, tumours

- Ear problems: labyrnthitis, Menière's disease
- Endocrine disorders: diabetic ketoacidosis, Addison's disease, hyper- and hypoparathyroidism
- Metabolic disorders: uraemia, hypercalcaemia, hyponatremia
- Medications: chemotherapy agents, analgesics, antiarrthymics, diuretics, hormonal drugs, antibiotics and antivirals, anticonvulsants, anti-parkinsonian drugs
- Alcohol
- Nicotine
- Psychological and psychiatric disorders: bulimia, depression, voluntary emesis, strong emotions such as disgust

Heartburn and reflux

Heartburn or acid indigestion is highly suggestive of gastro-oesophageal reflux. Most individuals have experienced this in their lifetime. It is typically aggravated by large meals, stooping over, lying down, straining on exercise and during pregnancy. It may be relieved by antacids. There may be an altered taste sensation or increased salivation (waterbrash). There may be associated swallowing difficulties due to oesophagitis. It must be differentiated from cardiac, respiratory and musculoskeletal causes of chest pain.

> **!RED FLAG**
>
> Alarm symptoms to exclude in patients with heartburn:
>
> - Progressive unintentional weight loss.
> - Progressive dysphagia.
> - Persistent nausea and vomiting.
> - Symptomatic gastrointestinal blood loss: haematemesis or melaena.

Predisposing factors

- Medications causing inflammation such as bisphosphonates or slow-release potassium.
- Medications causing motility problems such as theophylline-based tablets.
- Smoking.

Abdominal pain

Abdominal pain and discomfort is the most common gastrointestinal symptom. It needs to be defined further.

Features of history

There are ten characteristics that should be sought in any abdominal pain history:

- *Character*: dull ache, colicky spasms, deep or superficial. Colicky pain, occurring in waves, suggests coincidence with peristaltic waves in an obstructed hollow organ. Dull, constant and gnawing pain occurs in peptic ulcer disease, penetrating into the retroperitoneal tissue.
- *Location*: epigastric pain is said to be frequently due to disease of foregut structures such as the stomach or duodenum. Peri-umbilical pain is said to be due to midgut structures such as the small intestine or appendix. Lower abdominal pain may be the result of disease in hindgut structures such as the colon and rectum. The site of pain may not indicate the site of the problem.
- *Radiation*: radiation to back, loins, groin, chest, shoulder tip or other area of the abdomen. Disease of the liver or gallbladder is typically felt in the right upper quadrant, and may affect the lower chest or even the tip of the shoulder by irritating the diaphragm. Disease of the pancreas causes epigastric pain that may radiate into the back.
- *Onset*: sudden or gradual. Sudden onset severe pain may occur in pancreatic inflammation, obstruction of a bile duct by a gallstone or ischaemia of the intestine.
- *Progression*: is it becoming more severe and intense or constant?
- *Intensity*: estimate on a grading scale from 1 to 10, with 10 the worst pain imaginable.
- *Frequency*: this can be number of times in a day/week/month/year.
- *Duration*: when was it first noticed (this may be a prior episode)? The chronicity of pain is important; for example, the internationally agreed criterion for irritable bowel syndrome (IBS) is that abdominal pain should have been present for the majority of time for at least 6 months. Colicky pain from gallstone disease may occur intermittently in recurrent bouts over months before being diagnosed.
- *Aggravating and relieving factors*: posture, eating meals; worsened by movement, inspiration or coughing, better on lying still. Pain from peptic ulcers may be made worse by eating, or by fasting, causing so-called hunger pangs. Fatty meals, which stimulate contraction of the gallbladder, aggravate pain due to gallstones. Colonic disease may cause pain that precedes defecation and urges defecation. Typically in IBS, defecation relieves abdominal pain temporarily.

• *Associated symptoms*: a change in the pattern of symptoms should alert you to a change in pathology; consider the development of a new pathology, a complication of the original pathology or an incorrect initial diagnosis.

Box G Common causes of abdominal pain

Gastrointestinal causes
• Peptic ulcer
• Pancreatitis
• Biliary colic
• Renal colic
• Mesenteric ischaemia or arterial occlusion
• Volvulus
• Strangulated hernia
• Obstruction
• Perforation of stomach (peptic ulcer) or colon (carcinoma, diverticular)
• Appendicitis
• Diverticulitis

Non-gastrointestinal causes
• Myocardial infarction and arrhythmias
• Dissecting aortic aneurysm
• Pleurisy
• Vertebral prolapse or collapse
• Cord compression
• Diabetic ketoacidosis
• Ectopic pregnancy
• Testes or ovarian torsion
• Herpes zoster infection

Bloating or abdominal distension

Abdominal distension is caused by one of the 'five Fs':
• *Fat*: adipose deposition due to excess food consumed or alcohol.
• *Fluid*: consider ascites, bladder distension and ovarian cyst.
• *Faeces*: constipated stool and obstruction or Hirschsprung's disease.
• *Flatus*: obstruction and pseudo-obstruction.
• *Fetus*: could she be pregnant?
  Fluctuating abdominal swelling with diurnal variation is common in women and rarely caused by organic disease. It is a feature of irritable bowel syndrome.

Belching and flatulence

Repeated belching is of no major significance, indicating the swallowing of air, usually unintentionally. It may be associated with acid reflux or anxiety symptoms. Excessive flatus or rectal flatulence, which may be malodorous is troublesome, and may represent intestinal malabsorption or lactase deficiency. A full diet history should be taken and any intolerance documented. The absence of flatus is concerning and indicates intestinal obstruction.

Altered bowel habit

The normal bowel habit is different for every individual and should be defined. The normal bowel habit varies from three or so evacuations per day to one every 3 days. Changes in bowel habit may be an early sign of serious disease.

Features of history
• How does the current bowel habit differ from normal?
• Duration of symptoms: acute or chronic.
• Intermittent or persistent or alternating bowel habit change.
• Frequency day and/or night.
• Urgency.
• Nature of the stool: consistency, colour, odour, presence of mucus.
• Blood present: mixed in or separate.
• Specific characteristics, e.g. difficult to flush away is typical of steatorrhoea.
• Incomplete evacuation.
• Incontinence and leakage.
• Defecatory problems, such as prolonged straining, self-digitate or vaginal wall pressure.
• Alarm features, such as weight loss.
• Associated symptoms, such as abdominal pain.
• Aggravating and relieving factors, such as laxatives to relieve constipation.

Box H Abnormal stool colour

• Black tar: melaena from upper gastrointestinal bleeding or iron therapy
• Bloody: colitis, carcinoma, diverticulitis
• Pale: fat malabsorption (small intestinal or pancreatic)

Incomplete evacuation (tenesmus)

Incomplete evacuation with a persistent desire to pass stool may be caused by an infective, inflammatory or radiation-induced proctitis, rectal prolapse or rectal carcinoma.

Faecal incontinence

Constipation with faecal impaction, soiling and leakage may coexist, especially in the elderly. Poor anal sphincter tone may also lead to faecal soiling and seepage, leading to perianal itch and pain.

Diarrhoea

This may be defined as frequent defecation and/or loose or fluid stools. There may be associated urgency, a persistent desire to pass a stool and faecal incontinence.

Features of history
- Duration of altered bowel habit (acute or chronic).
- Nature of the stool: consistency, colour, odour, presence of mucus.
- Blood present: mixed in or separate.
- Stool frequency in a 24 h period: record on a stool chart.
- Urgency.
- Nocturnal symptoms.
- Faecal incontinence and leakage.
- Previous similar episodes.

Associated symptoms that may give a clue about aetiology
- Abdominal pain.
- Weight loss and anorexia.
- Tiredness, fatigue or listlessness.
- Inflammatory symptoms, such as arthralgia, skin rashes and ophthalmic abnormalities.
- Mouth pain and ulceration.

Possible risk factors
- Smoking: protective in ulcerative colitis but can exacerbate Crohn's disease.
- Alcohol consumption: pancreatic inflammation and atrophy may be caused by excessive alcohol use leading to exocrine dysfunction.
- Recreational drug use.
- Travel abroad and infection exposure.
- Ingesting food or drink that might harbor infection. Take a detailed food history.
- Consider sexually transmitted disease and pelvic inflammatory disease in sexually active patients.
- Medical history for autoimmune disorders such as thyroid disease, diabetes or cardiovascular disease.
- Family history of a similar disorder or any intestinal disorder.

- Prescription medications or over-the-counter substances.
- Anxiety and depressive illness.

> **Box I Causes of diarrhoea**
>
> **Acute diarrhoea**
> - Acute infective gastroenteritis
> - Medication induced, such as omeprazole, antibiotics, metformin, laxatives
>
> **Chronic diarrhoea**
> - Irritable bowel syndrome
> - Chronic parasitic infestation such as giardiasis
> - Inflammatory bowel disease
> - Intestinal infection such as tuberculosis, yersiniosis, amoebiasis
> - Microscopic colitis
> - Coeliac disease and malabsorption
> - Chronic pancreatitis
> - Colorectal cancer
> - Intestinal lymphoma
> - Bowel resection
> - Chronic laxative abuse
> - Autonomic neuropathy from diabetes
> - Thyrotoxicosis
> - HIV-related enteropathy
> - Neuroendocrine tumour such as Zollinger–Ellison syndrome

Constipation

This may be described as hard, pellet-like stools, infrequent defecation or excessive straining at stool with difficulties in evacuation.

Features of history
- Duration of symptoms.
- Frequency, nature and consistency of stools: pellets, hard.
- Obstructive problem: self-digitate, vaginal or perianal or lower abdominal pressure.
- Strain at stool.
- Sensation of incomplete evacuation.
- Perianal pain.
- Rectal bleeding.
- Faecal impaction or soiling of underwear.

Associated symptoms that may give a clue about aetiology

- Abdominal pain.
- Change in weight or appetite.
- Bloating and diurnal variation.
- Excessive flatulence or belching.
- Nausea and vomiting, and is this faeculent?

Box J Causes of constipation

- Diet: low fibre and low fluid intake
- Immobility or lack of exercise
- Pregnancy
- Elderly
- Drugs such as opiates, anticholinergics, iron
- Motility disorders such as idiopathic slow transit and irritable bowel syndrome constipation-predominant (IBS-C)
- Mechanical obstruction from hernia, tumour, stricture (e.g. Crohn's disease) or pelvic mass (e.g. fibroids)
- Anorectal pain from a fissure, anal ulcer or thrombosed haemorrhoid
- Anorectal strictures, mucosal prolapse, rectocele, descending perineum syndrome
- Metabolic disorder such as hypercalcaemia and hypokalaemia
- Endocrine disorder such as hypothyroidism
- Spinal cord lesion in multiple sclerosis or spinal metastasis
- Cerebral disease, including parkinsonism
- Absence of enteric nerves in aganglinosis (Hirschprung's disease, Chagas' disease)
- Pelvic nerve damage (e.g. trauma, autonomic neuropathy)
- Stress response if injured or unwell due to sympathetic overactivity

---

Defecation difficulty

Incomplete evacuation of stool, prolonged straining at stool, self-digitation or pressure on the perianal area or lower abdominal wall to help passage of a stool, are all features of defecation disorders. These require investigation with anorectal physiology and defecation studies.

Rectal bleeding

Rectal bleeding is rarely misreported by patients. However it is important to know if the bleeding is a manifestation of a local anal condition, such as haemorrhoids, which is

the common and benign condition, or of an intracolonic condition, such as a tumour, which is less common and more serious. Typically, bleeding from a local cause is bright red, noticed at the end of defecation and external to the stool, and frequently upon wiping the perianal skin. Bleeding from colon cancer or colitis is frequently mixed in with the stool, and the blood may be darker and partially digested.

Box K Causes of bright red rectal bleeding

- Haemorrhoids: profuse, on wiping and in toilet, after defecation
- Anal fissure: associated with anal pain pre- and post-defecation
- Colorectal polyps: blood mixed in with stool and mucus production
- Colorectal carcinoma: blood mixed in with stool and mucus production; may be associated with altered bowel habit and weight loss
- Inflammatory bowel disease: urgency and loose stool with blood mixed in
- Ischaemic colitis: blood mixed in with stool and associated vascular disease or fibrillation
- Diverticular disease: complicated disease, may be profuse bleeding

---

Anorexia and weight loss

Unintentional loss of weight is a serious alarm symptom, which has many causes. It may be the result of reduced energy intake or increased energy expenditure. There may be a loss of body fluid, adipose tissue and muscle mass. It may result from physical, social and psychological factors. Many patients find it difficult to quantify their weight loss, so describe it in terms of poorly fitting clothes or loose belts or ask them bring in old photographs for comparison. It is important to be as objective as possible. An accurate weight should be recorded in clinic and old weights checked in the medical case notes to establish a history of definite weight loss.

Box L Causes of weight loss

- Inadequate nutritional intake, which may be due to dieting or loss of appetite
- Malabsorption, which may a consequence of coeliac disease or pancreatic insufficiency
- Hypercatabolic state such as hyperthyroidism, systemic inflammation, febrile illness

- Carcinoma
- Increased physical exercise
- Medications, such as diuretics to remove body fluid or orlistat to reduce fat absorption
- Depressive illness
- Chronic alcohol abuse
- Psychiatric condition such as anorexia nervosa
- Social circumstances and lifestyle factors

Jaundice

This is the result of excess bilirubin in the blood. Causes are congenital, haemolytic, hepatocellular, drug-induced or obstructive in origin. The yellow discolouration may not have been noticed by the patient him/herself, but by relatives, close friends or the attending doctor.

Box M Causes of jaundice

Pre-hepatic (unconjugated bilirubin) causes
- Congenital defects: Gilbert's syndrome (common), Criger–Najjar syndrome (rare)
- Haemolysis: hereditary spherocytosis, sickle cell disease, glucose-6 phosphate dehydrogenase (G6PD) deficiency, thalassaemia, malaria, autoimmune haemolysis, hypersplenism and an incompatible blood transfusion

Hepatocellular causes
- Acute hepatocellular disease: viral hepatitis (such as hepatitis A, B, C and E, cytomegalovirus (CMV), Epstein–Barr virus (EBV)), infections (such as leptospirosis), liver abscess, alcoholic hepatitis, autoimmune hepatitis, drug-induced (such as paracetamol), toxins (such as carbon tetrachloride), Budd–Chiari syndrome
- Chronic hepatocellular disease: chronic viral hepatitis, chronic autoimmune hepatitis, cirrhosis (e.g. due to alcohol), hepatic metastases, hepatoma, lymphoma, Wilson's disease, haemochromatosis, cardiac failure

Cholestatic (conjugated bilirubin) causes
- Intrahepatic: drugs (such as chlorpromazine), primary biliary cirrhosis, viral hepatitis, pregnancy
- Extrahepatic (obstructive): gallstones in the common bile duct, benign stricture, cholangitis, sclerosing cholangitis, cholangiocarcinoma, pancreatic carcinoma, chronic pancreatitis, schistosomiasis infestation, porta hepatis lymph nodes, congenital biliary atresia, parenteral nutrition

---

Features of history

- Timing and sequence of events.
- Presence of abdominal pain.
- Dark urine, pale stools and itching of cholestatic jaundice.
- Fever and rigors of cholangitis, or a liver abscess.
- Prodromal flu-like illness with fever, malaise, arthralgia and myalgia of viral hepatitis.
- Weight loss and/or anorexia.
- Symptomatic anaemia.
- Haematuria, which may indicate haemolysis.
- Previous episodes of jaundice.

Possible liver insults

- Prior episodes of jaundice as a child or in adulthood, and trigger for this if known.
- Hepatobiliary surgery.
- Hepatotoxic medications and when taken.
- Herbal remedies and Chinese medicines.
- Occupational exposure to hepatotoxins, e.g. industrial exposure, animal handling.
- Contact with jaundiced individuals.
- Travel history, particularly to hepatitis endemic areas or countries with a high rate of malaria.
- Sexual activity and possible risk for hepatitis B/C exposure.
- Intravenous drug use and sharing of needles.
- Tattoos, and when/where.
- Blood or plasma transfusions, and when/where.
- Alcohol history.
- Dietary consumption and nutritional status.
- Alcohol consumption.
- Family history of jaundice, such as Gilbert's syndrome.

Markers of decompensated liver disease

- Evidence of gastrointestinal bleeding, especially variceal bleeding.
- Confusion, daytime sleepiness, alterations in the day/night sleep cycle, or personality change suggestive of encephalopathy.
- Abdominal distension with fluid and peripheral fluid.
- Bruise easily, due to thrombocytopenia and coaguloapthy.

Medical co-morbidity

Co-morbidity may have a role in the pathogenesis of the current condition.

Past medical illnesses should be documented. Common conditions such as diabetes mellitus, thyroid disease, vascular disease and asthma must be checked for. All have potential gastrointestinal correlates:

• Diabetes causing autonomic neuropathy may cause gastroparesis, diarrhoea or constipation.

• Thyroid disease may cause alteration in bowel habit and weight, and is associated with other autoimmune conditions such as coeliac disease.

• Extensive vascular disease may cause intestinal ischaemia manifesting as mesenteric angina or ischaemic colitis.

• Asthma is associated with an increased risk of eosinophilic oesophagitis.

Co-morbidity may also mean that the patient is using medications that might contribute to gastrointestinal symptoms. Asking about pre-existing illness means that the clinician can be more alert for such iatrogenic disease.

Previous surgical procedures should be documented. Previous appendicectomy is associated with a reduced risk of ulcerative colitis. Unless you ask specifically, the patient may forget to mention that they have had a hysterectomy or cholecystectomy, so asking can avoid an embarrassing mistake.

Medications

Much illness is a consequence of treatment for other conditions. This is particularly relevant to the gastrointestinal tract. Common culprits are:

• Anti-inflammatory drugs: gastritis, peptic ulcer, NSAID enteropathy.

• Antibiotics: diarrhoea, *Clostridium difficile* diarrhoea.

• Laxatives: diarrhoea.

• Metformin: diarrhoea.

• Proton pump inhibitors: diarrhoea.

• Opioid analgesics: constipation, loss of appetite, altered taste.

• Antipsychotics, especially olanzapine: weight gain.

• All drugs, including over-the-counter and herbal remedies: nausea and vomiting, loss of appetite, abnormal liver chemistry, pancreatitis.

Diet

This is an important contributory factor in many gastrointestinal diseases. A brief but thorough diet history can be taken in the outpatient clinic.

• Adequacy of diet in cases of loss of weight, anaemia or nutritional deficiency.

• Wheat and gluten sensitivity or intolerance in coeliac disease.

• Milk and dairy product intolerance in lactose insufficiency.

• Fibre intake may be inadequate, causing constipation, or excessive, which is a less common cause of constipation and bloating.

• Excessive intake of caffeine can contribute to diarrhoea.

• Ingestion of osmotically active substances such as non-absorbable sugar substitutes in chewing gum and drinks can cause diarrhoea.

• Exposure to pathogens, for example unpasteurised milk or undercooked poultry products, are important, particularly in cases of possible gastroenteritis.

Habits

• Eating habits affect gastrointestinal function, such as late-night eating, binging and bulimia. Contaminated food from home preparation or dining out can cause gastroenteritis.

• Exercise and lifestyle probably make a difference to symptoms of IBS.

• Smoking is a risk factor for Crohn's disease and colon cancer. Conversely, recently stopping smoking may precipitate the first presentation of ulcerative colitis.

• Excessive consumption of alcohol may cause gastritis, vomiting or diarrhoea and may precipitate acute pancreatitis. Long-term excessive use of alcohol is associated with liver disease and chronic pancreatitis.

• Recreational drugs such as cannabis, cocaine and heroin can affect intestinal function, and cause symptoms such as nausea and vomiting, constipation and intestinal dysmotility. The use of amphetamines may suppress appetite. The use of intravenous drugs is a risk for developing chronic viral hepatitis.

• Sexual activity may be important when determining risk factors in liver disease, especially hepatitis B and C and human immunodeficiency virus (HIV).

Travel

Travel, particularly to areas where infections are endemic, or where sanitation is inadequate, is associated with increased risk of bacterial and amoebic dysentery, gastroenteritis and parasitic infection including giardiasis. Exotic food and drink may precipitate symptoms such as heartburn and dyspepsia, and cause altered bowel habit, albeit transiently.

An episode of traveller's diarrhoea may lead to post-infectious IBS, characterised by diarrhoea, abdominal pain and bloating for months after the initial infection (apply the Rome III criteria for IBS).

Family background

Certain gastrointestinal disease can occur in families and have a genetic predisposition. In particular ask about:

- Coeliac disease.
- Inflammatory bowel disease.
- Colorectal cancer.
- Haemochromatosis.
- Wilson's disease.
- Autoimmune diseases.
- Vascular disease.

Colorectal cancer is common in the general population, so unless multiple members of the family are affected, or cancer occurred early in a relative, before the age of 50 years, a single occurrence is likely to be due to chance. Rarely, pancreatic, oesophageal and gastric cancer may run in families.

Liver diseases such as haemochromatosis, which is relatively common, and Wilson's disease, which is rare, may also emerge on careful questioning. Thyroid disease, diabetes mellitus and vascular disease have familial predisposition. IBS may run in families.

Examination

General examination

General end of the bed examination is helpful in determining if the patient is relatively well or rather unwell, and potentially in need of urgent diagnosis and treatment. There are many diagnostic clues found by looking around the bedside.

- Mood and manner of the patient: depression can cause poor appetite, loss of weight and be associated with constipation. Diarrhoea caused by thyrotoxicosis may occur in a patient who is overtly anxious, agitated or aggressive.
- Height and weight are used to calculate the body mass index.
- Look at the skin, sclerae and mucus membranes for pallor or jaundice. Look for skin rashes and document their features and distribution. Look for distribution of body hair and secondary sexual characteristics.
- Check for tremor in the outstretched hands: there may be a fine essential tremor, which is benign and without pathological significance, a thyrotoxic fine

tremor, or the flapping tremor or asterixis of hepatic encephalopathy.

- General observations in all patients include pulse rate, blood pressure, oxygen saturations, respiratory rate, temperature and blood sugar. Bradycardia may indicate hypothyroidism; tachycardia may indicate inflammation or infection. An elevated temperature suggests a fever that may have an inflammatory or infective source. Blood sugar may be raised in a poorly controlled or newly diagnosed diabetic, or low in infection or systemic illness among other causes.

Examination of the mouth and throat

These should be carefully examined for evidence of gastrointestinal disease:

- Lips for angular stomatitis from iron or riboflavine deficiency or from ill-fitting dentures.
- Teeth or dentures for adequate chewing and evidence of dental caries and discolouration.
- Gums for gingivitis, features of nutritional deficiency (scurvy causing hypertrophy and haemorrhagic gums) and systemic infection.
- Mouth for evidence of candida, mouth ulceration, apthous stomatitic and hydration of the mucus membranes.
- Tongue surface, colour and presence of furring. An atrophic tongue may be due to iron and vitamin B_{12} deficiency. Look for fasciculations suggestive of a neurological condition that may impair swallowing.
- Watch a swallow of liquids and solids if there is a complaint of dysphagia. If a bout of coughing immediately follows a swallow, consider neuromuscular causes or perhaps a fistula. If food is regurgitated in semisolid form, consider a pouch or high stricture.

Examination of the abdomen

Examination of the abdomen, as with any region, must be approached systematically. Examine in good light with warm surroundings for patient comfort. Position the patient comfortably in a supine position, with arms by their sides, on a single pillow if possible. Remove clothes to reveal the area of interest, maintaining dignity where possible. Ensure hands are clean and warm prior to examining.

Abdominal discomfort and pain are frequent presenting complaints, and it may be necessary to delineate the precise area is affected. Do so gently and avoid causing undue discomfort. Watch the patient's face as you palpate, to have early warning of a wince or groan.

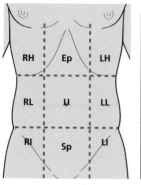

9 segments	
RH	Right hypochondric
Ep	Epigastric
LH	Light hypochondric
RL	Right lumbar
U	Umbilical
LL	Left lumbar
RI	Right inguinal
Sp	Suprapubic
LI	Left inguinal

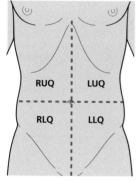

4 quadrants	
RUQ	Right upper quadrant
LUQ	Left upper quadrant
RLQ	Right lower quadrant
LLQ	Left lower quadrant

Fig. I The abdomen showing the abdominal quadrants and segments for examination.

Follow the nostrum of inspection, palpation, percussion and auscultation, as outlined in Table A.

Hernial orificies

Hernias are a protrusion of a viscus through an abnormal opening. External hernias occur at sites of defects in the abdominal wall. Internal hernias occur through defects in the mesentery or into the retroperitoneal space. The latter include femoral, indirect and direct inguinal hernia.
• Define the site.
• Check for a cough impulse.
• Reduction by gentle sustained pressure. Irreducible hernias may become obstructed and obstructed hernias may become strangulated, which is a surgical emergency.

Table A Technique for examining the abdomen.

Inspection	Shape – scaphoid abdomen due to wasting disease or starvation, distended abdomen from ascites or gaseous distension, visible masses
	Evidence of asymmetry
	Scars – define the natures of surgery
	Movements with respiration and peristalsis
	Vascular markings especially collateral veins
	Rashes such as erythema ab igne
	Hair distribution
	Iatrogenic drains, tubes or catheters
	Hernias – umbilical, epigastric, incisional, femoral, inguinal
Palpation	Superficial and deep tenderness by 'dipping' motion
	Organomegaly – gallbladder, liver, spleen, kidneys
	Masses – define their location in the abdomen (nine quadrants)
	Carnett's sign suggesting abdominal wall pain
	Murphy's sign suggesting acute cholecystitis
	Hernial orifices with cough reflex
	Testes if suspect torsion or atrophy
Percussion	Distinguish between gaseous, fluid filled ascites, cystic or solid
	Percussion tenderness
	Organomegaly to define borders of enlargement
	Shifting dullness and fluid thrill of ascites
Auscultation	Bowel sounds and quality
	Vascular sounds (bruits) over aorta, liver and kidneys
	Succession splash

Examination of the genitalia

The penis and scrotum should be carefully examined to look for swelling. The testes should be examined further for tenderness and swelling. Transillumination of the scrotum may be used to assess if the swelling is fluid or solid in nature.

Vaginal examination is not routine in the gastrointestinal work-up.

Rectal examination

The rectal examination is an integral part of the complete abdominal examination, although it may not be necessary in every case, and in every case must be approached sensitively and with due attention to the patient's feelings

Table B Procedure for examining the rectum.

Perineum	Scars
	Skin tags
	Fissure
	Fistula
	Abscess
	External haemorrhoids
Anal sphincter	Intact sphincter
	Tone on squeezing – normal, reduced, tight
	Pain and spasm, consider an anal fissure. May need local anaesthetic gel or examination under general anaesthesia
Rectum	Masses – position from anal verge, size of abnormal area
	Prostate in males
Stool	After withdrawal of the finger, examine the stool for consistency and colour. It may be loose, hard or blood-stained or there may be evidence of melaena

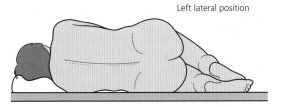

Left lateral position

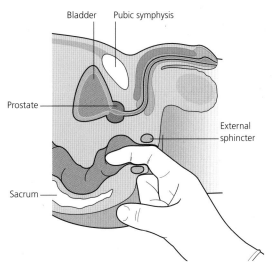

Bladder Pubic symphysis

Prostate

External sphincter

Sacrum

Fig. J Rectal examination.

about what is potentially embarrassing and threatening to them. It is always best to have a chaperone attending. Position the patient in the left lateral position, with the knees drawn to the chest. Lubricate the gloved examining finger. Check systematically as given in Table B.

Proctoscopy and sigmoidoscopy

Special equipment and training is necessary to safely perform these procedures without causing undue discomfort.
- *Proctoscopy*: allows examination of the anal canal to check for haemorrhoids and fissure.
- *Rigid sigmoidoscopy*: allows examination of the rectal mucosa to check for inflammation, bleeding or tumours. A stool specimen or rectal biopsy may be obtained at the time of sigmoidoscopy.

Investigations

When a diagnostic hypothesis is framed after careful history and examination, then there is a wealth of tests that can aid in establishing the exact diagnosis. These tests are frequently costly, often involve some inconvenience, discomfort or risk for the patient, and usually have limited specificity and sensitivity. Therefore clinical judgement is critical in choosing the appropriate test or tests, in limiting the number of tests, and interpreting the results of those that have been performed.

Blood tests

Blood tests are relatively cheap and non-invasive, and are frequently used early in the diagnostic pathway to determine if there is indeed a reason to be concerned about gastrointestinal disease. For example, in patients with typical symptoms of IBS, the absence of anaemia, normal liver chemistry, normal thyroid tests and negative serology for coeliac disease, together with the absence of other discernable pathology, allows one to make a positive diagnosis of IBS, without the need for invasive tests such as endoscopy.

Basic blood tests include the following:
- *Full blood count*: check for anaemia.
- *Haematinics* (ferritin, folate, B_{12}): check for deficiency.
- *Electrolytes*: ensure that sodium and potassium are normal.
- *Liver chemistry* (aspartate aminotransferase (AST), alanine aminotransferase (ALT), alkaline phosphatase (ALP), gamma glutamyl transferase (γ-GT), bilirubin):

check for hepatocellular damage, biliary damage and cholestasis.

- *Clotting tests* (prothrombin time): check hepatic synthetic function and for possible vitamin K deficiency.
- *Albumin*: check hepatic synthetic function, and for possible acute phase response, malnutrition and protein-losing enteropathy.
- *C-reactive protein (CRP)*: acute phase response.
- *Thyroid function test*: hypo- or hyperthyroidism.
- *Serological tests*: *Helicobacter pylori* and endomysial antibody for coeliac disease.

More specialised blood tests which are often more specific for particular disorders that may be ordered in the appropriate setting include, for example:

- *Serological tests*: antimitochondrial antibody, liver autoimmune tests.
- *Genetic tests*: HFE genotype, coeliac human leukocyte antigen (HLA) susceptibility alleles.
- *Copper and caeruloplasmin*: Wilson's disease.
- *Alpha-1 antitrypsin*: α_1-antitrypsin deficiency.
- *Fasting intestinal hormones*: gastrin, vasoactive intestinal polypeptide.

Urine tests

Special tests of the urine may be valuable in certain circumstances:

- *Urinary catecholamines and indoleamines*: carcinoid syndrome (a cause of diarrhoea and weight loss).
- *Urine sodium level*: reduced in chronic liver disease and reduced when total body sodium is depleted.
- *Urinary porphyrins*: screen for porphyria.

Stool tests

Examination of the stool is an integral part of the gastrointestinal assessment, particularly in patients with diarrhoea or malabsorption:

- *Microscopy, culture and sensitivity*: leukocytes and erythrocytes in inflammation; pathogenic parasites, bacteria or viruses in infection.
- *Faecal fat*: increased in malabsorption.
- *Faecal elastase*: decreased in pancreatic insufficiency.
- *Faecal calprotectin and lactoferrin*: increased in intestinal inflammation.

Breath tests

Gases such as H_2 or CO_2 rapidly diffuse into the blood stream even if they are elaborated in the intestinal tract, and can be measured in the expiratory breath. This phenomenon is exploited in tests where a test meal, which may contain an isotopic label, is administered, following which the proportion of H_2 or labelled CO_2 is measured in the breath.

Tests include the following, amongst others:

- *Urease breath test*: for *Helicobacter pylori* infection. Labelled urea is administered, if it is hydrolysed by urease from *H. pylori*, excess labelled CO_2 is detected.
- *Lactose breath test*: for lactose intolerance. A standard amount of lactose is administered. If the subject cannot digest lactose, it reaches the colon where it is digested by bacteria, producing excess H_2.
- *Lactulose breath test*: for small bowel bacterial overgrowth. A standard amount of lactulose is administered. Normally this is only hydrolysed to release H_2 when it reaches the colon. If there is bacterial overgrowth in the small intestine a premature rise in H_2 excretion is detected.

Physiological measurements

Many physiological measurements of the gastrointestinal system can be made. Certain tests are basic and self-explanatory, such as measuring the volume of stool produced, or the change in body weight. Others are more elaborate, and of these, some, such as oesophageal pressure manometry are well established and provide reliable diagnostic information in diseases such as achalasia, while others, such as electrogastrography, to determine if the gastric pacemaker is normal, are exploratory at the moment.

The following is a partial list:

- *Stool output (Bristol stool chart)*: to measure stool volume, frequency and content.
- *Stoma output*: to monitor stoma volume.
- Calorie intake and food diary: Nutritional intake
- *Body weight*: weight measured serially to chart nutritional progress.
- *Oesophageal manometry*: for dysmotility disorders.
- *Oesophageal pH measurement*: for reflux and acid disease.
- *Anal manometry*: for the investigation of defecatory disorders.
- *Electrogastrography*: to check gastric pacemaker.

Imaging tests

Radiological imaging of the gastrointestinal system includes all modalities, including ultrasound, X-rays, magnetic resonance imaging (MRI) and radio-isotope scanning. Certain simple tests such as *abdominal ultrasound* are extremely useful, particularly in liver and

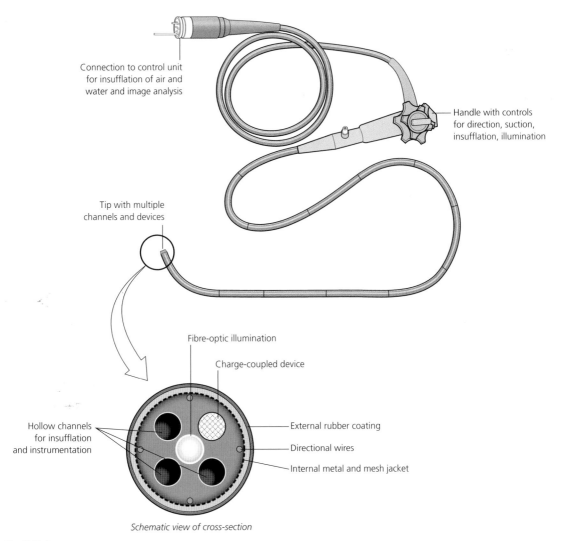

Connection to control unit
for insufflation of air and
water and image analysis

Handle with controls
for direction, suction,
insufflation, illumination

Tip with multiple
channels and devices

Fibre-optic illumination

Charge-coupled device

Hollow channels
for insufflation
and instrumentation

External rubber coating

Directional wires

Internal metal and mesh jacket

Schematic view of cross-section

Fig. K Endoscope.

biliary disease to detect abnormalities in the texture of the liver, to detect gallstones and to assess venous and arterial flow to the liver.

The *plain abdominal X-ray* is highly sensitive for evidence of intestinal obstruction, where dilated loops can be readily seen. Most gallstones are radiolucent, therefore this is a poor test for gallstones, in contrast to renal stones and pancreatic calcification, both of which are readily detected on plain abdominal X-ray. If a subject ingests a set of radio-opaque markers at intervals over a few days, a plain abdominal X-ray taken at the end of the period can detect if the markers have traversed the colon at an adequate rate, providing a simple *colonic transit study*.

Barium oral or anal contrast can be administered to delineate the lumen of the oesophagus, stomach, small intestine and colon. This forms the basis of tests such as the barium swallow, barium meal, small bowel series and barium enema.

Computed tomography (CT) and MRI scanning of the abdomen can also be enhanced with appropriate luminal contrast agents, which can also be supplemented with vascular contrast to provide greater detail. In the colon, luminal radio-opaque contrast such as barium can be followed with insufflation of air to provide double contrast – the resulting images can provide exquisite detail as the wall of the organ is outlined by a layer of barium.

Fluorography can provide dynamic images of intestinal function, for example in swallowing and defecation.

The liver and pancreas are particularly well visualised by *high-resolution or triple-phase CT scanning* and MRI scanning, and, with the appropriate software, the biliary and pancreatic ducts can be delineated with *magnetic resonance cholangiopancreatography* (MRCP).

Radio-nucletide scanning provides many special diagnostic uses:

• Gastric emptying scan: rate of gastric emptying after a test meal to check for gastroparesis.

• Octreotide scan: presence of aberrantly placed somatostatin receptors to detect neuroendocrine tumours.

• SehCAT scan: inadequate retention of a test dose of an exogenous bile salt to detect bile salt malabsorption, as seen in disease of the terminal ileum.

• White cell scan: abnormal concentration of labelled white cells in an area of inflammation.

• Red cell scan: abnormal accumulation of labelled red cells at a site of haemorrhage.

Endoscopy

Rigid instruments to examine the anus, rectum, pharynx and upper oesophagus have long been used, although the practice of gastroenterology was revolutionised in the 1970s by the advent of flexible instruments that could be inserted into the distal duodenum per orally, or to the terminal ileum via the anus. These endoscopes or colonoscopies were originally based on fibreoptic technology, and now typically contain an electronic camera with images transmitted electronically to a screen. They allow visualisation of the oesophagus, stomach, duodenum and colon, and allow the endoscopist to take diagnostic biopsies and perform therapeutic manoeuvres such as the injection of bleeding ulcers and removal of polyps.

Modern endoscopy can be safely and rapidly performed after administering a light sedative, or no sedative at all, to the patient. Instruments are specialised for various standard techniques with typical diagnostic or therapeutic uses:

• Upper endoscopy: to detect oesophagitis and peptic ulcer, and to treat upper gastrointestinal haemorrhage.

• Sigmoidoscopy: to assess distal colonic disease such as proctitis.

• Colonoscopy and ileoscopy: to assess the entire colon and potentially the terminal ileum, check for polyps or cancer, or Crohn's disease, and to remove polyps.

• Endoscopic retrograde cholangiopancreatography (ERCP): a special upper endoscope allowing cannulation of the ampulla of Vater, imaging of the biliary tree and pancreatic duct, and endoscopic removal of gallstones.

• Enteroscopy: special longer upper endoscope to visualise the distal duodenum and jejunum.

• Capsule endoscopy: swallowed electronic camera images are transmitted electronically to a detector, allowing a survey of the entire small intestine.

Histology

Endoscopy enables biopsies to be taken from the upper intestinal tract and the entire colon; consequently histopathology now can provide diagnostic information without the need for surgical resection. Histology is particularly helpful in the diagnosis of coeliac disease, where typical changes are seen in the number of intraepithelial lymphocytes and the size of villi in the distal duodenum, and in the diagnosis of inflammatory bowel disease, colorectal cancer and pre-cancerous changes in colonic biopsies and polyps.

Liver biopsy, which can be performed percutaneously, or via the jugular vein, is also essential for the modern management of liver disease. Cirrhosis is most accurately diagnosed on liver biopsy, and the cause of liver disease and extent of liver damage may not be apparent until a biopsy is taken and examined.

Special techniques, such as staining for deposits of iron or immunohistochemical detection of viral infection, allow rapid and accurate diagnosis. Abnormal areas in the liver can be sampled for histology by targeted liver biopsy using ultrasound guidance.

Case 1 A 61-year-old woman with progressive dysphagia

Mrs Sarah Whiston is a 61-year-old married secretary. She has a 6-month history of reflux and heartburn. Over the last few weeks she has found it more difficult to swallow certain foods. She has come to your clinic for further investigation.

What information should you elicit from the history?
History of dysphagia

1 *Level of dysphagia.* It is important to differentiate between oropharyngeal and oesophageal dysphagia:
  • Oropharyngeal dysphagia usually manifests in a difficulty *initiating* swallowing. There may be repeated attempts at swallowing or problems within a second of initiating swallowing.
  • Oesophageal swallowing manifests with a difficulty in swallowing *seconds after* initiating a swallow.
The level at which the patient points is not helpful in locating the site of the lesion.

2 *Type of dysphagia.* It is important to differentiate between dysphagia to solids, liquids or both:
  • Solids: suggests a mechanical cause.
  • Liquids: suggests a pharyngeal cause.
  • Both solids and liquids: suggests oesophageal dysmotility.
Exacerbation by hot or cold liquids is common in oesophagitis.

3 *Duration and pattern of dysphagia.* A short progressive history is more suggestive of malignancy. Intermittent symptoms occur in oesophageal dysmotility, eosinophilic oesophagitis or an oesophageal web. Progressive dysphagia suggests an organic cause.

Gastroenterology: Clinical Cases Uncovered, 1st edition.
© S. Keshav and E. Culver. Published 2011 by
Blackwell Publishing Ltd.

Associated features
  • Is there a history of swallowing a foreign body, such as fibrous or dry foods or tablets?
  • Is it painful to swallow (odynophagia)? This can occur in oesophageal candidaisis, oesophagitis, spasm and achalasia.
  • Is there a history of heartburn or reflux of acid? This suggests a peptic stricture or severe oesophagitis.
  • Has she unintentionally lost any weight? This may be more suggestive of malignancy.
  • Is there a history of regurgitation of solid or semisolid food? Is there nasal regurgitation or aspiration? Does she have bulging of the neck, gurgling or a nocturnal cough? A pharyngeal pouch must be considered.
  • Does she cough on swallowing or have an inability to initiate swallow? Consider a bulbar palsy.

Evidence of complications
  • Aspiration: evidence of a cough with sputum production and breathlessness.
  • Perforation: severe abdominal or chest pain or evidence of shock.

Predisposing factors
  • Past history of gastro-oesophageal reflux, Barrett's oesophagus, peptic stricture or oesophageal web.
  • Past history of systemic sclerosis.
  • Past history of a neurological disorder.
  • Medications known to precipitate swallowing problems. For example, bisphosphonates causes inflammation and stricturing, non-steroidal anti-inflammatory drugs (NSAIDs) causing oesophageal inflammation and ulceration, steroid inhalers for asthma may cause candidiasis or eosinophilic oesophagitis.
  • Corrosive substance swallowed, causing stricturing and inflammation.
  • Smoking history, which increases the risk of malignancy.
  • Alcohol consumption, which increases the risk of malignancy.

• Family history of gastrointestinal (GI) malignancy or familial tylosis.

She tells you she started the 'Lighter Life' diet 4 months ago in an attempt to lose weight. This consisted of soups and low fat chewy bars. She had lost 18 kg in the first 2 months. She was delighted by this but since trying to eat a normal diet she has had difficulty swallowing solid food. Swallowing has been a problem for the last 3 weeks, the food getting stuck at the mid sternum level a minute or so after swallowing. It is getting worse. She drinks fluid to dislodge this but has regurgitated water and at times undigested food into her mouth. This process is painful.

She has a 6-month history of reflux and heartburn, but has suffered from this intermittently in the past and takes Gaviscon as needed. She has never taken a protein pump inhibitor (PPI). She has no respiratory, neurological or other systemic symptoms.

Her past medical history was unremarkable with no chronic illnesses. She had two operations to strip varicose veins. She has used no regular or over-the-counter medications. She is a lifelong non-smoker and consumes little alcohol. She has a family history of ischaemic heart disease.

What findings are important on examination?

General examination

Inspect for evidence of dehydration or skin folds suggestive of weight loss. Look at the mouth, teeth and dentures for signs of acid erosion. Look in the eyes and at the skin for pallor of anaemia. Examine the neck for evidence of a pharyngeal pouch, palpable goitre or supraclavicular nodes from a carcinoma of the cardia.

• Is there evidence of scleroderma or systemic sclerosis evidenced by tight shiny skin (sclerodactyl), Raynaud's phenomenon, telangiectasia and calcinosis?

• Is there evidence of finger clubbing, Horner's syndrome or chest signs suggestive of a hilar bronchial carcinoma?

• Is there any focal neurology or evidence of bulbar palsy, tongue fasciculations or nasal speech?

• Is there evidence of thyroid disease: a palpable goitre, proptosis, sinus tachycardia and brisk reflexes (hyperthyroidism), or alopecia, weight gain and depressed reflexes (hypothyroidism)? If there a palpable goitre, percuss for evidence of retrosternal extension.

Abdominal examination

Inspect and palpate for an abdominal mass and organomegaly.

On examination she looks well. She weighs 60 kg with a body mass index (BMI) of 23.4. There are no signs of anaemia, lymphadenopathy or goitre. Respiratory and neurological examinations are unremarkable. There are no palpable masses or organomegaly of the abdomen.

KEY POINT

• It is important to establish the level (oesophageal or oropharyngeal), type (solids, liquids or both), duration and pattern (progressive nature) of dysphagia to guide further investigation and management.

List the possible differential diagnoses

In a woman in her 60s with progressive oesophageal dysphagia to solids over weeks, associated with weight loss, the most important cause to exclude is mechanical obstruction from a tumour.

The possible differential diagnoses include:
• Carcinoma of the oesophagus or cardia.
• External pressure from a bronchial tumour.
• Peptic stricture.
• Severe oesophagitis.
• Oesophageal web.
• Schatzki ring.
• Oesophageal dysmotility.

Box 1.1 Causes of oesophageal dysphagia

Oesophageal causes
• Oesophagitis
• Peptic stricture due to reflux
• Carcinoma of the oesophagus or cardia
• Oesophageal dysmotility
• Achalasia
• Diffuse oesophageal spasm
• Oesophageal web (Plummer–Vinson syndrome)
• Schatzki ring
• Caustic stricture due to acid/alkali
• Radiation stricture
• Foreign body in the lumen

External pressure
- Enlarged mediastinal lymph nodes
- Thoracic aortic aneurysm
- Bronchial carcinoma
- Retrosternal goitre
- Left atrial enlargement

Systemic conditions
- Systemic sclerosis
- Polymyositis
- Myaesthenia gravis
- Bulbar palsy
- Bulbar poliomyelitis
- Botulism[boxend]

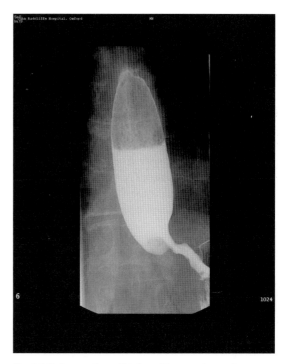

Fig. 1.1 Barium swallow: dilatation of the oesophagus above a narrow stricture. (Courtesy of the Gastroenterology Department, John Radcliffe Hospital.)

What are the most appropriate investigations to confirm your suspicions?

Blood tests

- Full blood count for anaemia. Iron studies should be done if anaemic. This may due to malignancy, bleeding or Plummer–Vinson syndrome (an oesophageal web causing iron-deficiency anaemia).
- Urea and electrolytes for evidence of dehydration and hyponatraemia. Hyponatraemia may occur in the syndrome of inappropriate anti-diuretic hormone (ADH) in bronchial tumours.
- Liver function for evidence of hepatic dysfunction from metastases, although this a poor discriminator for this.
- Calcium level for hypercalcaemia of malignancy.
- Thyroid function if there is evidence of thyroid goitre.

Chest X-ray

To look for a mediastinal fluid level and absent gastric bubble, large retrosternal goitre, mediastinal lymphadenopathy, thoracic aneurysm, hilar lung lesion or evidence of consolidation from aspiration.

Barium swallow

This is useful to exclude a large pharyngeal pouch prior to endoscopy if the history is suggestive. It shows evidence of oesophageal dysmotility, demonstrates compression from internal or external sources and oesophageal dilatation (Fig. 1.1). A smooth, tapering stricture is often benign. An irregular stricture is more alarming.

Upper endoscopy

An urgent endoscopy should be done to exclude a carcinoma (see Plate 1.1). This will also identify an oesophageal web, ring, stricture or severe oesophagitis. It may, however, miss small tumours not penetrating the mucosa. Biopsy and brushings (98% detection rate for tissue diagnosis) of any ill-defined area is therefore important. Narrow band imaging and confocal microscopy may help to target biopsies.

KEY POINT

- Urgent investigations are indicated when there is dysphasia for solids alone, if symptoms are progressive or when there is associated weight loss.

Mrs Whiston is booked on the 2-week wait referral system for urgent investigation. Her blood tests show an elevated C-reactive protein (CRP) of 19 mg/L (range 0–8 mg/L). There is no anaemia, renal or hepatic dysfunction. Her iron and ferritin are within the normal range. Her chest X-ray (CXR) is reported as normal.

Her barium swallow shows a significant hold up to the passage of contrast at the gastro-oesophageal junction and dilatation of the oesophagus above this. Upper GI endoscopy demonstrates a small polypoidal mass at 40 cm and a tight distal oesophageal narrowing suggestive of malignancy. Multiple biopsies are taken.

The barium swallow and endoscopic findings suggest a malignancy. What do you do now?

The upper GI nurse specialist should be available and present when you discuss the findings seen at endoscopy. Explain that there is an area that looks suspicious and you have taken tissue samples. Be honest, if she asks 'could this be cancer?' and share your concerns that it is likely but you will know more information when the biopsy results are available and after further scanning and tests. Organise a follow-up appointment and provide contact details.

What are your next investigations?

Contact the multidisciplinary team (MDT) coordinator for upper GI malignancy. The patient's barium and endoscopy investigations should be discussed at the next upper gastrointestinal MDT meeting. This consists of a team of gastroenterologists, GI surgeons, oncologists, radiologists, histopathologists, nurse specialists and palliative care physicians.

Other investigations could include:
• Computed tomography (CT) scan of the chest, abdomen and pelvis (staging scan) to look for extension and metastatic spread.
• Endoscopic ultrasound (EUS) is invaluable for staging mural invasion, nodal involvement and assessing operability.
• A positron emission tomography (PET) scan is indicated to further define extraluminal spread if there is uncertainty on imaging investigations, although it can yield false positives

Distal oesophageal biopsies show a poorly differentiated adenocarcinoma of the cardia. A staging CT scan confirms a heterogeneously enhancing lesion of the gastro-oesophageal junction that appears to be localised. There are indeterminate hypodense hepatic lesions.

A whole body PET scan with fluorodeoxyglucose (FDG) confirms a bulky 7 cm tumour in the cardia, with extensive retroperitoneal lymphadenopathy, and a small focus of increased uptake in the right liver lobe consistent with

metastases. There is a single focus of high uptake in the vertebrae L3 also suggestive of a solitary bone metastasis.

What are the management options?

The main aims of treatment are to relieve symptomatic dysphagia, prolong survival and, in a minority, provide a cure. The treatment options depend on the type of carcinoma, site of tumour, evidence of spread and the patient's age and general health.

1 *Surgery*. This is indicated if there is no local invasion and resection can be achieved. It is offered in less than a third of patients with oesophageal cancer. Operative mortality is reported at less than 10% in the hands of an experienced surgeon.
2 *Chemotherapy*. Adjuvant chemotherapy may be given prior to surgical resection.
3 *Radical radiotherapy*. This is only offered for sensitive squamous cancers, located post-cricoid or in the upper third of the oesophagus. It relieves symptoms in less than half of patients if used alone and has nasty side effects.
4 *Palliation of symptoms*. This is the option for over 70% of patients. This is most appropriate in this patient.

• Endoscopic dilatation of the malignant stricture is done immediately to help swallowing. Self-expandable metal stents can then be placed to prolong the swallowing benefits. There are risks of perforation on insertion, retrosternal pain after placement, occlusion by tumour or food and stent migration.
• Palliative chemotherapy may provide symptomatic benefit after tumour shrinkage in those with adenocarcinoma.
• Palliative photodynamic therapy may be used in advanced oesophageal carcinoma.
• Palliative radiotherapy can be used in sensitive squamous cancer to relieve pain.

Mean survival is usually 10 months after diagnosis and overall 5-year survival is about 5%.

Mrs Whiston's investigations were discussed at the local MDT meeting. She had evidence of metastases to the liver and bone and the disease was too advanced for surgery. She was referred for palliative chemotherapy and had four cycles of ECF (epirubicin, cisplatin and fluorouracil) / decitabine. There was no improvement of dysphagia. She underwent dilatation and oesophageal stent insertion with no complications. She was able to manage liquids and thin soups and maintained her weight with high calorie drinks.

CASE REVIEW

Dysphagia can be at the level of the oropharynx or oesophagus. It may be for solids, liquids or both. It may be of short duration and progressive or intermittent and static. Weight loss is an alarm symptom. Complications include aspiration and perforation. Investigations should be directed by the suspected underlying cause and patient co-morbidity. This includes blood tests, chest imaging, barium swallow and/or upper endoscopy with biopsies.

This woman had progressive dysphagia for solids over a short period with associated weight loss and a past history of reflux and heartburn. Barium confirmed a stricture and endoscopy demonstrated a mass lesion. This is classic for carcinoma.

Decisions as to the further investigation and management for suspected cancer are made at MDT meetings by teams of specialists. The aim of treatment is to relieve symptoms, improve survival and cure if possible. The majority receive palliation of symptoms through dilatation and stenting. Prognosis is poor with a 5-year survival of 5%.

KEY POINTS

- The history is crucial in detecting dysphagia, and determining if it is intermittent or continuous, progressive or variable.
- You must determine the duration, type (solid, liquid or both), pattern and associated features of dysphagia.
- Barium swallow is the first line investigation for disorders of motility, to detect a pharyngeal pouch and in elderly patients with intermittent dysphagia.
- Urgent endoscopy should be done for dysphagia at any age with alarm symptoms, for solids alone or when symptoms are progressive.
- Carcinoma of the cardia may mimic carcinoma of the lower third of the oesophagus or achalasia.
- There is a multidisciplinary team approach to cardia and oesophageal cancer.
- CT staging, EUS and PET scans are used to determine if the tumour can be resected and whether an operation may be potentially curative.

Case 2 A 52-year-old man with atypical chest pain

Mr Fred Drunson is a 52-year-old man who describes chest pain related to meals and exertion. He was seen by his general practitioner 3 months ago who referred him to the cardiologists for investigation of possible angina. His electrocardiogram was described as showing sinus rhythm with no ST abnormalities. An exercise tolerance test reproduced his symptoms without electrocardiograph changes. He had a diagnostic angiogram with normal coronary arteries.

His chest pain persists. A chest X-ray showed normal lung fields and no bony abnormalities. Thyroid function tests and an autoimmune screen were normal. He has been referred to you to exclude a gastrointestinal cause of his chest pain.

List the gastrointestinal causes of atypical chest pain

- Gastro-oesophageal reflux disease.
- Oesophageal spasm or motility disorder.
- Oesophagitis.
- Barrett's oesophagus.
- Hiatus hernia (large and/or complicated).
- Benign oesophageal stricture.
- Oesophageal malignancy.

What questions will help to identify a gastrointestinal cause of this chest pain?
Presenting complaint
Describe his chest pain:
- Is it a retrosternal burning sensation?
- Is there reflux of acid or bile into the mouth? Is there an altered taste sensation? This is often described as a bitter taste.

Gastroenterology: Clinical Cases Uncovered, 1st edition.
© S. Keshav and E. Culver. Published 2011 by
Blackwell Publishing Ltd.

- Does he have increased salivation (waterbrash) in the mouth associated with the pain?
- Is it aggravated by meals, lying down, stooping or straining and exercise? Chest pain that is postural or exertional, both of which increase intra-abdominal pressure, can be hard to distinguish from angina.
- Is there relief with antacids?
- What is the duration of his symptoms? Has he had similar symptoms in the past? Did they resolve spontaneously or require treatment? What is the frequency and severity of these symptoms? Are they getting progressively worse?

Associated symptoms
- Does he have upper abdominal pain or discomfort associated with early satiety and post-prandial fullness (dyspepsia)?
- Does he have intermittent dysphagia? This is usually due to dysfunctional peristalsis or a peptic stricture. Is there pain on swallowing? This is often attributed to severe oesophagitis, typically reflux or candidiasis.
- Does he suffer from a dry cough or hoarseness? This may be due to aspiration of gastric contents into the mouth and larynx. This may also be due to bronchial or upper respiratory tract disease.
- Does he have nocturnal asthma-like symptoms of cough or wheeze? This can be caused by reflux of gastric acid at night.

!RED FLAG

The following are alarm symptoms at any age:

- Progressive unintentional weight loss
- Progressive dysphagia
- Persistent nausea and vomiting
- Symptomatic gastrointestinal blood loss (haematemesis or melaena)

Past medical history

Ask about previous gastrointestinal disease, especially oesophageal irritation, inflammation and ulceration. Ask about previous gastrointestinal investigation, including endoscopy or barium studies. What were they for and what did they show?

Medications

In particular focus on the use of NSAIDs, bisphosphonates and slow-release potassium tablets that may inflame or stricture the oesophageal mucosa. Antidepressants, anticholinergics or theophylline-based tablets may cause dysmotility.

Ask if he has tried any medication to treat his chest pain, such as Gaviscon or antacid medication. Has anything improved his symptoms? Glyceral trinitrate (GTN) spray for angina may also relieve oesophageal spasm.

Social history

Ask about smoking, alcohol and caffeine consumption as well as dietary habits. Do any of these aggravate his symptoms? Eating large meals, and eating at erratic times of the day or late at night, often aggravates reflux symptoms.

Family history

Establish if there is a family history of oesophageal carcinoma.

On further questioning, Fred describes his pain as retrosternal and burning in quality, which is aggravated by meals and by exertion. The pain occurs a few times a week. He has had symptoms for the last 4 months. He gets reflux of acid with pain on lying flat and has a sour taste in his mouth. He has no problem with swallowing solids and liquids. He has a nocturnal cough but no other respiratory symptoms. There are no alarm symptoms.

Fred has a past medical history of irritable bowel syndrome, hypertension and hepatitis A. He had an endoscopy 10 years ago for persistent abdominal pain and weight loss. He was diagnosed with a gastric ulcer. Biopsies of the ulcer showed no evidence of dysplasia. The ulcer was thought secondary to ibuprofen that he was taking for tension headaches. He did not have Helicobacter pylori eradication treatment as his breath test was negative.

His only medication is ramipril 10 mg daily. He no longer takes NSAIDs. He works as a sales manager, drinks alcohol

in moderation and is a non-smoker He has a family history of one uncle (on his mother's side) with carcinoma of the oesophagus, although he is uncertain as to the age of diagnosis.

What are the important features on examination?

Examination is undertaken to look for evidence of serious gastrointestinal pathology, systemic disease and to guide investigations.

• Look for evidence of weight change, especially weight loss.

• Look for conjunctival pallor of anaemia.

• Inspect the mouth for evidence of acid erosion on his teeth and smell of halitosis.

• Inspect for white plaques of *Candida* in the mouth (see Plate 2.1).

• Palpate for cervical lymphadenopathy and goitre of hyperthyroidism.

• Examine the chest for evidence of cardiovascular or respiratory disease.

• Palpate for evidence of musculoskeletal tenderness over the sternum and ribs.

• Examine the upper abdomen for scars and hernias, palpate for tenderness, organomegaly or a mass, and auscultate for bowel sounds.

On examination, he is overweight. There is no conjunctival pallor or lymphadenopathy. There is no evidence of acid erosion of the teeth. He has a soft, non-tender abdomen with an appendicectomy scar. There is a small right inguinal hernia which is reducible.

What investigations, if any, are required?

These symptoms are typical of gastro-oesophageal reflux. He has no alarm symptoms. He is overweight, which may exacerbate his symptoms. Investigation is only needed in the presence of alarm symptoms or if they are frequent and severe or progressive.

What treatment should be offered in this case?

General measures should be suggested as first line as they are more effective and more readily accepted than drugs. Medication should be offered if general methods do not relieve symptoms.

General measures

• Dietary intervention: reducing fat intake (fat delays gastric emptying and promotes reflux by relaxation of the lower oesophageal sphincter), smaller and regular meals, eating earlier in evening (to reduce intra-abdominal pressure and to promote gastric emptying before lying in bed), and avoiding spicy or irritant foods.

• Lifestyle changes: raising the head of the bed or sleeping on multiple pillows (gravitational), avoiding hot drinks and alcohol before bed (promotes reflux by relaxation of oesophageal sphincter), stopping smoking, and reducing alcohol and caffeine intake.

• Promote weight loss through regular exercise and healthy eating (to reduce intra-abdominal pressure). In women, pregnancy increases intra-abdominal pressure and promotes reflux symptoms.

• Avoid medications that may aggravate symptoms: NSAIDs, antidepressants, anticholinergics and theophylline-based treatments.

Medication

• Use antacids as needed for symptomatic relief.

• A therapeutic trial of a protein pump inhibitor (PPI) such as omeprazole 20–40 mg or lansoprazole 15–30 mg is reliable to confirm the diagnosis of gastro-oesophageal reflux when doubt exists. PPIs irreversibly block acid production by parietal cells.

Ensure a back-stop appointment to review the patient's response to general measures and medication in 4–6 weeks.

> Fred tries to loose weight by diet modification and increasing his daily exercise but fails. He finds it difficult to cut out the alcohol from his daily routine. In the meantime, he uses Gaviscon liquid as needed with some improvement in symptoms.
>
> He returns 4 weeks later for a prescription of PPI therapy. He has a 4-week course of omeprazole 20 mg daily. He returns to the surgery and describes relief of his chest pain and acid reflux. He is happy to discontinue the medication.
>
> He returns 4 months later describing a recurrence of atypical chest pain.

He re-presents with atypical chest pain. What do you do now?

• Re-take the history and ensure there are no new alarm symptoms.

• Reinforce the general measures of dietary modification and lifestyle advice as before.

The intermittent treatment of recurrent symptoms is safe in the absence of any alarm symptoms. You should aim to use the smallest dose of PPI to control symptoms.

> Fred describes retrosternal burning and acid reflux on most days of the week. This is aggravated by bending over and associated again with noctural cough. He is given a further 4-week course of omeprazole 20 mg daily. This provides partial relief of his symptoms only. The dose is escalated to omeprazole 40 mg daily for a further 4 weeks. This settles his daily symptoms but he still has acid and excess salivation in the mouth on stooping over or after a large meal.
>
> He returns to see you, concerned that the symptoms are not completely controlled. He is anxious.

The symptoms have not resolved on high dose PPI for 4 weeks. What do you do now?

• Check compliance with his medication. Patients may not be compliant with medication due to side effects, including gastrointestinal upset, nausea and loose stools. Compliance may also be an issue due to busy working schedule, lack of education as to the importance of a daily regimen, and lack of instant benefit.

• If he is compliant, consider endoscopy to look for other organic causes.

Endoscopy

This is indicated for atypical symptoms, those that are persistent and severe, or progressive, on adequate therapy. There is no correlation between the severity of reflux symptoms and findings on endoscopy; it is common to get symptomatic reflux and a normal endoscopy.

The patient must stop his PPI 2 weeks before the procedure so oesophageal inflammation and abnormal mucosa can be seen.

Biopsies are taken to distinguish histologically between reflux oesophagitis and Barrett's oesophagus (see Plates 2.2 and 2.3). They are also done to look for evidence of dysplasia or carcinoma. Techniques such as narrow band imaging, confocal microscopy and chromoendoscopy allow for targeted biopsies to detect dysplasia. *H. pylori* is negatively associated with reflux oesophagitis.

Box 2.1 Findings at endoscopy in patients with reflux symptoms

- Oesophageal inflammation
- Oesophageal ulceration
- Barrett's oesophagus
- Hiatus hernia (sliding or rolling)
- Oesophageal stricture (benign or malignant) (see Plate 2.4)
- Oesophageal carcinoma

Box 2.2 Reflux oesophagitis and Barrett's oesophagus

Reflux

Reflux is predominantly caused by transient relaxation of the lower oesophageal sphincter, which leads to prolonged exposure of the distal oesophageal mucosa to an acidic pH. This damages the mucosal barrier and leads to inflammation and ulceration called oesophagitis. Prolonged reflux increases the risk of oesophageal adenocarcinoma by eight-fold. The severity of symptoms correlates with the increased risk of carcinoma.

Barrett's oesophagus

Barrett's oesophagus is a pre-malignant condition that may undergo dysplasia and develop into adenocarcinoma. Chronic acid reflux can induce metaplastic changes in the distal oesophagus, transforming squamous epithelium to columnar epithelium with gastric or small intestinal features. Barrett's is a histological diagnosis and can look similar to oesophagitis down the endoscope. Once confirmed, segments over 5 cm long require endoscopic surveillance with quadrantic biopsies every 2 cm. The risk of carcinoma is related to the length of Barrett's metaplasia. Narrow-band imaging, confocal microscopy and dye spraying with targeted biopsies are being utilised to increase diagnostic yield in specialist centres.

KEY POINT

- Histology is needed to differentiae between Barrett's oesophagus and reflux oesophagitis. This is important as it guides the needs for long-term PPI therapy and surveillance endoscopy, which is appropriate in the latter.

Fred discontinued his PPI therapy for 2 weeks and was booked for endoscopy. Upper endoscopy revealed oesophageal inflammation with patchy ulceration and a small 3 cm sliding hiatus hernia (see Plate 2.5). The stomach was normal and CLO test was negative. The distal oesophagus was biopsied to confirm oesophagitis with no evidence of dysplasia.

He was re-started on omeprazole 40 mg for a further 4 weeks to allow mucosal healing. He was advised to lose weight, reduce his alcohol consumption and modify his diet. He was reminded to avoid medications that could flare his symptoms.

He returns to your clinic with a few questions.

How should you answer your patient's questions?

Firstly, how long should he continue to take his PPI?

PPI maintenance treatment should be continued for patients with refractory symptoms on discontinuation, confirmed Barrett's oesophagus (with increased risk of adenocarcinoma), peptic strictures or confluent oesophagitis with ulceration. Fred should continue PPI treatment at the lowest dose for symptomatic benefit.

Secondly, what are the risks of taking long-term PPI?

There has been an association with PPIs and increased risk of *Clostridium difficile* infection, intestinal bacterial overgrowth and interference with vitamin B_{12} absorption, although the true significance remains uncertain.

Thirdly, what about the hiatus hernia, does it need treatment?

Hiatus hernia is present in a third of people in those over 50 years. It forms when part of the stomach herniates through a space in the diaphragm up into the oesophagus. Reflux can be aggravated by this hernia. There are two types of hiatus hernia:
- A sliding hernia is the most common type. It causes no symptoms itself and requires no treatment.
- A rolling hernia is uncommon and may lead to a gastric volvulus and become strangulated, causing episodic pain and vomiting. This is a surgical emergency.

Lastly, if medication is ineffective, is surgery an option?

Fundoplication may be an option in intractable reflux despite medication, in the presence or absence of a hiatus hernia. This is attractive in young patients who do not wish to take lifelong medication but can be associated with mortality as high as 1%. Some patients require PPI therapy again even after surgical intervention. It is important to choose patients for surgery carefully.

Investigations prior to consideration of surgery

• *Oesophageal manometry* (or a marshmallow barium swallow): to differentiate between reflux and dysmotility. Pressure transducers are placed over the lower oesophageal sphincter to evaluate function. It is used to diagnose diffuse oesophageal spasm and achalasia.

• *pH studies*: these are conducted if it is difficult to distinguish symptomatic reflux from other causes of chest pain or if manometry is normal. It measures the frequency and severity of acid reflux and its relationship to the patient's symptoms. pH electrodes are passed down the nose or mouth, where they remain for 24h to investigate how sleeping, activity and eating influences acid production. Catheter-free bravo capsules are also available; they can help to guide treatment recommendations (Fig. 2.1).

CASE REVIEW

Atypical chest pain can be a symptom of gastro-oesophageal reflux disease. Associated symptoms include excess salivation (waterbrash), altered bitter taste in the mouth, retrosternal burning sensation, pain aggravation by stooping and bending, and a nocturnal cough or wheeze. There may also be cardiovascular, respiratory, musculoskeletal and endocrine causes of chest pain that must be excluded.

Initial management should include general lifestyle measures, such as weight loss, dietary intervention, reduction of alcohol and caffeine and stopping smoking. Medication should be introduced if these measures fail to control symptoms, with a 4-week trial of PPI. Endoscopy is only indicated in the presence of alarm symptoms, or persistent and severe symptoms not controlled by the above measures. Surgical intervention for intractable reflux symptoms should only be considered after evaluation by manometry and pH studies to identify those who may benefit from this procedure.

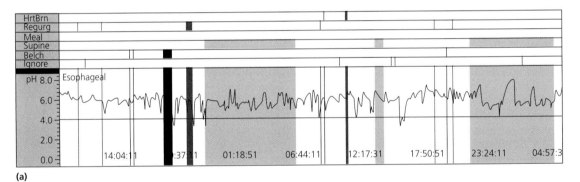

(a)

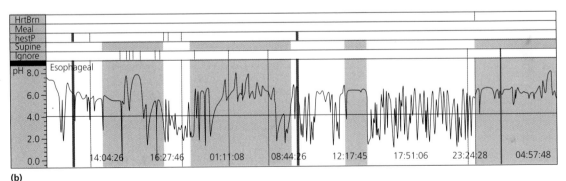

(b)

Fig. 2.1 Bravo capsule pH study: (a) tracing of a normal oesophageal pH study; (b) tracing of an abnormal oesophageal pH study demonstrating severe reflux.

KEY POINTS

- Gastro-oesophageal reflux symptoms occur frequently, although reflux oesophagitis may be asymptomatic. There is no clear relationship between symptomatic reflux and the endoscopic severity of oesophagitis.
- Reflux is usually caused by transient relaxation of the lower oesophageal sphincter causing prolonged exposure of the distal oesophageal mucosa to an acidic pH and causing oesophagitis.
- Prolonged reflux increases the risk of oesophageal adenocarcinoma, and acid suppression may reduce this risk.

- Most patients with gastro-oesophageal reflux do not need investigation; endoscopy is indicated for atypical symptoms or persistent and severe symptoms despite adequate PPI therapy.
- Manometry and/or barium swallow can distinguish between reflux and dysmotility.
- pH studies are reserved for those with normal endoscopy and manometry to correlate symptoms with low pH and to guide further management.

Case 3 A 57-year-old woman with upper abdominal discomfort

Mrs Abby Gaunt is a 57-year-old shop worker who describes a 1-year history of intermittent upper abdominal discomfort. It has become more severe and more frequent over the last month. She is concerned that something serious is underlying it. She wants to know if she could have cancer.

What are the possible causes of this woman's upper abdominal pain?

• Peptic ulcer disease, caused by *Helicobacter pylori* or NSAIDs.
• Non-ulcer dyspepsia.
• Gallstone disease (cholelithiasis).
• Gastro-oesophageal reflux disease.
• Coeliac disease.
• Pancreatitis.
• Pancreatic cancer.
• Gastric cancer.
• Mesenteric ischaemia.
• Myocardial ischaemia.

What information should you elicit from the history to narrow the diagnosis?
Presenting complaint

A full description of abdominal discomfort should be elicited. This includes its character, location, intensity and severity, radiation, frequency and associated factors. The exact duration of symptoms is important to guide further investigation. Onset over weeks or months is

more concerning than pain that has been present for many years. Define previous episodes of abdominal pain or discomfort and if they resolved spontaneously or were treated, and how.

Specific aggravating factors include eating (gallstones, mesenteric ischaemia, peptic ulcer), nocturnal symptoms (reflux), bending/stooping (reflux) and exertion (cardiac). Specific relieving factors include food (peptic ulcer), milk and antacids (reflux, ulcer and non-ulcer dyspepsia). Ask about certain food intolerances, for example to dairy or wheat-based foods (lactose intolerant, coeliac disease).

Associated features

• Acid reflux or a retrosternal burning sensation: consider gastro-oesophageal reflux disease.
• Anorexia, nausea and vomiting: consider peptic ulceration, gallstones and, if persistent, gastric outlet obstruction.
• Post-prandial fullness and early satiety: this may suggest peptic ulcer, *H. pylori* infection or non-ulcer disease. You must also consider an obstructive or motility cause.
• Bloating and abdominal distension, excessive flatulence, belching or borborygmi: consider obstructive causes, gallstones or malabsorption. Irritable bowel remains a diagnosis of exclusion in this age group.
• A change in bowel habit: consider malabsorption due to coeliac disease or pancreatic insufficiency.

Alarm symptoms

The presence of any of these features *at any age* warrants urgent referral for further investigation. Retrospective studies have found that cancer is rarely detected in patients under the age of 55 years without alarm symptoms and, when found, is usually inoperable.

Gastroenterology: Clinical Cases Uncovered, 1st edition.
© S. Keshav and E. Culver. Published 2011 by Blackwell Publishing Ltd.

Alarm symptoms/features at any age:

- Symptomatic gastrointestinal blood loss
- Progressive unintentional weight loss
- Progressive dysphagia
- Persistent nausea and vomiting
- Epigastric mass
- Iron-deficiency anaemia (unless pre-menopause female)
- Consumption of ulcer-inducing medication, such as NSAIDs and steroids
- Previous gastric ulcer
- Concomitant disease with possible gastrointestinal involvement

Medical background

A history of gastric or duodenal ulceration, gallstones, pancreatic inflammation and abdominal surgery is important. There may have been prior investigations such as a barium meal or endoscopy; the date and findings of such tests should be sought.

Non-gastrointestinal disease is also important. Ischaemic heart disease or peripheral vascular disease may be suggestive of mesenteric ischaemia. Late-onset diabetes may be a marker of pancreatic insufficiency and support a diagnosis of chronic pancreatic inflammation or neoplasia. A history of other autoimmune conditions may suggest celiac disease.

Medications

A drug history is essential. In particular, ask about NSAIDs, steroids, salicylates, nitrates, bisphosphonates, theophyline and calcium antagonists, which may have caused oesophageal or gastric inflammation and ulceration. Ask about medication taken to relieve the abdominal discomfort. This includes analgesics and antacid medication. If so, what were they, what dose was used, and did they have any positive effect?

Social history

Elicit a history of smoking tobacco, alcohol use and caffeine consumption. All of these may exacerbate ulcer disease. Excessive alcohol intake may cause pancreatic inflammation. A history of hot spicy foods or citrus-containing foods may suggest gastro-oesophageal reflux, ulcer and non-ulcer dyspepsia. Establish food intolerances and eating habits. Does she eat late at night and eat large portions of food? Body weight and fluctuations are important. Is she overweight and has she noticed any recent increase in body weight, which may exacerbate reflux symptoms?

Family history

A family history of gastric malignancy should be elicited.

Mrs Gaunt describes her symptoms as a heaviness and unease in her upper abdomen with a feeling of fullness after meals. It is worse at night and after eating large meals. She denies any alarm symptoms. She has no history of ulceration. She has tried Gaviscon, taken as required, and a 2-week trial of ranitidine with no effect.

She has a history of hypercholesterolaemia, for which she takes a statin, and is an ex-smoker with a 20 pack year history. She consumes 30 units of alcohol a week. Her diet is poor, with lots of ready-made meals and late night take aways. She finds exercise difficult and usually drives to her work, which is 2 km from her home.

What are the important features on examination?

General examination

Look for signs suggestive of organic and serious gastrointestinal disease. Look for evidence of weight change – weight loss suggested by loose skin folds and loose clothes, weight gain by stretch marks and tight fitting clothing. Look in the eyes for signs of anaemia, such as conjunctival pallor, and for scleral icterus (jaundice) suggesting biliary or liver disease. Feel for lymphadenopathy, especially supraclavicular lymph nodes of gastric carcinoma (Virchow's node). Look for signs of malabsorption and vitamin/mineral deficiency.

Abdominal examination

Inspect for skin discolouration from the use of a hot-water bottle to relieve pain (erythema ab igne), especially found in pancreatic inflammation. Inspect for abdominal scars from prior surgical procedures. Inspect for abdominal distension or the impression of a mass. Palpation for abdominal tenderness is usually non-specific. Hepatomegaly may be a benign, enlarged lobe or indicate hepatic metastases. If a mass is felt, its location, size and character should be assessed. Auscultation for a 'succussion splash' suggestive of outlet obstruction should be undertaken, and for bowel sounds, which are 'tinkling' in obstruction.

On examination she is overweight, with a BMI of 29. There is no conjunctival pallor or scleral icterus. There are no palpable lymph nodes. Abdominal exam reveals some non-specific epigastric tenderness with no guarding or rebound. There is no palpable organomegaly or masses and bowel sounds are normal.

What is the most likely cause of this woman's symptoms?

This patient gives a classic description of dyspepsia: a central upper abdominal or retrosternal discomfort with heaviness, unease, post-prandial fullness and early satiety. The discomfort is often related to eating, hunger, certain foods and time of day. There are no alarm symptoms.

How would you investigate and manage this woman?

Not all patients need investigation. Routine endoscopy in patients with dyspepsia and without alarm symptoms is not indicated. As she has no alarm symptoms, general measures, testing and treating for *H. pylori* and a trial of therapy are appropriate.

General measures

Explain the symptoms of dyspepsia and reassure her that in the absence of alarm symptoms the risk of cancer is very low.

- Give lifestyle advice. Tell her to stop smoking, consume less alcohol and loose some weight to help improve symptoms.
- Give dietary advice. Encourage healthy eating, limit spicy and acidic foods and avoid those foods that exacerbate symptoms.
- Provide access to educational material on dyspepsia, including website details and leaflets to read.
- Review medications that may be aggravating her symptoms, either prescribed or over-the-counter.
- In the first instance, advise self-treatment with antacids or alginates as needed.

Trial of PPI and 'test and treat'

If general measures are not effective give a trial of full dose PPI (e.g. omeprazole 40 mg od or lansoprazole 30 mg od) for 1 month *and* test for *H. pylori* via a breath test and treat with triple therapy if positive. A minimum of 2 weeks should be given between a trial of PPI therapy and a breath test for infection with *H. pylori*.

Addition of other agents

The addition of a H_2-receptor antagonist (H_2RA) such as ranitidine 150 mg bd or a prokinetic such as domperidone 10 mg tds for a further month may be advised if the above are ineffective.

Once symptoms are controlled, there should be a stepwise reduction of medications to take the lowest dose required.

Mrs Gaunt stopped smoking, reduced her alcohol intake and started walking to work. Unfortunately, she didn't manage to loose any weight despite this. She tried a 4-week course of omeprazole 40 mg daily, and although the symptoms improved they did not entirely settle. She had a negative H. pylori breath test. She remained concerned that her symptoms persisted and came back to your clinic asking for advice.

What should you tell her now?

Most patients with dyspepsia without alarm symptoms, who do not respond to lifestyle advice, acid suppression and *H. pylori* eradication, if breath test positive, have non-ulcer dyspepsia. However, as she is over the age of 55 years and symptoms have persisted despite the above, referral for endoscopy should be considered to look for organic causes of dyspepsia.

Box 3.1 Organic causes of dyspepsia

- Peptic ulcer (duodenal or gastric ulcer)
- Reflux oesophagitis
- Gastritis or duodenitis
- Gallstone disease
- Gastric cancer

KEY POINT

- In the absence of alarm symptoms, general lifestyle measures, testing and treating for *H. pylori* and a trial of acid suppression therapy are appropriate for typical dyspepsia. In those who do not respond to the above measures, further investigation may be warranted to look for organic causes of dyspepsia.

What investigations are appropriate?
Blood tests

A full blood count should be taken to look for anaemia and thrombocytopenia. Liver function tests and coagulation studies should be taken for gallstone and hepatic disease. C-reactive protein is a marker of inflammation and infection. Amylase may be elevated in pancreatitis, but may also be normal. Immunoglobulin A (IgA) anti-endomysial antibody or tissue transglutaminase have high sensitivity and specificity in detecting coeliac disease. Tumour markers are not indicated as a screening tool.

Upper gastrointestinal endoscopy

Endoscopy should be done to look for peptic ulceration, inflammation and malignancy (see Plates 3.1 and 3.2). Biopsies should be taken for *H. pylori*. Patients should be free from PPI and H_2RA for 2 weeks prior to investigation, as acid suppression can mask the detection of oesophageal and gastric carcinoma.

Barium meal

This can be done if it is difficult to define the anatomy at endoscopy and to look for evidence of pyloric obstruction.

Abdominal ultrasound

This should be done to identify the presence of gallstone disease and any evidence of pancreatic inflammation, atrophy or a mass. If pancreatic abnormalities are detected, further imaging by CT or magnetic resonance scanning of the pancreas/bile ducts will be necessary.

> *Mrs Gaunt had blood tests, which were normal including coeliac serology. She proceeded to gastroscopy, which was entirely normal, and abdominal ultrasound, which was also normal. Biopsies taken at endoscopy did not show any evidence of malignancy or H. pylori. She returned to the clinic a little confused. She continued to have the upper abdominal discomfort.*

She is confused that all her investigations are normal but she continues to have upper abdominal discomfort. How do you manage her?

Non-ulcer dyspepsia is defined as upper abdominal discomfort related to meals, lasting for more than 4 weeks and for which no cause can be found after investigation.

Reassurance

She needs an empathetic explanation emphasising the benign nature of her dyspepsia. There is no evidence of cancer and this will not progress to cancer.

General measures

Once again, general measures including lifestyle advice, diet modification, access to educational material and self-treatment with antacids or alginates should be enforced.

Discontinue ineffective medication

All ineffective medications should be stopped, and she should use medications as required or the lowest possible dose to control her symptoms.

Additional therapies

These are recommended by clinicians in resistant cases:
• Trial of domperidone 10 mg tds (prokinetic for symptoms of dysmotility).
• Trial of amitriptyline at 10 mg daily at night.
• Trial of an antispasmodic such as buscopan.
• Combination of above treatments.
• Dietary referral to explore restricting starch intake.
• Complementary therapies may be considered such as aromatherapy, hypnotherapy and cognitive-behavioural therapy.

CASE REVIEW

Dyspepsia is a central, upper abdominal or retrosternal discomfort with heaviness, unease, post-prandial fullness and early satiety. The discomfort is often related to eating, hunger, certain foods and time of day. Alarm symptoms, such as gastrointestinal blood loss, unintentional weight loss, progressive dysphagia and persistent nausea and vomiting, should prompt referral for early investigation. Other alarm features include an epigastric mass on examination, consumption of ulcer-inducing medications and a prior history of gastric ulcer.

Dyspepsia without alarm symptoms should be managed through general lifestyle advice, dietary intervention and education. A 1-month trial of PPI *and* a breath test for *H. pylori* is appropriate. Additional medications such as H₂RAs and prokinetics may be added.

Organic disease should be excluded in anyone with alarm symptoms, in those over the age of 55 years, and in those whose symptoms are refractory to the above measures. Blood tests should be done to look for coeliac disease. Endoscopy is indicated to look for ulceration, inflammation and malignancy. Abdominal ultrasound will exclude gallstone disease and look for pancreatic pathology, if the history and examination is suggestive.

This woman had typical dyspepsia with no alarm symptoms or signs. Symptoms were refractory to general measures and PPI therapy. Blood tests, endoscopy and abdominal ultrasound were normal and the benign nature of her disease was reinforced and general measures reinstituted.

KEY POINTS

- Dyspepsia is defined as chronic or recurrent pain or discomfort centred in the upper abdomen. It should be differentiated from gastro-oesophageal reflux disease as management differs.
- Dyspepsia due to organic disease must be differentiated from functional or non-ulcer dyspepsia.
- Patients with alarm symptoms should have an urgent referral for endoscopy.

- If no alarm symptoms are elicited, lifestyle advice, general measures and a therapeutic trial of acid suppression for 1 month *and* a test and treat for *H. pylori* are indicated.
- Most patients with no alarm symptoms, who do not respond to lifestyle advice, acid suppression and *H. pylori* eradication, have non-ulcer dyspepsia. Endoscopy does not usually alter management in these patients.

A 36-year-old man with upper abdominal discomfort and heartburn

Graham Clo is a 36-year-old mechanic who comes to you complaining of upper abdominal discomfort for the last few weeks. Unlike previous episodes of what he would have called 'indigestion', this feeling has persisted. He has not experienced this discomfort before.

What questions would help to establish the cause of these symptoms?

Abdominal discomfort

It is important to identify symptoms of dyspepsia (upper abdominal discomfort or pain), and distinguish these from cardiac-, musculoskeletal- or respiratory-related illness. The key distinguishing questions are:

• Is there a relationship to eating; is it either worsened by or is there temporary relief after a meal?
• Are the symptoms related to exertion? Is there associated breathlessness or palpitations?
• Has there been unaccustomed exertion or injury? Is it worsened on movement?
• Has there been a recent respiratory infection? Is there associated cough, sputum or breathing difficulty?

Associated symptoms

Dyspepsia and heartburn and/or reflux symptoms often occur together. The bowel habit may be altered in coeliac disease, often with loose or frequent bowel motions. Weight loss may be the result of food avoidance; weight gain may occur because he eats more to assuage pain.

Alarm features

A set of 'alarm features' should be checked to guide the need for prompt investigation. These include progressive unintentional weight loss, progressive dysphagia, persistent nausea and vomiting, presence of an abdominal mass on examination and iron-deficiency anaemia on blood testing.

Medical history

A history of previous gastric or duodenal ulceration is important. Any surgical operations of his abdomen, or previous endoscopic or abdominal imaging may help to guide investigations.

Drug history

Non-steroidal anti inflammatory drugs (NSAIDs) and aspirin can cause intestinal inflammation and peptic ulceration, so should be actively sought in the drug history. It is worthwhile establishing if he has tried any over-the-counter analgesia or antacids to relieve his symptoms, and if they have been effective.

Social history

Cigarettes, alcohol and certain eating habits, such as eating spicy foods or eating late at night, may exacerbate symptoms of dyspepsia and heartburn. Milk-based drinks, which are alkaline, may help to relieve symptoms.

Family history

Ask if there is a family history of peptic ulcer disease or gastric cancer at a young age.

> **KEY POINT**
>
> • Life-threatening upper gastrointestinal disease is unlikely in young person, i.e. younger than 55 years old. To aid in the early detection of serious illness, a set of 'alarm features' should be checked.

Gastroenterology: Clinical Cases Uncovered, 1st edition.
© S. Keshav and E. Culver. Published 2011 by
Blackwell Publishing Ltd.

> **!RED FLAG**
>
> Alarm symptoms/features or 'red flags' at any age are features in the presentation that should trigger prompt investigation for upper intestinal disease such as peptic ulcer or malignancy:
>
> - Progressive unintentional weight loss
> - Progressive dysphagia
> - Persistent nausea and vomiting
> - Symptomatic gastrointestinal blood loss
> - Epigastric mass
> - Iron-deficiency anaemia

Mr Clo describes heartburn and upper abdominal discomfort that are exacerbated by eating and alcohol. He denies any alarm features. He has no previous medical history apart from occasional cold and flu-like symptoms. He takes no regular medication. He has not tried antacids, although he noticed that milky drinks sometimes relieve his symptoms.

He smokes 10 cigarettes a day, consumes at least 5 units of alcohol per week and has a healthy diet. He is active and his capacity for exercise is not diminished in any way.

List the most likely causes for this man's abdominal discomfort

In a young man with no other medical problems and typical dyspepsia, the following should be considered:
- *Helicobacter pylori* infection.
- Gastritis secondary to alcohol excess or NSAIDs.
- Peptic ulceration.
- Gastro-oesophageal reflux disease.
- Non-ulcer dyspepsia.
- Coeliac disease.
- Gallstone disease.

What do you look for on examination to aid your diagnosis?
General examination
Examination is important to look for signs of serious gastrointestinal pathology.
- Look for evidence of weight loss, such as loose skin or loose-fitting clothing, and record the body mass index.
- Look for signs of anaemia, such as conjunctival and skin pallor.
- Look for evidence of lymphadenopathy, such as in the supraclavicular fossa (Virchow's node) suggestive of gastric malignancy.

- Look for evidence of icteric sclera (jaundice), which may suggest biliary disease.

Examination may also help to exclude other non-dyspeptic causes of pain:
- Assess for evidence of musculoskeletal tenderness.
- Assess for signs of lower respiratory tract infection or cardiovascular disease.

Abdominal examination
Important signs on inspection include:
- The presence of skin discolouration from the use of a hot-water bottle to relieve pain – erythema ab igne.
- The presence of abdominal scars from prior surgical procedures.
- The impression of a mass in the abdomen.

Palpate each of the four quadrants of the abdomen for:
- Abdominal tenderness, and document the location and association with scars and other pathology.
- Organomegaly, note size and which organs.
- An abdominal mass and its size, shape and depth.

Auscultation for a 'succussion splash' suggestive of outlet obstruction should be undertaken.

On examination there is no anaemia, lymphadenopathy or evidence of weight loss. On abdominal examination, deep palpation in the epigastrium reminds him of his symptoms. There are no abdominal masses.

Now review the possible causes again
- *Helicobacter pylori infection.* This is extremely common worldwide, although the population rate of infection is lower in the UK than in some communities. Testing for infection is relatively cheap and readily available. Furthermore, effective treatment to eradicate infection is available if the test were positive.
- *Gastritis secondary to alcohol excess or NSAIDs.* This man drinks at least 5 units of alcohol per week and smokes tobacco. Changes in lifestyle, such as moderation of alcohol and stopping smoking, may therefore be helpful. Are you certain that he is not using NSAIDs? These are present in many over-the-counter medications such as cold remedies and compound analgesics. It is worth going over this again.
- *Peptic ulceration.* The most common causes for ulceration are *H. pylori* infection and NSAID use. Smoking also increases the risk of peptic ulceration as well as many other diseases. Once an ulcer forms it is less likely to heal and more likely to have complications if smoking continues.

- *Gastro-oesophageal reflux disease* (GORD). This affects up to 30% of the general population. The main symptoms are those of heartburn and regurgitation, provoked by bending or lying, often accompanied by excess salivation (waterbrash). This can be aggravated by eating dietary fat, chocolate, alcohol or coffee, which relaxes the lower oesophageal sphincter, eating late meals, bending over after eating and possibly smoking. Antacids and proton pump inhibitors are the treatments of choice.
- *Non-ulcer dyspepsia.* This is defined as chronic dyspepsia with no evidence of organic disease on investigation. Other symptoms may include early satiety, bloating, fullness and nausea. Endoscopy is essential in this instance to exclude organic cause.
- *Coeliac disease.* This can manifest in many different ways. Symptoms can include abdominal discomfort, bloating, nausea and altered bowel habit. Other features include vitamin deficiency, anaemia and osteoporosis. It is readily detected by a single blood test, either an IgA anti-endomysial antibody or tissue transglutaminase.
- *Gallstone disease.* This is the most common disorder of the biliary tree. In those under 40 years there is a female predominance. In developed countries there is an increasing incidence and they occur at an earlier age. There presence can be investigated in the first instance by an abdominal ultrasound. Liver function tests may show a cholestatic picture if a gallstone obstructs the common bile duct.

What tests should be done?

- Blood tests should include a full blood count to detect anaemia, one of the 'alarm features' identified above.
- Coeliac serology, such as IgA anti-endomysial antibody or tissue transglutaminase, has a high sensitivity and specificity for detecting coeliac disease.
- Liver function tests may be done if considering gallstone disease, but it is unlikely in this case.
- *Helicobacter pylori* testing is discussed below.

Do you think an endoscopy is necessary?

Most clinicians believe that endoscopy is only required if the patient is older than 55 years or if one of the alarm features is present. This approach avoids unnecessary discomfort and risk to patients, and conserves resources, because dyspepsia is an extremely common symptom.

Mr Clo has normal full blood count and liver function tests. An endomysial antibody test is negative, in the context of a

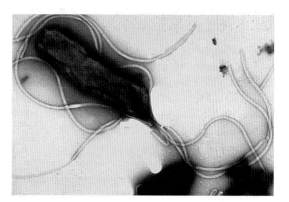

Fig. 4.1 Electron micrograph of *H. pylori* with multiple flagella.

normal IgA, making coeliac disease highly unlikely. He went on to have H. pylori testing.

What is *H. pylori* infection?

The link between chronic infection with *H. pylori* (Fig. 4.1) and peptic ulcer disease and gastritis was first described by Warren and Marshall in the 1980s. Despite initial scepticism, that has now been overturned, they won the Nobel Prize for this work in 2006. *H. pylori* infection is distributed worldwide, with a high prevalence in developing countries (up to 90% colonised by their late teens). Possible routes of infection in early childhood include oral–oral, gastro–oral and faecal–oral routes. Iatrogenic infection may occur from nasogastric tubes or endoscopes that have been inadequately sterilised.

Helicobacter survives in the gastric mucosa, producing a urease enzyme that neutralises stomach acid by producing alkaline ammonia and volatile CO_2 from urea. Consequently, it depends on the presence of stomach acid for survival and the number of bacteria in the stomach is markedly reduced when patients use acid suppressants such as PPIs and H_2 receptor antagonists.

Helicobacter pylori is a causal factor in many upper gastrointestinal conditions from minor dyspepsia to gastric cancer, so eradication is worthwhile. Therefore, *H. pylori* testing should be discussed with the patient. The British Society of Gastroenterology recommends a 'test and treat' approach, testing for its presence and then offering treatment to eradicate the infection.

How would you diagnose *H. pylori* infection in this patient?

There are both non-invasive and invasive tests for the detection of *H. pylori* and its subsequent eradication after treatment.

PART 2: CASES

Non-invasive tests

^{13}C urea breath test

This is the one of the most reliable tests and can also be used to determine if eradication has been successful. It depends on the activity of the urease enzyme from *H. pylori*. ^{13}C-labelled urea is incorporated into a drink, which the patient ingests after an overnight fast. If the patient has *Helicobacter* in their stomach the ^{13}C-labelled urea is split by urease into NH_4 and CO_2, and the proportion of ^{13}C-labelled $_{CO2}$ in the expired air indicates the presence of the bacteria. ^{13}C is a stable, non-radioactive isotope, and therefore the patient is not exposed to any risk. Concurrent use of acid suppressants, such as PPIs or H_2RAs, or even antibiotics that might reduce the number of *Helicobacter* organisms, might give rise to a false-negative test.

Serology

Circulating antibodies to *H. pylori* are formed in response to infection. They persist even after infection is eradicated; therefore antibody testing is best used as a screening tool and in epidemiological studies. High false-negative rates occur in children and in those over 55 years.

Stool antigen enzyme immunoassay

This detects *H. pylori* antigen in those with active colonisation, and is both sensitive and specific (90%). It is mainly used in children, as it avoids the need for a blood test.

Invasive tests

Endoscopy and biopsies are highly sensitive and specific although false-negative results can arise with concurrent use of acid suppressants and antibiotics:

Urease test

Freshly taken biopsies are immediately placed in a medium containing urea and a pH indicator. A change in colour, which may develop in minutes or hours, indicates that the *H. pylori* urease enzyme has hydrolysed neutral urea to alkaline NH_4 and volatile CO_2. The test is also known colloquially as the CLO test, for *Campylobacter*-like organism, reflecting the original classification of *H. pylori* as a *Campylobacter*-like species.

Histology

Patchy infection in the stomach may also lead to false negatives, and if the infection is sparse then special stains and multiple biopsies are necessary.

Culture of *H. pylori*

This s rarely used unless antibiotic sensitivity needs to be determined.

> **KEY POINT**
>
> - The ^{13}C urea breath test is the most appropriate test in general practice, with a high sensitivity and specificity for *H. pylori*.

Mr Clo has a ^{13}C urea breath test that is positive for H. pylori. He returns to you for advice about what to do next.

How do you eradicate *H. pylori*?

Helicobacter pylori infection can be readily eradicated with a combination of antibiotics and acid suppressants. The success rate of most eradication regimens is usually high (>85%), and reinfection is rare. Once infection has been diagnosed, treatment is worthwhile even if it does not influence symptoms. *H. pylori* infection is associated with gastritis, gastric and duodenal ulceration, gastric carcinoma, Ménétrièr's disease and mucosal-associated lymphoid tissue (MALT) lymphoma. It may also be associated with functional dyspepsia and NSAID-related ulcers.

Many treatment regimens have been devised. Most recommend treatment for 7–14 days. Eradication failure is usually due to poor compliance. Other reasons include bacterial resistance, inadequate acid suppression or, rarely, early reinfection.

Give the patient a thorough explanation regarding the reasons for treatment, dosing regimen and possible side effects.

Low-risk patients

- Patient with non-ulcer dyspepsia in the community.
- Those with antral or body gastritis (diagnosed from endoscopic biopsies) with no ulcers or complications.

  The treatment regimen is outlined in Table 4.1.

High-risk patients

High-risk patients include those with:
- Atrophic gastritis, associated with increase risk of progression to gastric cancer.
- Peptic ulcer disease, especially if there is bleeding or it is associated with other risk factors such as NSAID use.

Table 4.1 Treatment of patients with low-risk *H. pylori* infection.

First line for 7 days	Omeprazole 20 mg bd	Metronidazole 400 mg bd *or* amoxicillin 1 g bd	Clarithromycin 500 mg bd
Second line for 14 days (if first line fails)	Omeprazole 20 mg bd	Amoxicillin 1 g bd	Metronidazole 400 mg bd

Table 4.2 Treatment of patients with high-risk *H. pylori* infection.

First line for 7 days (as above)	Omeprazole 20 mg bd	Metronidazole 400 mg bd *or* amoxicillin 1 g bd	Clarithromycin 500 mg bd	
Second line for 14 days (if first line fails)	Omeprazole 20 mg bd	Metronidazole 400 mg bd	Amoxicillin 1 g bd *or* clarithromycin 500 mg bd	De-Noltab 2 tabs bd
Third line for 14 days	Omeprazole 20 mg bd	Metronidazole 400 mg bd	Tetracycline 500 mg tds	De-Noltab 2 tabs bd
If MALT lymphoma	Omeprazole 20 mg bd	De-Noltab 2 tabs bd	*Plus* two antibiotics not used before: rifambutin 300 mg od and levofloxacin 250 mg bd	

- MALT lymphoma (75–95% of patients are infected with *H. pylori*). Eradication alone is said to induce regression in 70–80% of cases.
- Post-resection of gastric cancer.
- First-degree relatives of gastric cancer patients.
- Low risk patients in whom future use of NSAIDs is essential.

The treatment regimen is outlined in Table 4.2.

Mr Clo received omeprazole 20 mg bd, clarithromycin 500 mg bd and metronidazole 400 mg bd for 1 week. He returned to the surgery 4 weeks later to ask if his infection has been cleared.

Does he require follow-up and retesting after treatment?

After *H. pylori* eradication for dyspepsia over 60% of people experience persistent or recurrent symptoms. Approximately 40% become asymptomatic. If symptoms persist or recur and there are no alarm symptoms, treatment for functional dyspepsia is recommended.

Lifestyle modifications must be emphasised in addition to eradication therapy. Reduction of alcohol intake, stopping smoking, weight loss in some individuals and dietary changes are important.

Box 4.1 Retesting for H. pylori

- Routine retesting is unnecessary
- A breath test is indicated when the patient has suffered a complicated duodenal ulcer (an ulcer that bled or perforated), gastric ulcers or has MALT lymphoma. It may also be helpful if symptoms persist after eradication
- Retesting should occur 4–8 weeks after treatment has been completed and acid suppressant drugs and/or antibiotics stopped
- Serology is inappropriate for retesting as it remains positive even after successful eradication

KEY POINT

- Routine retesting for *H. pylori* after eradication therapy is unnecessary.

Mr Clo has stopped smoking and reduced his alcohol intake. His symptoms resolved after eradication therapy.

CASE REVIEW

Helicobacter pylori is a widespread infection that is easily tested for and treated in the community. It can be detected non-invasively by a urease breath test and patients do not require endoscopy in the absence of alarm features and in uncomplicated cases.

The treatment to eradicate the bacteria is two antibiotics and a protein pump inhibitor for 1 week. Retesting is not appropriate unless there are severe recurrent symptoms, complicated peptic ulcer disease or MALT-lymphoma. Up to 60% of patients have persistent symptoms despite eradication and should be treated for functional dyspepsia unless there are alarm symptoms.

KEY POINTS

- Dyspeptic symptoms should prompt testing for *H. pylori* infection, and treating once found.
- *Helicobacter pylori* is an endemic human infection that is distributed worldwide.
- It is strongly associated with gastritis, gastric and duodenal ulceration, gastric cancer and MALT lymphoma.
- Spontaneous eradication of *H. pylori* infection is rare.
- Infection can be detected by reliable, cost-effective and non-invasive tests. The most reliable is the ^{13}C urease breath test.
- Infection can be eradicated by reliable and cost-effective therapy. Two antibiotics and a protein pump inhibitor are given for 1 week.
- Eradication failure is usually due to poor compliance. Reinfection with *H. pylori*, once eradicated, is rare.
- Retesting is usually unnecessary unless there are severe recurrent symptoms, complicated peptic ulcer disease or MALT-lymphoma.

Case 5　A 27-year-old woman with nausea and vomiting

Emily Gallen is a 27-year-old teaching assistant. She has been referred to your clinic with an 8-week history of persistent nausea and vomiting. She initially thought it may be acid related, so cut out acidic fruits and drinks with no improvement. She has had a trial of Gaviscon and ranitidine twice daily for 4 weeks with no improvement. She is taking a regular antiemetic, cyclizine three tablets daily, to help to control some of her symptoms.

What questions should you ask her?
Presenting compliant
Take a full history of the nausea and vomiting.
• Timing and frequency of symptoms. What time of day or time of the week does the nausea or vomit occur? Is there any pattern? Are the episodes becoming more severe or frequent or just the same?
• Are there specific precipitants or stimuli?
• Are there any relieving factors or medications?
• The contents and amount of vomit: is it faeculent, bile-stained or altered food? Is there any blood (fresh or coffee ground)?
• Duration of symptoms: have they been present for just 8 weeks or is there a prior history of similar symptoms? How did the prior episode evolve and what settled it?
• Has she been off work because of her symptoms?

Associated symptoms
Isolated nausea and vomiting are rarely organic. The associated symptoms usually narrow the differential diagnosis. The timing of these symptoms and their relationship to the nausea and vomiting should be worked out.

Gastroenterology: Clinical Cases Uncovered, 1st edition.
© S. Keshav and E. Culver. Published 2011 by
Blackwell Publishing Ltd.

• Is there any menstrual or mood disturbance? Could she be pregnant?
• Does she suffer from abdominal pain? If so, describe the type of pain and its location, radiation, frequency, intensity and relieving and intensifying factors. Is the pain related to eating? This could be peptic ulcer related. Is the pain relieved by defecation? There may be an element of constipation.
• Does she have reflux of acid or heartburn? This may suggest acid-related disease.
• Does she feel bloated or suffer excessive belching and flatulence? There may be malabsorption. There may be a functional component.
• Does she have dysphagia to solids or odonyphagia? She may have a peptic stricture, or perhaps an oesophageal ring or web.
• Has she experienced a change in bowel habit? Is this loose or solid stool? Diarrhoea and vomiting in short duration suggest an infective or obstructive aetiology. Inflammation is more likely in illness longer than this.
• Has her appetite or weight changed? If she has lost weight, how much over how long?
• Has she become jaundiced or itchy? Does she have pale stools or dark urine? Has she been feverish or had rigors? Consider gallstone disease.
• Does she have any neurological symptoms such as headaches, visual disturbance, neck stiffness, weakness or parenthesis or vertigo? Is there a rash? Consider meningeal irritation or inflammation.
• Does she suffer from other symptoms of diabetes such as excessive thirst, excessive urination, weight loss or skin infections?
• Does she suffer from other symptoms of thyroid disease such as temperature dysregulation, weight change, mood disturbances, tremors or palpitations; is there a new goitre?
• Does she suffer from any psychiatric symptoms such as delusions, hallucinations, etc?

Past medical history

• Does she suffer from diabetes or thyroid disease? Is this well controlled?

• Is there an underlying psychiatric disorder or psychological problems?

Medications

• Causative: is she taking any new medication (prescribed or over-the-counter)? Specifically, non-steroidal drugs, opioids, antiarrythmic medication, diuretics, hormonal drugs, antibiotics and antivirals, anticonvulsants?

• Treatment: has she tried any medication for the nausea and vomiting? What doses, for how long and did they help?

Social history

• Sexual history: is she sexually active and using contraception? Could she be pregnant?

• Travel: has she travelled abroad in the last few months? Where did she travel, for how long and was she exposed to anyone with an infection?

• Does she drink alcohol to excess? Does this have an impact on her symptoms?

• Does she use recreational drugs?

• Is she in contact with any children in her school who are unwell?

• Any depressive or anxiety issues? Is she enjoying her work?

She confirms an 8-week history of nausea, with intermittent vomiting over the last 2 weeks, especially in the morning. She describes a vague abdominal discomfort in the upper epigastrium with no radiation. She has been experiencing acid reflux since the vomiting started. She has noticed her stool has become harder and less frequent but considered this due to her reduced appetite and oral intake. Her weight is unchanged.

She has no known medical problems. She started taking diclofenac a few months ago for a knee injury that she sustained whilst on a school trip, although only takes one per day. She is sexually active and on the oral contraceptive pill. She had her last withdrawal bleed 1 month ago. There has been no recent travel or contact with infection. She drinks a glass of wine every night and has never smoked. She is overweight and feels rather low in mood about it.

She has worked at the same school for the last 3 years. Her job is busy but she enjoys her work and has no concerns related to this.

What is your differential diagnosis at this stage?

The differential diagnosis of nausea and vomiting can be broad. The abdominal discomfort and drug history may narrow the possibilities.

• Pregnancy (intrauterine or ectopic). Despite being on the oral contraceptive pill and having withdrawal bleeds, this must be excluded before more invasive tests are organised. A simple urinary test can be done in the first instance.

• Peptic ulcer disease. Given the history of reflux, an ulcer should be excluded.

• Drug induced from her NSAIDs. NSAID-related gastric and small bowel ulceration and inflammation may occur. This responds to discontinuation of medication.

• Gallstone disease. This may also cause abdominal discomfort, reflux, nausea and vomiting. It is less common in younger individuals.

• Functional disorder such as irritable bowel or non-ulcer dyspepsia.

• Metabolic disorder such as hypercalcaemia. Symptoms include constipation, nausea and vomit, renal stones, mood disturbance and abdominal pain. The most common cause in this age group is related to the parathyroid.

• Endocrine disorder such as Addison's disease. This is an important cause in young patients and can be easily missed if not considered.

• Psychological disturbance. Consider once organic pathology is excluded and if there is a corroborative history. Referral to a psychologist for cognitive and behavioural therapy may be needed.

What examination findings may help to confirm a cause?
General examination

• Look for signs of dehydration such as dry mucus membranes and loss of skin turgor. This may be due to poor oral intake or an inability to keep fluids down.

• Look at her teeth for signs of dental enamel loss. Does she have halitosis from severe reflux or bulimia?

• Look at her body habitus for signs of rapid weight gain or loss. Does she look malnourished?

• Look at her skin for pigmentation. This is a sign of Addison's disease.

• Look at her neck and eyes. Does she have a goitre or proptosis of thyroid disease?

• Look for focal neurological signs or localising signs.

Abdominal examination

- Look for visible peristalsis. Can you elicit a gastric succussion splash of obstruction?
- Feel for abdominal tenderness. Is there guarding or rebound?
- Feel for an abdominal hernia or mass. Is there a palpable uterus or ovarian mass?
- Consider intrauterine or ectopic pregnancy. Consider ovarian cysts and uterine fibroids.
- Listen for bowel sounds. Are they hyperactive?

She looks well from the end of the bed. There are no signs of clinical dehydration. Abdominal examination reveals abdominal distension and generalised tenderness. There are no masses and no evidence of a prominent uterus. She has a normal neurological examination.

KEY POINTS

- There are many causes of nausea and vomiting so a detailed history is important.
- Do not forget neurological, endocrine and metabolic causes.
- Do not forget pregnancy in women of childbearing age.

Box 5.1 Causes of nausea and vomiting

This depends on the clinical picture:
- Mechanical obstruction such as pyloric stenosis and small intestinal strictures
- Motility disorders such as achalasia
- Functional disorders such as gastroparesis, irritable bowel syndrome, non-ulcer dyspepsia or pseudo-obstruction
- Gastrointestinal infections and food poisoning
- Organic disease such as peptic ulcer disease, pancreatitis, hepatitis, cholecystitis, mesenteric ischaemia or gastric cancer
- Drugs such as chemotherapy agents, analgesics, antiarrhymics and diuretics, hormonal drugs, antibiotics and antivirals, anticonvulsants and anti-parkinsonian medications
- Alcohol and nicotine
- Intracranial pathology such as raised intracranial pressure, meningitis, migraine, seizures or tumours
- Ear problems such as labyrnthitis or menders

- Endocrine disorders such as diabetic ketoacidosis, Addison's disease or hyper/hypoparathyroidism
- Metabolic such as uraemia, hypercalcaemia or hyponatraemia
- Pregnancy
- Psychological and psychiatric disorders including bulimia, depression, voluntary emesis and strong emotions such as disgust

What investigations would you do?
Urine sample

- Beta-human chorionic gonadotrophin (β-HCG) to exclude an intrauterine or ectopic pregnancy.
- Dipstick for ketones (starvation and ketoacidosis), glucose, leucocytes and nitrites (urine infection).

Blood tests

- Urea (uraemia) and electrolytes (hyponatraemia).
- Liver function (hepatitis, cholecystitis) and amylase (pancreatitis).
- Glucose (impaired glucose tolerance and diabetes) and calcium (hypercalcaemia).
- Bicarbonate level for evidence of metabolic alkalosis in severe vomiting.
- Short synacthen test for Addison's disease. A random cortisol is not sufficient for diagnosis.

Endoscopy

- To look for peptic ulcer, gastritis and other upper gastrointestinal causes.
- A CLO test for *Helicobacter pylori* should be done if inflammation is present.

Abdominal ultrasound

To look for gallstones causing cholecystitis or pancreatic inflammation

What are your management options whilst you await test results?

- Stop the NSAID and replace with paracetamol for the knee pain.
- Give an antacid medication for symptomatic reflux and dyspepsia. She has already tried ranitidine with no success. A trial of omeprazole 20–40 mg daily, with Gaviscon as needed. This should be started after the endoscopy (or discontinued for 1 week prior to endoscopy to get a representative *H. pylori* test).

Table 5.1 Characteristics of different antiemetics.

Type of antiemetic	Examples	Action	Use
Acetylcholine (ACh) receptor antagonists	Hyosine	Target the vomiting centre and vestibulocochlear nuclei	Motion sickness and vestibulocochlear dysfunction
Histamine (H_1) receptor antagonists	Cyclizine 50 mg tds	Target the vestibulocochlear nuclei	Labyrinthine disorder, e.g. motion sickness, vertigo, migraine
Dopamine (D_2) receptor antagonists	Metoclopramide 10 mg tds, prochlorperazine 5 mg tds, domperidone 10 mg tds	Act centrally – antiemetic Act peripherally – prokinetic effects	Metabolic, opioid induced, postoperative or vestibular sickness
Serotonin ($5HT_3$) receptor antagonists	Ondansetron 4 mg tds	Block stimuli from the chemoreceptor trigger zone	Drug-induced nausea

• Supportive measures to replace fluid and electrolyte losses, preferably oral rehydration sachets.
• Antiemetics can be given for symptomatic nausea, even when the causative agent remains (Table 5.1).

What are the consequences of recurrent vomiting?

The consequences of vomiting include:
• Haematemesis from a superficial tear in the oesophageal mucosa (Mallory–Weiss tear).
• Fluid and electrolyte disturbance (hypokalaemia, hyponatraemia, metabolic alkalosis or acidosis).
• Renal impairment.
• Risk of aspiration (if reduced consciousness or inebriated) and pneumonia.
• Acid damage to teeth and gums over a chronic period of time.
• Psychological distress and impaired quality of life.

Emily is called back to see you to discuss the results of investigations. She continues to be symptomatic with nausea and vomiting despite stopping the NSAID and using the oral rehydration sachets. She has taken a 4-week course of high dose omeprazole. Her reflux symptoms have been controlled.

She had a negative pregnancy test and normal urinalysis. Blood tests showed elevated corrected calcium of 3.18 (albumin 37), with normal electrolytes and renal function. Abdominal ultrasound was normal. Upper endoscopy showed some mild gastritis, likely secondary to NSAID use and no ulceration or obstruction. She was CLO negative. Biopsies of the duodenum were normal.

What do you do now?

Her nausea and vomiting, abdominal discomfort and constipated stool are likely due to hypercalcaemia, as these symptoms continued despite stopping the NSAID and starting antacid medication for gastritis. The calcium level should be repeated to confirm elevation (alongside albumin to calculate corrected calcium). If it remains elevated a parathyroid level should be sent.

She should be referred to an endocrinologist for ongoing management.

Her calcium level remained elevated on repeat sampling and her parathyroid hormone was elevated. She was discussed with the endocrinologists who arranged a parathyroid scan to investigate hyperparathyroidism. A parathyroid adenoma was seen and later excised. Her symptoms resolved after surgery.

CASE REVIEW

There are many causes of nausea and vomiting. In a woman of child-bearing age, pregnancy must be excluded at an early stage. Gastrointestinal causes are the most common and include peptic ulceration and obstructive pathology. Endocrine and metabolic causes are often forgotten. A detailed history and supportive examination should narrow the differential diagnosis and guide subsequent investigation.

Patients with hypercalcaemia due to hyperparathyroidism should be referred to the appropriate specialist for advice about subsequent investigations and management. In this case surgery to remove a parathyroid adenoma gave symptomatic relief.

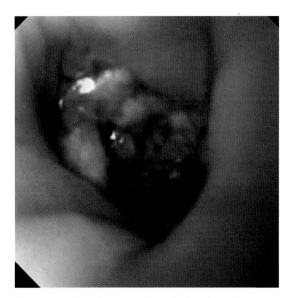

Plate 1.1 Gastric malignancy projecting up into the cardia at endoscopy. (Courtesy of the Gastroenterology Department, John Radcliffe Hospital.)

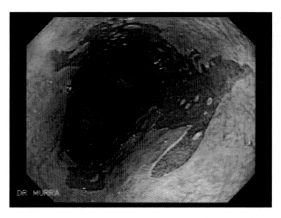

Plate 2.2 Barrett's oesophagus. The Prague classification is used to classify length of circumferential and tongues of Barrett's mucosa. (Reproduced from Talley NJ (ed.) 2010 *Practical Gastroenterology and Hepatology: Esophagus and Stomach.* Wiley-Blackwell, Oxford.)

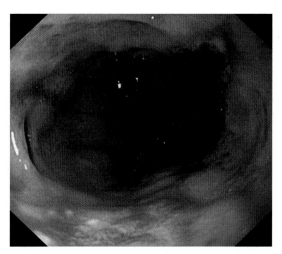

Plate 2.3 Reflux oesophagitis. Inflammation and ulceration may be present.

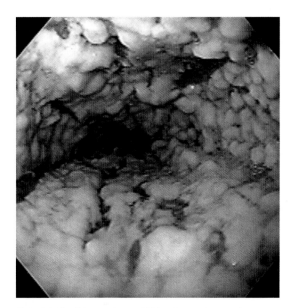

Plate 2.1 *Candida* oesophagus. White plaques that may be discrete or confluent, and are not washed away. (Reproduced from Talley NJ (ed.) 2010 *Practical Gastroenterology and Hepatology: Esophagus and Stomach.* Wiley-Blackwell, Oxford.)

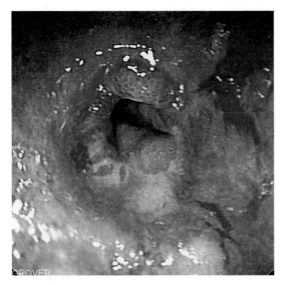

Plate 2.4 Oesophageal stricture: a benign inflammatory stricture due to chronic reflux disease. An endoscope will pass easily through this stricture, although dilatation may be required for persistent symptoms. (From Wikipedia, en.wikipedia.org.)

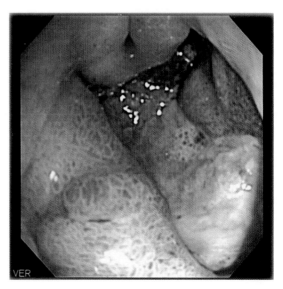

Plate 3.1 Benign gastric ulcer. Gastric ulcers should be biopsied to look for evidence of malignancy. (From Wikipedia, http://en.wikipedia.org/wiki/Image:Deep_gastric_ulcer.png.)

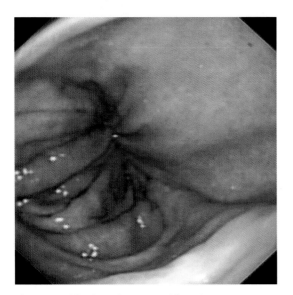

Plate 2.5 A sliding hiatus hernia viewed from above.

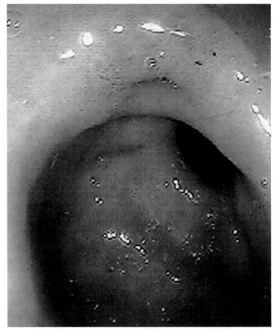

Plate 3.2 Antral gastritis. This is probably due to NSAID use. The diagnosis of gastritis should be confirmed by biopsy and histological correlation.

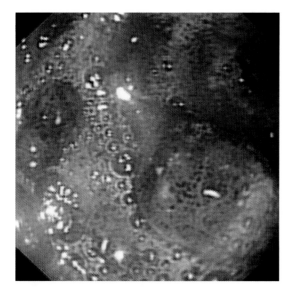

Plate. 6.1 Erosive duodenitis showing inflammation and superficial erosions of the mucosa.

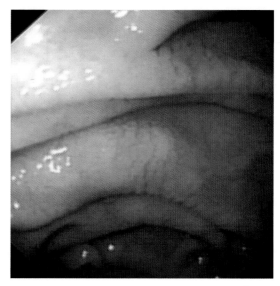

Plate 7.1 Scalloping of duodenal folds and granulation suggestive of coeliac disease.

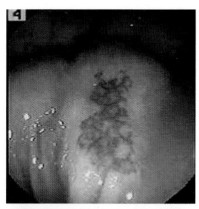

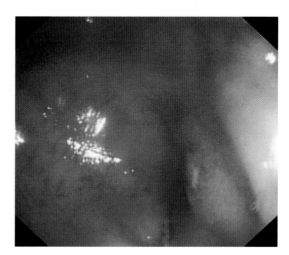

Plate 9.1 Apthous ulcer in the terminal ileum.

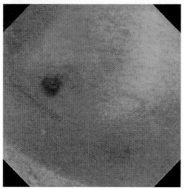

Plate. 6.2 Angiodysplastic lesions in the small bowel at capsule endoscopy. (Courtesy of the Gastroenterology Department, John Radcliffe Hospital.)

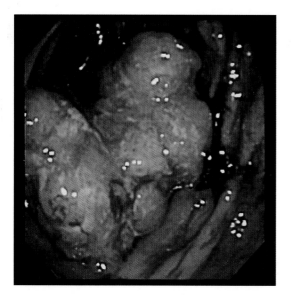

Plate 11.1 Colonoscopy demonstrating a malignant lesion of the colon.

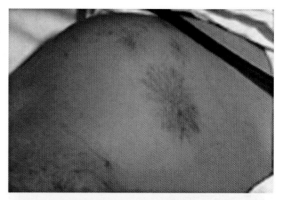

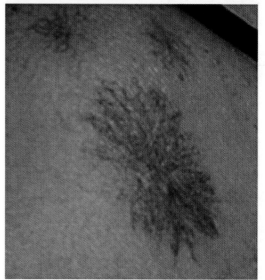

Plate 14.1 Spider naevi. (From Herbert Fred, Hendrik van Dijk. Images of Memorable Cases: Case 114, http://cnx.org/content/ m14900/latest/.)

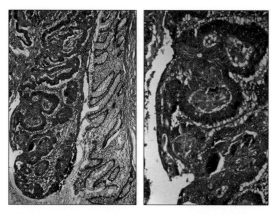

Plate 11.2 Histology demonstrating a moderately differentiated adenocarcinoma. (Reprinted with permission of the Department of Pathology, Virginia Commonwealth University and the VCU Health System.)

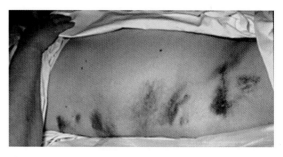

Plate 20.1 Grey Turner's sign: large ecchymosis of the right flank.

KEY POINTS

- Vomiting is the forceful expulsion of luminal contents out of the mouth, coordinated by signals from the intestine, body and brain. It is a protective mechanism designed to expel noxious material from the gastrointestinal tract.
- There is a wide differential to consider when assessing any patient with nausea and vomiting. This includes gastrointestinal, endocrine, metabolic, neurological, cardiac, psychiatric and drug-induced causes. Pregnancy must not be forgotten in women of child-bearing age.
- Investigations should be tailored to the individual patient and guided by associated symptoms and signs.

- Management includes fluid and electrolyte replacement, antiemetics and treatment of the underlying cause.
- In those with intractable nausea and vomiting, the history should be re-taken and diagnosis reviewed. Combination therapy may help when a single drug fails.
- In chronic unexplained nausea and vomiting consider psychological causes and cyclical vomiting syndrome, which responds to antimigraine therapy.

Case 6 A 73-year-old man with haematemesis and melaena

Mr Atkins is a 73-year-old man who presented to the accident and emergency department with a 5-day history of black tarry stools and abdominal pain. Just before admission he felt sick and vomited some dark-stained material that looked like coffee grounds. He is moved to resus by the triage team. You are called to assess him.

What do you do on arrival to the resus department?

This man has had a witnessed upper gastrointestinal bleed. He requires haemodynamic monitoring and needs active resuscitation.

Measurement of vital signs

Blood pressure and pulse are essential guides to haemodynamic stability in patients who are bleeding. They need to be monitored regularly, every 15 min if actively bleeding, as they may change quickly.

Respiratory rate, oxygen saturations, Glasgow coma score and blood glucose measurement are important other vital signs that make up the 'early warning score'. These factors determine the need for early intervention by the medical team.

Resuscitation

Venous access is essential. Two large bore cannulas should be placed proximally, e.g. in the antecubital fossa or other large vein. Immediate intravenous fluids should be administered. Colloid such as gelofusin, Hartman's solution or 0.9% saline (not dextrose) is used to stabilise blood pressure until blood arrives. This should be given

Gastroenterology: Clinical Cases Uncovered, 1st edition.
© S. Keshav and E. Culver. Published 2011 by
Blackwell Publishing Ltd.

quickly unless there is a history of cardiovascular disease or evidence of fluid overload.

In an emergency, O Rhesus-negative blood can be used until grouped and cross-matched.

Blood tests

A sample of blood should be sent to the blood bank, and to the haematology and biochemistry departments.
• Blood gas analyser: in most accident and emergency departments, a blood gas analyser will enable an arterial or venous sample to be analysed within seconds/minutes to give a guide as to acid–base status, lactate, haemoglobin level and electrolytes.
• Blood bank: group and save or cross-match. As a guide:
  • Group and screen if there is no evidence of fresh bleeding and the patient is haemodynamically stable.
  • Cross-match for 4 units if there is fresh melaena per rectum or the systolic blood pressure is less than 100 mmHg.
  • Cross match 6 units for a suspected variceal bleed.
• Haematology: full blood count and coagulation screen. Haematinics including iron studies (B_{12} and folate if clinically indicated).
• Biochemistry: urea, creatinine, electrolytes and liver function.

Electrocardiogram

Look for evidence of a tachyarrhythmia and ischaemia. This may be corrected with adequate fluid and blood product resuscitation.

Erect chest X-ray

• Look to exclude free air under the diaphragm as a sign of perforation.
• Look for cardiomegaly or evidence of interstitial fluid, which will determine the rate of fluid resuscitation.
• Look for any evidence of aspiration if vomiting.

PART 2: CASES

KEY POINT

- Early resuscitation in gastrointestinal bleeding is crucial to patient survival.

What do you need to know from the full history and examination?
Upper GI blood loss
- Check he definitely vomited up blood. This can be confused with haemoptysis or epistaxis by some patients, families and even doctors!
- The appearance of coffee grounds is often due to altered blood, although it may indicate faeculent material associated with intestinal obstruction.
- The appearance of bright red blood suggests an upper gastrointestinal cause for bleeding.

If there was prolonged vomiting, without any indication of bleeding, followed by some bright red blood, this may indicate that there had been some damage to the oesophageal lining causing superficial bleeding – a so-called Mallory–Weiss tear. Occasionally these can bleed severely, although usually they cause only minor, self-limiting haematemesis.

If the vomit was prolonged and voluminous, with blood from the start, consider oesophageal or gastric varicies, large gastric or duodenal ulcer or a spurting vessel as a cause.

Lower GI blood loss
- Melaena stool is black, tar-like and often malodorous. This suggests an upper gastrointestinal cause of bleeding with altered blood being passed.
- Fresh red blood or plum-coloured stool suggests a lower GI source of bleeding. However, in some patients the blood may pass so quickly though the GI tract that an upper GI cause must be excluded.

Alternative explanations for black stool
- Dietary causes: the consumption of prune juice or liquorish can turn the stool black.
- Medication: iron tablets can cause black-green loose or solid thick stool.

Severity indicators
- Symptoms suggestive of shock: dizziness, especially postural, collapse or loss of consciousness.
- Symptoms of anaemia: extreme lethargy, shortness of breath on exertion or chest pain.

Abdominal pain
- Location, type and radiation of pain are key factors. The duration and frequency are important when determining the relationship to bleeding.
- Epigastric aching, associated with food consumption, is typical of a peptic ulcer.
- Retroperitoneal pain radiating to the back should make you consider pancreatic inflammation and perforation of a posterior ulcer.

Associated symptoms
- History of indigestion/heartburn or acid reflux. This may suggest gastric erosions or peptic ulceration.
- Weight loss or systemic illness indicating an underlying gastric malignancy.
- Dysphagia or odonyphagia (and chronicity). This may mean an oesophageal stricture which could be due to reflux with ulceration or it could be malignant.

Past medical history
- *Liver disease.* Does he have a history of liver disease or cirrhosis? If not, may he have undiagnosed liver disease? An alcohol history, a risk factor screen for hepatitis and examination findings that suggest chronic liver disease are key. If he has liver disease he may have varices, putting him at higher risk and changing the management algorithm.
- *Peptic ulcer.* Has he had a prior peptic ulcer? Did he bleed in the past? Was he eradicated for *Helicobacter pylori*?
- *Malignancy.* Is he known to have malignancy? Where is the lesion? What is the current treatment plan?
- *Co-morbidities.* In particular, does he have renal disease or cardiovascular disease, which worsen prognosis in bleeding?
- *Gastrointestinal or abdominal surgery.* Has he had a prior gastric resection? This is particularly important when considering anatomy at endoscopy and location of ulcers. Has he had a recent or previous aortic aneurysm repair? A CT angiogram and/or aortogram may be needed urgently as the first line investigation to define a leak or fistula for repair. These patients bleed severely and decompensate rapidly.

Medications
Causative
- NSAIDs: increased risk of inflammation and gastric ulceration.

- Antiplatelet drugs, such as aspirin or clopidogrel: increased risk of inflammation and bleeding.
- Anticoagulants: need reversal of anticoagulant agents to stop the bleeding. The methods for doing this will depend on the reason for anticoagulation, target international normalised ratio (INR) and severity of bleeding.
- Bisphosphonates: increased risk of oesophagitis and stricturing.

Protective

- Protein pump inhibitor: important when considering ulceration risk and when interpreting the CLO test at endoscopy for *H. pylori*.

Confounding factors in the interpretation of shock

- Beta-blockers, rate-controlling or antihypertensive medications: important to look for the use of these agents when predicting risk.

Social history

- Alcohol: does he drink alcohol and how much does he consume?
- Smoking: does he smoke or is he an ex-smoker, and when did he stop?
- Occupational exposure: what is his occupation and would it put him at risk of bleeding? For example, a publican who drinks alcohol to excess and has undiagnosed liver cirrhosis; or a mechanic who takes NSAIDs for his arthritic shoulder.
- Level of function: what is his usual level of functioning? Would he be a candidate for intensive care if he became really unwell? Who does he live with and who do you call in the case of an emergency?

Family history

Is there a family history of gastrointestinal cancer?

He has been passing black tarry stools for 5 days. He describes postural dizziness over the last few days but no history of collapse or blackouts. He has longstanding indigestion, for which he takes Gaviscon as needed. His stools are usually normal in colour and consistency but he suffers from constipation intermittently. He has lost weight, over 6 kg in the last year.

He has a history of transient ischaemic attack and peripheral vascular disease for which he takes a daily aspirin. He drinks up to 40 units of alcohol per week

and smokes 20 cigarettes per day, with a 50 pack-year history. He lives alone and had no next of kin or relatives. He was able to walk 500 m to the shops prior to admission, limited by claudication.

What to look for on examination?

- Vital signs: blood pressure, pulse rate, presence of postural hypotension, respiratory rate, oxygen saturation, Glasgow coma scale and blood sugar. Look for shock.
- Venous pressure and level of filling to assess fluid balance before resuscitation.
- Evidence of anaemia, and facial and conjunctival pallor.
- Ejection systolic murmur (consider Heyde's syndrome: angiodysplasia and aortic stenosis, an uncommon clinical entity).
- Stigmata of chronic liver disease (see Case 14).
- Evidence of encephalopathy (if liver disease), slowed mentation, disorientation, liver flap and stigmata of chronic liver disease.
- Abdominal tenderness and signs of peritonism to exclude a perforated viscus.
- Evidence of melaena on digital rectal examination to confirm history and active bleeding.

KEY POINT

- Digital rectal examination should be done in all patients with suspected gastrointestinal bleeding to confirm melaena or plum-coloured stool. This may help determine the site of bleeding.

On examination he was confused but cooperative. Vital signs were checked and he was tachycardic with a pulse of 120 beats/min and hypotensive with a blood pressure of 90/60 mmHg. There was a postural drop of over 20 mmHg. He was underfilled and had conjunctival pallor of anaemia. There was a loud ejection systolic murmur radiating to the carotid arteries.

He had epigastric tenderness but no signs of peritonism or abdominal mass. He had no stigmata of chronic liver disease. A rectal exam revealed an enlarged prostate and there was fresh melaena on the glove. There was no fresh red rectal bleeding.

What do you need to know to determine his need for intervention and predicted mortality from a bleed?

The 'Rockall score' is a validated mortality risk assessment score for patients admitted with upper gastrointestinal bleeding (Table 6.1). It is simple and practical, helping identify those at highest risk of dying and needing active intervention. It also identifies those for safe, early discharge (initial score 0, final <2).

His Rockhall score pre-endoscopy is 3, giving a predicted mortality of 11%.

KEY POINT

- Use the 'Rockall score' as a validated mortality risk assessment for patients admitted with upper gastrointestinal bleeding.

Table 6.1 (a) Factors to assess to work out a patient's Rockall score; (b) predicted mortality of different scores.

(a)

	Rockall score (max. score 11)			
Factors	**0**	**1**	**2**	**3**
Age	<60 years	60–79 years	>80 years	
Shock	None	Pulse >100 (and systolic BP >100)	Systolic BP <100	
Co-morbidity	None		Cardiac failure Ischaemic heart disease Major co-morbidity	Renal failure Liver failure Disseminated malignancy
Endoscopic diagnosis	Mallory–Weiss tear or no lesion *and* no sign of bleeding	All other diagnoses	Malignancy of upper GI tract	
Major stigmata of recent haemorrhage	None or dark spot only		Blood in upper GI tract Adherent clot Visible or spurting vessel	

(b)

Initial risk score, pre-endoscopy (max. score 7)		Final risk score, post-endoscopy (max. score 11)
0	0.2%	0.0%
1	2.4%	0.0%
2	5.6%	0.2%
3	11.0%	2.9%
4	24.6%	5.3%
5	39.6%	10.8%
6	48.9%	17.3%
7	50.0%	27.0%
8+	–	41.1%

What is the differential diagnosis of upper gastrointestinal bleeding in this man?

- Peptic ulceration.
- Oesophageal varices.
- Malignancy.
- Angiodysplasia.

What medication should be given?
Protein pump inhibitors pre-endoscopy

There remains controversy as to the indication for intravenous or oral PPIs for upper GI bleeding. In practice, in a hospital where upper endoscopy will not be possible within 12 h of admission, intravenous PPIs should be used pre-endoscopy in those who are shocked or with evidence of fresh melaena. If endoscopy is possible within this timeframe, there is no indication for giving intravenous PPIs before endoscopy.

Antiplatelet agents, anticoagulants and NSAIDs

Stop aspirin and NSAIDs. The need to continue clopidogrel (e.g. after coronary stent insertion or myocardial infarct) is made on an individual basis depending on the degree of shock and in conjunction with the cardiology department. Reversal of warfarin or heparin agents will depend on the reason for such medication, the causes and amount of bleeding, and the risk:benefit ratio. Haematologists will guide the use of vitamin K, fresh frozen plasma and the need for beriplex or protamine in most departments.

Antihypertensive or rate-controlling drugs

Stop any medication that may interfere with the interpretation of haemodynamic status.

Mr Atkins was resuscitated with 4 L of intravenous saline and gelofusin. He was transfused 4 units of red blood cells. His blood pressure stabilised to 120/60 beats/min and his pulse rate decreased to 88 beats/min.

His blood tests confirmed a haemoglobin of 5.4 g/dL and macrocytosis (predominantly reticulocytes). He had an elevated urea of 17.4 mmol/L with a normal creatinine. He had an isolated elevated alkaline phosphatase (ALP) of 700 U/L with normal gamma glutamyl transferase (γ-GT) and other liver tests. His clotting was normal.

An electrocardiogram (ECG) showed a sinus tachycardia with left ventricular hypertrophy and no evidence of ischaemia. A CXR showed no signs of fluid overload.

His aspirin was discontinued. He did not receive a PPI.

Which interventions will determine the cause of bleeding and treat the problem?

Upper gastrointestinal endoscopy should be done within 12 h of admission. Endoscopy is important to diagnose the source of blood loss and for therapeutic intervention if there is evidence of stigmata of recent haemorrhage. It should never be done until the patient is fully resuscitated. Blood must be available at request. Sedation is often needed if therapy is considered.

Gastroscopy demonstrated inflammation and superficial erosions only in the duodenal cap (see Plate 6.1). There was no convincing ulceration, visible vessel or stigmata of bleeding. There was no altered or transmitted blood. No biopsy or CLO test was done. He was started on oral PPI omeprazole 40 mg daily. He was not eradicated for H. pylori.

What do you recommend now?

Melaena comes from the upper GI tract. There are three possible reasons:

1 The source of blood loss was missed at initial endoscopy.
2 The source of blood loss is high in the colon, such as the caecum.
3 The source of blood loss is in the small bowel and not seen at endoscopy.

Repeat upper gastrointestinal endoscopy

This should be done to have another look for a missed source of bleeding at the initial endoscopy. A Dieulafoy lesion is a large tortuous arteriole in the submucosa of the stomach, typically in the fundus, that erodes and bleeds intermittently. This may not be seen at the initial procedure.

Colonoscopy

Colonoscopy should be done to look for bleeding in the proximal colon or caecum. This may be from angiodysplastic lesions, a polyp or tumour.

Repeat upper endoscopy showed no further source of bleeding. Colonoscopy after full preparation was unremarkable in the caecum. There was no evidence of further blood loss and he remained haemodynamically stable. His haemoglobin was 9.7 g/dL after transfusion. He was started on ferrous sulphate tablets 200 mg three per day to replete his iron stores. He continued the omeprazole 40 mg daily. He was discharged.

However, he is readmitted 7 days later with recurrent black stools, abdominal pain and dizziness on standing. On examination he is tachycardic and there are fresh melaena (not iron stools). His blood count has dropped to 7.5 g/dL.

You are called to assess him. What do you do now? What is the next investigation of choice?

He requires resuscitation with intravenous fluid and further cross-match and transfusion.

• *Repeat upper endoscopy*: this is the first investigation of choice. However, a source of bleeding is not found in 10% of cases.

• He has had a colonoscopy a week ago, which was normal, and this should not be repeated again unless there were uncertainties as to the views obtained or pathology seen.

• *CT angiography*: this can detect the source with bleeding rates as low as 0.5 mL/min. Its accuracy in the detection of acute upper GI bleeding is 90%, and it is helpful in assessing occult bleeding. Once a bleeding vessel has been identified, it can be embolised. If no active bleeding is identified, prophylactic embolisation of the left gastric artery or the gastroduodenal artery may be performed in some patients to control gastric or pyloroduodenal bleeding, respectively.

Repeat upper gastroduodenoscopy is unremarkable. There is no visible bleeding lesion or new ulceration. A CT angiogram shows evidence of small bowel bleeding. There is no identifiable vessel. No vessel is embolised. Incidental note is made of a bulky prostate, small mesenteric lymphadenopathy and patchy bone changes.

The small bowel has been identified as the source of blood loss. How do you investigate this further and treat the bleeding?

• *Capsule endoscopy* identifies the source of bleeding in up to 70% of cases if done within 48 h of bleeding. It is not possible to perform therapy with a capsule. Antifibrinolytics such as tranexamic acid may be given to stop bleeding.

• *Enteroscopy* can be done in specialised centres to isolate and potentially treat a source of bleeding. This procedure is time consuming and labour intensive.

• *Surgical laparotomy* is invasive and associated with operative morbidity and mortality. It is the quickest method to identify and stop a bleed by clipping or resection (Table 6.2).

He proceeded to inpatient capsule endoscopy. This was done within 48 h of the bleeding. It revealed multiple angiodysplastic lesions of the proximal, mid and distal small intestine (see Plate 6.2). There was evidence of active bleeding. No tumour was seen. Tranexamic acid was started. There was no further bleeding. He did not require enteroscopy or surgery.

Table 6.2 Indications for surgery (age dependent).

Age <60 years	Age >60 years
Transfusion >8 units in 24 h	Transfusion >4 units in 24 h
One or two re-bleeds	One re-bleed
Spurting vessel at gastroscopy, not controlled	Spurting vessel at gastroscopy
Continued bleeding	Continued bleeding

KEY POINTS

• Endoscopy is the first line diagnostic examination and treatment option for upper gastrointestinal bleeding. Findings can be non-diagnostic in about 10% of cases.
• Angiography is limited by the rate of bleeding, which usually must be at least 0.5 mL/min before it is detected. Bleeding vessels can be embolised once detected.

CASE REVIEW

Upper gastrointestinal bleeding is a medical emergency. Early and adequate resuscitation is vital with fluids and blood products as needed. This should happen prior to any endoscopic or radiological intervention. The Rockhall score should be calculated for each patient as a mortality risk assessment. It helps to define those at need of early intervention and to predict mortality from bleeding.

The presentation of bleeding depends on the amount and location of haemorrhage. Haematemesis, coffee ground vomiting and/or melaena is common. There may also be complications of anaemia including syncopy, fatigue, shortness of breath and chest pain. Examination concentrates on the vital signs to determine the severity of bleeding and the timing of intervention, abdominal and rectal exam, and assessment for stigmata of chronic liver disease and portal hypertension to determine if there may be a variceal source of bleeding.

Upper endoscopy is the first investigation of choice to detect and treat upper gastrointestinal bleeding. If no source of bleeding is found and re-bleeding occurs, a repeat upper endoscopy is advocated to detect missed lesions. Colonoscopy with full preparation should be considered to look for caecal or proximal colonic bleeding. A CT angiogram is advocated, where available, when there is active bleeding and haemodynamic compromise. Bleeding vessels can be embolised. Emergency surgery may be needed in a subgroup of patients if a bleeding source can not be identified or endoscopic/radiological therapy fails.

KEY POINTS

- The Rockall score is a good predictive tool for the need for urgent intervention and 30-day mortality after a bleed.
- Endoscopy should only be done after full resuscitation of the patient.
- Surgical intervention may be necessary and should be considered at an early stage.
- Endoscopy may miss a bleeding source and repeat endoscopy should be done in the event of a re-bleed.
- Colonoscopy may be the second line investigation, depending on the history.
- A CT angiogram is invaluable when the patient is actively bleeding.
- Capsule endoscopy gives a high diagnostic yield if the patient is actively bleeding but does not allow for treatment.

Case 7   A 68-year-old woman with fatigue, weight loss and altered bowel habit

Mrs Gladys Brown is a 68-year-old retired lawyer. She has been referred to your outpatient clinic complaining of tiredness and loss of energy. She initially thought this was due to looking after her grandchildren twice a week, but since stopping this, the symptoms have persisted. She describes loose bowel motions for the last few months and has lost 12.5 kg in weight.

What questions should you ask?
Fatigue (tiredness)

Fatigue or tiredness are very non-specific symptoms and can occur for many reasons, both organic and functional. Find out the duration of her symptoms, and its relationship to stopping work. Ask about a preceding infection, intense exertion or stressful life event that could account for the tiredness.

Loose stool

A change in bowel habit is more concerning. Certain features should be asked about:

• Stool colour, consistency and odour: stools that are pale, oily, malodorous and difficult to flush (steatorrhoea) are suggestive of malabsorption of fat. Stools that are watery and liquid with high frequency may suggest bacterial overgrowth or microscopic colitis. Black stools that are tarry and malodorous suggest upper gastrointestinal blood loss.

• Urgency, frequency and nocturnal defecation: this may be suggestive of inflammatory bowel disease or malignancy.

• Presence of blood mixed in with or separate to the stool (fresh red or clot)s: the presence of blood should be

investigated. Haemorrhoids may cause visible fresh red blood on wiping, but so too can an anal or rectal carcinoma. Non-visible blood (faecal occult blood) is relatively non-specific for any condition causing inflammation or trauma to the surface of the bowel mucosa.

• Presence of mucus or discharge rectally.

• Feeling of incomplete evacuation of stool (tenesmus): this may suggest a degree of obstructive defecation, especially when combined with self-digitalisation and straining and is more usual in patients suffering from constipation. Urgency with incomplete evacuation may suggest rectal inflammation or a rectal mass.

• Faecal incontinence: ask about precipitants, if any.

Weight loss

Intentional and non-intentional weight loss and the methods by which intentional weight loss has been achieved should be established, dietary or other. There may be overlap between these. Quantify the weight loss – how much over how long? An associated loss of appetite is important.

Associated symptoms

• Abdominal pain or discomfort. Describe the character, location, radiation, intensity, frequency and associated factors. An upper abdominal unease is suggestive of dyspepsia. Radiation to the back may suggest pancreatic or spinal pathology. A colicky nature is consistent with biliary pain.

• Bloating, distension and excessive passage of flatus. Think of malabsorption. Irritable bowel is not consistent with the presentation.

• Heartburn or reflux symptoms, suggesting upper GI pathology.

Systemic enquiry

• Ask about features associated with inflammatory bowel or coeliac disease, recurrent mouth ulcers, arthritis

Gastroenterology: Clinical Cases Uncovered, 1st edition.
© S. Keshav and E. Culver. Published 2011 by
Blackwell Publishing Ltd.

or arthralgia, and rash. The rash may be intensely itchy and on the elbows or buttocks (dermatitis herpetiformis is associated with celiac disease), or there may be tender, palpable, erythematous nodules typically on the shins (erythema nodosum may occur in inflammatory bowel).
• Ask about systemic symptoms of an endocrine disorder, thyroid disease or diabetes. This includes temperature dysregulation, palpitations, tremors, irritability (thyroid disease), polyuria and polydipsia (diabetes).
• Also ask about menstrual history and gynaecological problems. This should not be forgotten in women in this age group.

Past medical history

A history of autoimmune disease, such as type 1 diabetes, thyrotoxicosis or Addison's disease, would be relevant. These conditions may produce these symptoms and are also more common in coeliac disease. Previous gastrointestinal or gynaecological surgery may help to narrow the differential.

Medications

Take a drug history to evaluate if she started any new drug treatment in the last few months, and when this was in relationship to her symptoms. Did this coincide with the onset of loose bowel motions? For example, the use of laxatives, metformin, orlistat or proton pump inhibitors.

Social history

• Ask about recent travel abroad. Could she have a chronic parasite infestation causing chronic diarrhoea, such as *Giardia*?
• Ask about smoking; is she a recent ex-smoker? Smoking has a negative impact in Crohn's disease, but is believed to afford a degree of protection in ulcerative colitis. The first presentation of ulcerative colitis may be associated with recent discontinuation of smoking.
• Ask about drinking of alcohol to excess, and a daily intake in units. Pancreatic insufficiency may be the result of alcohol misuse causing chronic inflammation and atrophy.
• Ask about her diet. Does she have a healthy diet? Is she intolerant of any foods such as wheat or milk?
• Ask about health-compromising behaviours. Consider immune compromise. Human immunodeficiency virus (HIV) enteropathy can cause all the features in the presenting complaint but is infrequently considered in this patient group.

• Ask about a history of depression and anxiety. Explore her mood, anxiety issues and stress-related problems. Is she starving herself?

Family history

Is there anyone in her family with coeliac disease, inflammatory bowel or colorectal cancer?

Mrs Brown has been tired and lethargic for the last month. She describes a 6-month history of watery loose stools, up to three times per day, associated with bloating and flatulence. There is no blood. She has had abdominal cramps intermittently for the last few years, usually epigastric, on most days. She has lost 12.5 kg in weight over the last 6 months which was not intentional. She suffers from mouth ulcers every winter but not regularly. There have been no new rashes or other symptoms.

Her medical history includes hypertension, hypothyroidism and asthma. She takes daily aspirin, lisinopril and levothyroxine tablets and beclametasone and salbutamol inhalers. She is compliant with her medications. She has never used laxatives. She worked as a lawyer and is now retired, drinks 2 units of alcohol per month and has never smoked. There is no recent travel history. She has a family history of colorectal cancer, with her father dying in his 60s. This is her main reason for consultation.

What are the important signs on examination?
General examination

Look for signs of malabsorption or malnutrition, including angular stomatitis, cracked nails and alopecia. Look for signs of anaemia, conjunctiva pallor and glossitis of iron deficiency. Look for mouth ulceration, poor dentition or evidence of acid erosion. Look for features of thyroid disease, such as a goitre, exophthalmos, tachycardia and tremor (hyperthyroid). Palpate the cervical region for a supraclavicular lymph node, suggestive of gastric malignancy, or generalised cervical lymphadenopathy.

Abdominal examination

Examine for abdominal tenderness, organomegaly or a mass lesion. A digital rectal examination (DRE) must be done to exclude a rectal carcinoma.

Examination reveals angular stomatitis and a few mouth ulcers. The abdominal exam was unremarkable with no palpable organomegaly or mass. The DRE was normal with good anal tone and no masses.

List the differential diagnosis based on the history and examination findings

- Coeliac disease.
- Chronic pancreatitis and pancreatic insufficiency.
- Thyrotoxicosis.
- Colorectal cancer.
- Inflammatory bowel disease, especially Crohn's disease.
- Microscopic colitis.
- Pancreatic cancer.
- Small bowel bacterial overgrowth.
- Small intestinal lymphoma.
- Bile salt malabsorption.
- Neuroendocrine tumour.

What investigations should be done?
Standard blood tests

- A full blood count can identify anaemia and thrombocythaemia in inflammatory disease. Haematinics should be done for iron, folate or B_{12} deficiency.
- Urea, creatinine and electrolytes are taken as a baseline of renal function.
- Liver tests and coagulation studies: raised aspartate aminotransferase (AST) and alanine aminotransferase (ALT) can occur in coeliac disease. Raised ALP and ALT can occur in biliary and metastatic disease. The prothrombin time may be prolonged due to vitamin K deficiency in malabsorption.
- C-reactive protein (CRP): elevated levels are a marker of inflammation.

Specific blood tests

- Amylase may be elevated in chronic pancreatitis, although it is usually normal unless the patient has acute exacerbations of inflammation on a background of chronic disease.
- Thyroid tests (thyroid-stimulating hormone (TSH), free T_4 (thyroxine) and free T_3 (tri-iodothyronine)) to check for thyrotoxicosis.
- Calcium and vitamin D levels should be checked in malabsorption.
- Blood film detects hyposplenism, target cells and Howell–Jolly bodies in coeliac disease.
- Coeliac serology should be sent, either immunoglobulin A (IgA) endomysial antibodies or IgA tissue transglutamase antibodies. These should be interpreted in the context of IgA levels as deficiency causes a false-negative result. In patients with IgA deficiency, histological confirmation is needed.

> **Box 7.1 Coeliac tests**
>
> - IgA endomysial antibodies are 85–98% sensitive and 97–100% specific
> - IgA tissue transglutamase antibodies are more sensitive but less specific
> - IgA antigliadin antibodies are used in children less than 2 years old and are moderately sensitive but poorly specific, and so are not used in adults

Stool sample

Send a sample for estimation of faecal elastase, a level below 200 g/L suggesting pancreatic insufficiency. A sample for parasites, ova and cysts should only be sent in chronic diarrhoea if giardiasis is a possible diagnosis.

Endoscopy and biopsies

This should be done to exclude an upper GI malignancy and to look for features of untreated coeliac disease. Biopsies of the third portion of the duodenum are the gold standard to confirm the diagnosis of celiac disease. Changes are patchy so four biopsies should be taken. Typical histology shows increased numbers of intraepithelial lymphocytes, villous atrophy (Fig. 7.1) and crypt

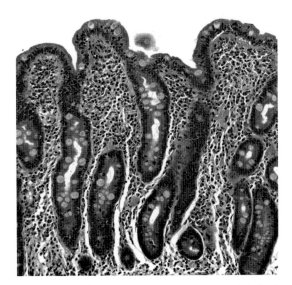

Fig. 7.1 Subtotal villous atrophy. (Reproduced from *Journal of Clinical Pathology*, Dickson, Streutker and Chetty, 59(10),1008–1016, copyright BMJ 2006 with permission from BMJ Publishing Group Ltd.)

hyperplasia. This must be done whilst consuming gluten in the diet, for at least 4 weeks prior to the procedure.

Colonoscopy and biopsies

This is indicated to exclude colorectal cancer and look for evidence of inflammatory bowel disease. Even if the mucosa is normal, biopsies should be taken to check for microscopic colitis with loose stools.

Abdominal ultrasound

Look for pancreatic inflammation, atrophy or a mass. If an abnormality is identified or the history is highly suggestive of a pancreatic cause, a CT scan of the abdomen is more appropriate.

Blood tests confirmed a microcytic anaemia (haemoglobin 10.4 g/dL, mean corpuscular volume (MCV) 68.1 fL) and low ferritin and transferrin saturation (ferritin 6 ng/mL, transferring saturation 5%). She had a strongly positive endomysial antibody and normal range IgA. Her liver tests were abnormal (ALT 222 U/L, ALP 562 U/L, γ-GT 79 IU/L, bilirubin 7 μmol/L, albumin 42 g/L). Clotting was normal.

Gastroscopy showed scalloping and loss of folds in the third part of the duodenum (see Plate 7.1). Biopsies confirmed widespread partial and subtotal villous atrophy associated with increased intraepithelial lymphocytes and lymphoplasmacytic cells in the lamina propria. These features were consistent with a diagnosis of coeliac disease. Colonoscopy was macroscopically normal and biopsies of the colon and terminal ileum were normal.

Abdominal ultrasound showed evidence of a fatty liver with no pancreatic inflammation or atrophy.

She has been diagnosed with coeliac disease. She wants to know more information about this disease. What do you tell her?

She should attend a specialist coeliac clinic to discuss her diagnosis, get focused dietetic information and advice, and begin treatment.

Disease presentation

Coeliac disease can present at any age, most commonly in childhood or middle age. There is a female preponder-ance. Many adults are asymptomatic and the diagnosis is discovered incidentally. Others present with one or a combination of the following:

• Symptoms of malabsorption, such as diarrhoea, steat-orrhoea, weight loss, lethargy, bloating and abdominal discomfort.
• Chronic or recurrent iron-deficiency anaemia.
• An isolated nutritional deficiency, including iron and calcium (absorbed in the proximal small intestine), folic acid and vitamins C and B_{12} (absorbed in the jejunum and ileum). The latter are deficient in more advanced disease.
• An intensely itchy and blistering rash over the elbows and buttocks called dermatitis hepetiformis. Up to 90% of individuals with this have villous atrophy.
• Reduced fertility or oligo/amenorrhoea can occur in women.
• Bone pain from fractures due to osteoporosis from vitamin D and calcium deficiency.
• Neurological disease such as peripheral neuropathy and cerebellar symptoms and signs are a rare presenta-tion. Symptoms can resolve with treatment of the under-lying cause.
• Abnormal liver biochemistry, whilst investigating other causes of liver disease.

Genetic susceptibility

Susceptible individuals develop an immunological reaction to gluten-derived gliadin peptides upon dietary exposure. There is 10% prevalence in first degree relatives. These individuals carry HLA-DQ2 (the major-ity) or DQ8.

Treatment

A gluten-free diet is currently the only treatment for coeliac disease. You should arrange a consultation with a dietician to discuss the components of a gluten-free diet and the importance of strict adherence. She can have a prescription for gluten-free products. Symptoms often improve within 2 weeks of dietary restriction (in three-quarters of patients).

Serology should be rechecked to confirm response after 3–6 months. Some clinicians advocate repeat endos-copy and biopsy to ensure histological resolution of the disease with reversal of villous atrophy. However, histol-ogy can take up to 12 months to resolve.

She should be given iron tablets for her iron-deficiency anaemia, which may resolve on the gluten-free diet but should be treated as she is symptomatic with lethargy.

Folic acid supplementation may be needed also (if there is evidence of folate deficiency).

She requires a DEXA (dual energy X-ray absorptiometric scan) scan as she is at risk of osteoporosis. Half of all patients on a gluten-free diet become osteoporotic due to malabsorption of calcium and secondary hyperparathyroidism. They require calcium and vitamin D supplementation and a bisphosphonate.

If symptoms suggest intolerance to milk products, a lactose breath test should be done. Fifty percent of patients have secondary hypolactasia at diagnosis.

The Coeliac Society UK provides educational material, contact information and organises social events for patients to learn more about the disease and on-going research.

KEY POINT

- Coeliac disease is a gluten-sensitive enteropathy defined as small intestine villous atrophy that resolves with the elimination of gluten from the diet.

What if her symptoms do not resolve on a gluten-free diet?

Gluten sensitivity persists for life. Poor compliance with a gluten-free diet is the most common reason for persistent and recurrent symptoms. Other causes include untreated nutritional deficiencies, unrecognised hypolactasia or complications of the disease. Severe refractory disease may respond to a course of oral corticosteroids.

There is an increased risk of a small intestinal T-cell lymphoma, adenocarcinoma and possibly oesophageal malignancy in patients with celiac disease. Good compliance with a gluten-free diet reduces these malignant complications.

She attends the clinic and sees the dietician for advice on a gluten-free diet. She reports good dietary compliance and

her symptoms resolve within a few weeks. At 3 months her repeat blood tests confirm her endomysial antibodies are undetectable and her anaemia has resolved. Her liver function is persistently abnormal. Her ALT has risen to 360 U/L, ALP to 562 U/L, γ-GT to 79 IU/L and bilirubin to 7 μmol/L. The albumin, prothrombin time and platelets are normal.

The DEXA scan confirms a spinal T score of –3.6 and total hip T score or –2.1 consistent with osteoporosis. She is given lifestyle advice, started on vitamin D 800 U/day and calcium 1000 mg/day supplementation and a bisphosphonate drug once weekly.

What is the cause of her abnormal liver tests?

The presence of abnormal liver tests is well recognised in coeliac disease and may occur in up to 40% of patients. If they are caused by coeliac disease then they will resolve with good adherence to a gluten-free diet.

Liver abnormalities persisted despite compliance with a gluten-free diet, what should you do now?

As for any patient with abnormal liver function, an abdominal ultrasound and full liver screen is warranted. She has already had an abdominal scan that showed evidence of fatty liver disease. She was advised to exercise, eat healthily and abstain from alcohol. Her fasting glucose was checked to confirm she was not diabetic.

Blood glucose was normal. Serology for hepatitis B and C were negative. Electrophoresis showed elevated IgG and IgA with a polyclonal hypergammaglobulinaemia. An autoimmune hepatitis screen showed a positive anti-SM antibody of 1/40. Other tests including α₁-antitrypsin, ferritin, caeruloplasmin and α-fetoprotein (AFP) were normal.

She proceeded to liver biopsy which confirmed autoimmune liver disease. She was started on steroids with improvement of liver function.

CASE REVIEW

Coeliac disease is a gluten-sensitive enteropathy. It may present in many different ways: malabsorptive symptoms, iron-deficiency anaemia, nutritional deficiencies, a rash of dermatitis herpetiformis, reduced fertility, osteoporotic fractures, neurological manifestations or abnormal liver biochemistry.

Investigation aims to exclude other causes of symptoms, including malignancy, and diagnose the gluten enteropathy. Upper endoscopy is the gold standard, revealing scalloped distal duodenal folds. Histology shows subtotal villous atrophy and intraepithelial lymphocytosis. Treatment is with a gluten-free diet. Steroids may be con-sidered in refractory patients if compliance with diet is confirmed and there is no evidence of other disease pathology, including a search for small bowel lymphoma.

This patient had symptomatic coeliac disease with evidence of malabsorption and iron-deficiency anaemia. Diagnosis was made from positive serological tests and confirmed by endoscopy and distal duodenal biopsies showing subtotal villous atrophy. Symptoms responded to a gluten-free diet and serology became negative. Despite compliance with a gluten-free diet, her liver function was persistently abnormal, biopsies confirming autoimmune liver disease.

KEY POINTS

- Coeliac disease is a gluten-sensitive enteropathy defined as small intestine villous atrophy that resolves with the elimination of gluten from the diet.
- The gold standard for diagnosis is endoscopy and duodenal (D2 or d3) biopsies showing subtotal villous atrophy.
- Resolution of symptoms, serological tests, and endoscopic and histological abnormalities occur when compliant with a gluten free diet.

- Coeliac disease may be asymptomatic, or may present with gastrointestinal symptoms, isolated iron-deficiency anaemia and nutritional deficiency.
- Less frequent presentations include reduced fertility, bone disease and fractures, abnormal liver function, and neurological and psychiatric symptoms.
- Abnormal liver function related to coeliac disease should resolve with gluten withdrawal.

Case 8 A 23-year-old woman with constipation

Miss Daphne Potts is a 23-year-old woman who has come to see you with severe constipation. She feels bloated, has gained weight and has crampy abdominal pain. She has tried laxatives with no relief. She asks for another medication to help with her symptoms.

What do you want to know from the history?
Constipation
• Define the frequency, nature and consistency of her stools. How long has she suffered from these symptoms?
• Is there an obstructive problem? Does she have difficulty with evacuation of stool? Does she experience an urge to defecate?
• Is there any unusual posture on defecating? Does she need to digitate the rectum or apply posterior vaginal pressure to allow defecation?
• Does she strain whilst passing stool? Are there prolonged and unsuccessful attempts? Does she have a sensation of incomplete evacuation?
• Is there any perianal pain?
• Is there any rectal bleeding?
• Has she ever been faecally impacted or soiled her underwear?
• Does she have a preoccupation with her bowel habit?

Abdominal pain
Describe her abdominal pain – the character, location, radiation, intensity, frequency and associated factors. Specifically ask about aggravating and relieving factors.

Weight
Define her weight gain – how much weight over how long?

Gastroenterology: Clinical Cases Uncovered, 1st edition.
© S. Keshav and E. Culver. Published 2011 by
Blackwell Publishing Ltd.

Bloating
• Does she suffer from bloating, and does this have diurnal variation?
• Does she have excessive flatulence or belching?

Nausea or vomiting
Does she suffer from nausea or vomiting? Is this ever faeculent? How does this related to food or bowel motions?

Systemic enquiry
• Is there any generalised muscular weakness (myopathy) to suggest Cushing's syndrome?
• Are there symptoms of hypothyroidism, such as slowness, lethargy, alopecia and cold intolerance?
• Are there extraintestinal manifestations of Crohn's disease such as mouth ulceration, rashes, arthritis and eye inflammation?
• Are there any neurological symptoms?

She describes a 1-year history of difficulty opening her bowels, with a frequency of once per week of hard, pellet-like stool. Her previous bowel habit was once every 3 days. There was no blood or mucus, no straining at stool and no urge to defecate. She describes a nagging discomfort in her left lower abdomen, which is not relieved by defecation. Over the last few months she developed nausea and a bloated sensation, especially after eating. There have been a few episodes of vomiting. She has a poor appetite but claims to have gained 10 kg in weight in the last 4 months.

What other history is important?
Past medical history
• Does she suffer from depression or is there a history of sexual abuse?
• Could she be pregnant? Does she have children; was there a traumatic childbirth?
• If the patient is older, has she had a hysterectomy?

• Is there a history of thyroid disease (hypothyroidism)? Is she diabetic (autonomic neuropathy)?

Medications

Detail the laxatives she has tried, the dose taken and effect, if any. Chronic stimulant laxative use can cause a cathartic megacolon, hypokalaemia and melanosis coli. Ask about constipating agents prescribed or over-the-counter, such as opioid analgesia, anticholinergics, tricyclic antidepressants or iron.

Social history

• Ask about her diet: fruit and fibre content.
• Does she exercise regularly or is she relatively immobile?

Family history

• Is there a family history of colorectal cancer affecting a first degree relative under the age of 50 years?
• Is there a history of inflammatory bowel disease?

She has a past history of depression and migraines. She takes fluoxetine daily. The only laxative she has tried is lactulose 10 mL up to three times daily, which had no effect after 2 weeks. She is taking regular paracetamol and codeine for the abdominal pain. She lives with her partner, smokes two cigarettes per day and drinks occasional alcohol. She works as an administrator in an office, which is a rather sedentary job.

She describes her diet as poor, low in fibre with little fruit or vegetables. Her uncle had bowel cancer in his 60s and her grandmother had a diabetic autonomic neuropathy with constipated bowel. Her mother suffers from hypochondriasis and anxiety.

What features do you look for on examination?

General examination

• Look for conjunctival pallor of anaemia.
• Look for extraintestinal manifestations of Crohn's disease such as mouth ulcers, rashes, arthritis and eye inflammation.
• Look for signs of thyroid disease such as a goitre, alopecia and depressed reflexes.

Abdominal examination

• Inspect and palpate for abdominal masses including faeces.

• Listen for active bowel sounds and evidence of obstruction.

Rectal examination

• Inspect the perianal area for scars, fistula and external haemorrhoids.
• Perianal sensation should be assessed to exclude saddle anaesthesia of spinal cord pathology.
• Palpate for fissures, internal haemorrhoids, masses, strictures and faecal impaction.
• Assess the sphincter tone at rest and on contraction.
• Test perineal descent; ask the patient to bear down on your gloved finger. Excessive descent is defined as greater than 3.5 cm or below the plane of the ischial tuberosity. This indicates laxity of the perineum due to excessive straining or childbirth. Limited descent indicates an inability to relax the pelvic floor muscles during defecation.

Neurological examination

• Look for evidence of a spinal cord lesion such as sensory level, altered gait, hyper-reflexia and upgoing plantars.
• Look for signs of cerebral disease and parkinsonian features in older patients.

Examination revealed a distended abdomen, tender left flank with palpable faeces in the colon and sluggish bowel sounds. There was a normal sphincter tone with no faeces in the rectum. There was evidence of exaggerated perineal descent. Neurological examination was normal.

KEY POINT

• Rectal examination is crucial to identify obstructive defecation, in particular sphincter tone and perineal descent. This will guide the need for further investigations.

What are the differential diagnoses?

• Drug-induced cause, such as codeine.
• Lifestyle factors, such as a low fibre diet and lack of exercise.
• Pregnancy.
• Motility disorder, such as slow transit constipation.
• Defecation disorder.

- Mechanical problem, such as a stricture causing partial obstruction.
- Metabolic cause, such as hypercalcaemia.

> ### Box 8.1 Causes of constipation
>
> - Diet: low fibre and low fluid intake
> - Immobility or lack of exercise
> - Pregnancy
> - Older age
> - Drugs such as opiates, anticholinergics or iron
> - Motility disorders such as idiopathic slow transit and irritable bowel syndrome constipation-predominant (IBS-C)
> - Mechanical obstruction from hernia, tumour, stricture (e.g. Crohn's disease) or pelvic mass (e.g. fibroids)
> - Anorectal pain from a fissure, anal ulcer or thrombosed haemorrhoid
> - Anorectal strictures, mucosal prolapse, retrocele, descending perineum syndrome
> - Metabolic disorder such as hypercalcaemia and hypokalaemia
> - Endocrine disorder such as hypothyroidism
> - Spinal cord lesion in multiple sclerosis or spinal metastasis
> - Cerebral disease, including parkinsonism
> - Absence of enteric nerves in aganglinosis (Hirschsprung's disease, Chagas' disease)
> - Pelvic nerve damage, e.g. trauma or autonomic neuropathy
> - Stress response if injured or unwell due to sympathetic overactivity

What investigations should you arrange?

This woman is young and there are no alarm features of weight loss, tenesmus or rectal bleeding. Simple non-invasive investigations should be done.

Urine

- Beta-HCG (pregnancy test).

Blood tests

- Full blood count for anaemia.
- Electrolytes for hypokalaemia.
- Calcium and albumin to identify hypercalcaemia.
- Thyroid function (TSH and free T_4) for hypothyroidism.
- C-reactive protein may be elevated in an inflammatory condition.

What general advice do you give?

- Advise her to stop taking drugs that cause constipation. Replace the codeine with non-opioid analgesia.
- Advise a high fibre diet with more fruits, leguminous vegetables and wholemeal bread.
- Drink an adequate fluid intake (at least 8 glasses of water per day) and take regular exercise (at least 20 min three times per week).
- Identify psychological and emotional factors. Empathise with her and discuss expectations of a normal bowel habit.
- Re-educate and retrain her bowel. Tell her to avoid prolonged sitting on the toilet, avoid excessive straining, not to ignore the urge to pass stool and to get into a regular routine.
- Consider drugs only if these measures fail and try to give them for short periods only.

What treatment options are there?

- If electrolyte abnormalities are identified, these should be corrected.
- If thyroid dysfunction is identified, it should be treated.
- A trial of laxatives is indicated if general measures are unsuccessful. The type depends on the underlying cause (Table 8.1). A combination is sometimes useful.

Daphne returns to your surgery 4 weeks later. She has changed her diet to increase the fibre content, drinks more fluids and has started cycling every day to work. She stopped taking the codeine and used paracetamol only with some improvement in her abdominal pain. She has tried Movicol 2 sachets daily and senna 2 tablets at night for the last 3 weeks with no improvement in her bowel habit. The stool is softer and sometimes watery but the frequency is still once per week and abdominal distension persists.

She is not pregnant and her blood tests are unremarkable with normal electrolytes, calcium and thyroid function.

What further investigations are indicated?

General measures and a trial of osmotic and stimulant laxatives have not been effective. This will work in the majority of young women with constipation.

The options include:

- Offering a further course of stronger laxatives including enema treatment
- Performing investigations to exclude underlying pathology.

The latter is preferred by most clinicians.

PART 2: CASES

Table 8.1 Different types of laxatives and their uses.

Type of laxative	Example	Action and use
Stool bulking agent	Fibre supplements (bran) Ispaghula husk (fybogel) Methylcellulose	Increase faecal mass, which stimulates peristalsis
Osmotic laxative	Lactulose and Movicol Phosphate enema for rapid bowel evacuation Magnesium salts	Retain fluid in the bowel
Stool softeners	Liquid paraffin Arachis oil enemas	Lubricate and soften impacted faeces Useful in painful haemorrhoids or anal fissure
Stimulant laxatives	Bisacodyl tablets or enema and senna Docusate sodium has stimulant and softening actions Glycerine suppositories are a rectal stimulant	Increase intestinal motility and are contraindicated in intestinal obstruction
Specific receptor antagonists	Tergaserod	Used in IBS-C

Colon investigation

• Flexible sigmoidoscopy and biopsies of the mucosa are indicated if the patient is less than 50 years old and has no alarm features.

• Colonoscopy is the preferred method if the patient is older than 50 year or alarm features are present at any age.

Radiological studies

• An abdominal X-ray will show any evidence of faecal loading in the colon, will identify megacolon/rectum and will show small bowel or large bowel obstruction.

• Colon transit studies ('shape' studies) involve the ingestion of radio-opaque markers with abdominal radiography performed 3 and 5 days after ingestion. They are useful in differentiating slow transit and normal transit constipation.

Anorectal physiology

• Anorectal manometry detects pressure changes in the anus and rectum.

• Defecating proctograms are done to identify defecation disorders.

Histological investigation

Full-thicknesss rectal biopsy and silver stain (to show mesenteric plexus) for aganglionosis is only needed if anorectal manometry shows inhibited sphincter relaxation.

Magnetic resonance imaging of the spine

This can be done to exclude a spinal cord lesion in the presence of neurology.

Investigations were organised to determine the cause of her persistent constipation. Abdominal X-ray confirmed faecal loading of her entire colon with prominent bowel loops but no evidence of obstruction. Flexible sigmoidoscopy and biopsies were normal. Colonic transit studies confirmed global slow transit, with 6 markers in the right colon, 17 in the left colon and 21 in the rectosigmoid at 5 days (Fig. 8.1). Anal manometry was normal.

The defecating proctogram confirmed a tight pelvic floor and no pelvic floor descent. There was no urge to defecate and the anal canal failed to open during evacuation.

What do you tell her and what are the treatment options?

She has slow transit constipation and a defecation disorder, which are managed in different ways.

Slow transit constipation

• Picolax (between 1 and 3 sachets) is used to empty the bowel.

• Osmotic laxatives are then started in high doses, for example Movicol 2 sachets twice daily.

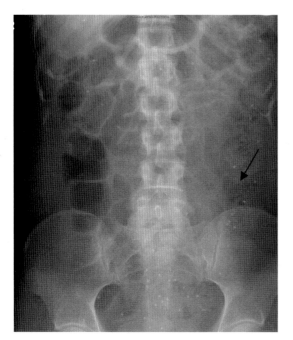

Fig. 8.1 Colon transit study showing slow colonic transit with radio-opaque markers (arrow) still in the right colon. (Courtesy of the Gastroenterology Department, John Radcliffe Hospital.)

• Stimulant laxatives should not be used daily (there is a risk of colonic atony and hypokalaemia) but can be used intermittently in times of crisis.

Defecation disorder

• Psychological distress and anxiety management are important.

• Biofeedback uses psychological retraining alongside anorectal manometry catheters.

• Botulium toxin can be injected into the puborectalis muscle if the pelvic floor does not relax during defecation. This can be associated with urgency and minor faecal leakage.

She received picolax and took regular osmotic laxatives as recommended for her slow transit constipation. She used senna occasionally only.

She was assessed by the colorectal surgeons. They performed a local anaesthetic block and injected botulium toxin into the puborectalis and external anal sphincter. She was seen at the colorectal pelvic floor clinic 2 weeks later. Post-injection she developed an urge to defecate and opened her bowels every 3 days with complete evacuation and no incontinence.

CASE REVIEW

Constipation can be described as a decrease in the frequency of stool passage and/or change in the consistency of the stool to a hard, pellet-like stool. The duration of symptoms, presence of alarm features and systemic symptoms help to direct further tests.

General lifestyle advice is first line management in the absence of alarm symptoms. Laxatives should then be given. If a combination of the above is unsuccessful, investigations should be directed according to the history to look for colonic, rectal or anal abnormalities. Management is individualised depending on the underlying disorder.

KEY POINTS

• Normal passage of stool varies greatly amongst individuals.

• Constipation is characterised by reduced frequency and volume of stool, straining, pain and incomplete evacuation.

• A careful history and examination helps to determine the possible cause.

• Most constipation does not need investigation, especially in young, otherwise well individuals.

• Indication for investigation includes age over 40 years, recent change in bowel habit, loss in weight, tenesmus, rectal bleeding and mucus discharge.

• Treatment of the underlying cause, diet and lifestyle interventions are usually all that is needed to restore normal bowel habit.

• Drugs should be used if theses measures fail.

• Colonoscopic evaluation, transit studies and anorectal physiology are indicated to exclude specific conditions before escalating treatment further.

PART 2: CASES

Case 9 A 24-year-old woman with chronic diarrhoea

Ms Emma Ritchie is 24 years old and recently moved from Glasgow to London. She has suffered with increased frequency of bowel opening, up to five times a day, abdominal pain and feeling generally unwell for the last 6 months. Before coming to London, her GP had found her to be slightly anaemic, and recommended that she increase the amount of iron in her diet. Her condition seems to be worsening, and she is keen to know what the problem is, and how you propose to treat her.

What would you like to determine from a detailed history?
Presenting complaint
• Bowel habit: define exactly how the bowel habit has changed. Although five times a day is more frequent than for most people, what was it before? What is the nature of the stool: loose, watery, blood-stained, containing mucus? Is it fatty, pale, odoriferous and difficult to flush (steatorrhoea)? Is there urgency? Does it wake her from sleep?
• Abdominal pain: what is the nature? Is it localized at all?
• Anaemia: why might she be anaemic? Does she have excessive menstrual bleeding? What does her diet comprise? Is there visible blood from the gastrointestinal tract?
• Prior symptoms: is this the first occasion on which she has experienced these symptoms, or have they been recurrent?

Associated symptoms
• Body weight: constant or reduced?
• Inflammatory symptoms, such as arthralgia, skin rashes, ophthalmic abnormalities, fever or sweating?
• Tiredness, fatigue, listlessness?

Gastroenterology: Clinical Cases Uncovered, 1st edition.
© S. Keshav and E. Culver. Published 2011 by
Blackwell Publishing Ltd.

Potential risk factors
• Smoking: does she smoke? Has she recently stopped smoking? Smoking is protective in ulcerative colitis and can exacerbate Crohn's disease.
• Alcohol: amount consumed and weekly units? Pancreatic inflammation and atrophy may be caused by excessive alcohol use. Steatorrhoea and malabsorption may result.
• Recreational drugs: current or past use?
• Travel abroad: could she have picked up an infection?
• Ingesting food or drink that might transmit infection: take a detailed food history.
• Is she sexually active? Consider sexually transmitted disease and pelvic inflammatory disease.
• Any family history of a similar disorder or any intestinal disorder?
• Prescription medications or over-the-counter substances. Take a full drug history for those that could cause diarrhoea.

Her motions are definitely more frequent than previously, when she went once a day, and they are loose, with flecks of mucus. There is no obvious blood in them. Her weight has decreased by about 5 kg, despite doing her best to eat healthily. She has enjoyed the change in weather in London compared to Scotland, as she has recently found the cold hard to withstand. The pain in the abdomen is most frequently localised to the right lower quadrant, and it is constant and moderate in intensity. Opening her bowel has no effect on the pain, and she has not tried any analgesics.

When she thought carefully about her symptoms, she thinks that she is more tired than usual, and has aching joints, particularly the ankles, wrists and elbows. She has not noticed any skin rash, although she thinks she has very frequent ulcers in the mouth that seem to heal slowly.

She has no family history of note, and in particular no member of the family has coeliac disease or inflammatory bowel disease. She does not smoke, and drinks very rarely. She is a devout Jehovah's Witness, and is appalled at the idea of using recreational drugs.

She married last year, which is why she has moved to London, as her husband is originally from Streatham, and wanted to return home. They took a honeymoon in Ireland, and have not travelled abroad apart from this. They have a conventional diet, and are aware of the risk of salmonellosis from undercooked poultry and eggs. Apart from taking a few over-the-counter iron supplements, the patient has not taken any medications, and has never been seriously ill.

What is the differential diagnosis?

The problem is one of chronic diarrhoea, and there is a wide differential diagnosis:

- Irritable bowel syndrome.
- Chronic parasitic infestation, e.g. giardiasis.
- Inflammatory bowel disease.
- Intestinal infection, e.g. tuberculosis, yersiniosis, amoebiasis.
- Microscopic colitis.
- Coeliac disease.
- Chronic pancreatitis.
- Thyrotoxicosis.
- Chronic laxative abuse.
- HIV-related enteropathy.
- Colorectal cancer.
- Intestinal lymphoma.
- Neuroendocrine tumour, e.g. Zollinger–Ellison syndrome.

What does the history tell you? What can be ruled out?

The loss of weight, anaemia and sustained ill health in a previously asymptomatic and uncomplaining individual make irritable bowel syndrome unlikely. The lack of an appropriate travel history makes chronic giardiasis unlikely. There is no family history of pancreatitis and no alcohol history to support chronic pancreatitis. There is little evidence of dietary indiscretion and no history of laxative abuse. She is unlikely to have thyrotoxicosis, as she prefers warm weather and has no other features to support this. She has no risk factors for HIV-related disease.

Coeliac disease and inflammatory bowel disease (IBD) are distinct possibilities, particularly with the history of anaemia, joint pains and likely apthous ulceration.

Where would you direct your examination?

General examination

- Look for signs of anaemia.
- Look for signs of nutrient deficiency such as koilonychia and angular stomatitis.

- Look for finger-end clubbing. This can occur in inflammatory bowel disease.
- Look for a skin rash or evidence of previous rash – coeliac disease is associated with dermatitis herpetiformis; IBD may be accompanied by pyoderma gangrenosum or erythema nodosum.
- Look in the mouth for ulceration or healed ulcers.
- Look in the eyes for inflammation.
- Look for evidence of active joint inflammation and swelling.
- Feel for lymphadenopathy – a lymphoma might present in many different ways.
- Weigh her and determine her BMI – is she underweight? This could be a consequence of malabsorption or chronic inflammation.

Abdominal examination

In many gastrointestinal diseases there is little to find on abdominal examination.

- Feel for palpable masses such as an inflamed terminal ileum and caecum in Crohn's disease, or a thickened loop of distal colon in ulcerative colitis.
- Feel for enlargement of intra-abdominal organs, especially liver and spleen, which may indicate liver disease or a lymphoproliferative process.

Anorectal examination

- Look for signs of perianal Crohn's disease – fissures, skin tags, abscesses. Look for evidence of perianal excoriation possibly due to frequent watery diarrhoea.
- Digital rectal examination and proctoscopy can reveal anal fissures, haemorrhoids and anal or distal rectal cancer.
- Rigid sigmoidoscopy can visualise the rectal mucosa, which is almost always affected in cases of ulcerative colitis.

On close inspection, she is thin, pale and has clubbed fingers. She has a few apthous ulcers under her tongue. The skin is normal, although her elbows are tender when you move them. Her BMI is 17, which is below the normal range.

Abdominal examination reveals a tender, vaguely defined mass in the right iliac fossa. Rectal examination is normal, and you elect not to perform a rigid sigmoidoscopy.

What should be done next?

The patient is clearly unwell – she is pale, underweight, passing loose stool and with a painful mass in her abdomen. The likelihood that she has pathology affecting her caecum and ileum is high, and Crohn's disease is the probable diagnosis.

However, other conditions can mimic this, including caecal cancer, ileocaecal tuberculosis and rare infections with organisms such as *Yersinia enterocolitica* and *Entamoeba histolytica*. These must be excluded.

What tests would you order?

Tests are required to establish the correct diagnosis, determine the severity and extent of disease, and initiate appropriate treatment.

Examination of the stool

• *Stool chart*: document the frequency and consistency of the stool, and the presence of blood in the stool. The Bristol stool chart is a medical aid designed to classify the form of human faeces into seven categories (Fig. 9.1). Types 1 and 2 indicate constipated stool; types 3 and 4 are the 'ideal stools', especially the latter, as they are the easiest to pass. Types 5–7 are tending towards diarrhoea or urgency.

• *Stool volume*: the usual volume is about 200 mL per day.

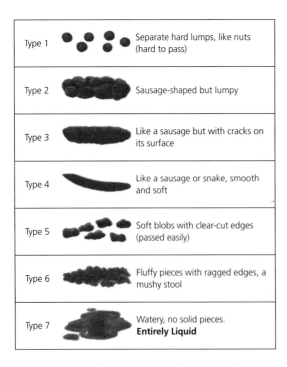

Type 1		Separate hard lumps, like nuts (hard to pass)
Type 2		Sausage-shaped but lumpy
Type 3		Like a sausage but with cracks on its surface
Type 4		Like a sausage or snake, smooth and soft
Type 5		Soft blobs with clear-cut edges (passed easily)
Type 6		Fluffy pieces with ragged edges, a mushy stool
Type 7		Watery, no solid pieces. **Entirely Liquid**

Fig. 9.1 Bristol stool chart.

• *Macroscopic examination*: determine if there is blood or mucus in the stool, which may indicate inflammation or neoplasia.

• *Microscopic examination*: look for traces of blood and excessive numbers of inflammatory (white blood) cells. The presence of fat globules suggests malabsorption of fat (steatorrhoea), which may indicate pancreatic insufficiency or coeliac disease. Microscopy can also detect trophozoites of invasive amoebi, and the oocytes and cysts of other parasites that can cause diarrhoea.

• *Stool culture*: to detect bacterial pathogens such as *Salmonella*.

Standard blood tests

These should include a full blood count, electrolytes, liver chemistry and C-reactive protein level.

• A blood count can confirm anaemia and determine if it is microcytic, possibly due to iron deficiency, which may be a feature of coeliac disease, chronic IBD or colorectal cancer. If it is macrocytic, this may indicate folic acid or vitamin B_{12} deficiency, possibly indicating jejunal disease (e.g. chronic giardiasis), gastric disease (pernicious anaemia, Zollinger–Ellison syndrome) or ileal disease (Crohn's disease, tuberculosis, yersiniosis).

• An elevated white cell count may suggest infection, and an elevated platelet count may be an indication of chronic inflammation or of hyposplenism associated with coeliac disease.

• Chronic diarrhoea may cause electrolyte abnormalities that may need urgent correction.

• Mildly abnormal liver chemistry is often seen in coeliac disease and Crohn's disease. A biliary pattern of enzyme abnormalities (i.e. disproportionately elevated ALP and γ-GT levels) may indicate biliary or pancreatic disease.

• The C-reactive protein is typically elevated in inflammatory conditions such as Crohn's disease and intestinal infection. It is usually normal in coeliac disease. It may be normal in cases of ulcerative colitis and colon cancer unless the disease is severe or advanced.

Specialised blood tests

• There is no single diagnostic blood test for Crohn's disease, although in many patients antibodies to enteric microorganisms such as *Saccharomyces cerevisiae* (anti-*S. cerevisiae* antibody – ASCA) can be detected.

• Antibodies to gliadin peptides (antiendomysial antibody) and to the autoantigen tissue transglutaminase (anti-tTG antibody) are virtually diagnostic of coeliac disease.

- The serum amylase is markedly raised in acute pancreatitis; however, in chronic pancreatitis, which may cause malabsorption, the levels may be normal or only marginally elevated.
- Tumour markers such as carcinoembryonic antigen, which may be used to monitor the progress of treatment of colorectal cancer, are *not* used to make the diagnosis in the first instance.

Radiological tests

- *Abdominal ultrasound:* this may help to delineate the mass felt in her abdomen. Is it an abscess? Does it invade tissues like the psoas muscle? In other cases, ultrasound is useful to determine if there are gallstones, and if the pancreas is damaged.
- *Plain abdominal radiographs:* these help to determine if there is obstruction, when widened loops of bowel might appear, or in cases of colitis to determine if the colon is dangerously dilated, when it might perforate and cause peritonitis (megacolon, toxic megacolon).
- *Contrast studies of the bowel:* for example barium meal and follow-through are used widely to examine the jejunum and terminal ileum (Fig. 9.2).
- *CT and magnetic resonance imaging (MRI) scanning:* these are often combined with the ingestion of oral contrast medium to delineate abnormal areas of the intestine, as in Crohn's disease, ulcerative colitis and colon cancer.

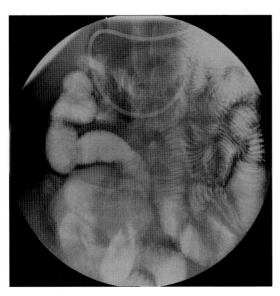

Fig. 9.2 Barium study: distal ileal stricture of Crohn's disease. (Courtesy of the Gastroenterology Department, John Radcliffe Hospital.)

Endoscopic tests

- *Upper endoscopy with distal duodenal biopsy:* this can be used to confirm or exclude the diagnosis of coeliac disease and demonstrate inflamed duodenal tissue with granulomas in Crohn's disease.
- *Colonoscopy with biopsies:* these can establish or exclude Crohn's disease, intestinal tuberculosis, colorectal cancer and ulcerative colitis. Histological examination of biopsies can be used to determine the diagnosis unequivocally. Biopsies may also be sent for microbiological testing and culture to detect bacterial and viral infection.

Emma has a mild microcytic anaemia. She is iron deficient and has borderline levels of vitamin B_{12}, with normal levels of folic acid. Her CRP is elevated at 30 mg/L. The rest of her blood tests are normal. The tTG level is normal. ASCA antibody testing is not available in this hospital. An ultrasound scan of the abdomen shows a possible mass in the right iliac fossa. The rest of the examination is normal.

Barium X-rays were considered, and then abandoned in favour of urgent upper endoscopy and colonoscopy with biopsies. Upper endoscopy shows a normal stomach and duodenum. Colonoscopy shows a normal colon, with some inflammatory changes in the caecum. The ileum is inflamed with shallow and deep ulcers (see Plate 9.1) and a mucopurulent exudate.

Biopsies suggest the diagnosis of Crohn's disease, with a few granulomas noted in the submucosa. There are no acid-fast bacilli detected. Cultures for mycobacteria are negative after 6 weeks.

What is the likely diagnosis?

The likely diagnosis is Crohn's disease of the ileum. It is possible; although unlikely, that chronic infection is present and has not been detected.

Treatment

The treatment of Crohn's disease is multifaceted.

Stop smoking

Smoking tobacco makes Crohn's disease more severe, and reduces the efficacy of treatment. In contrast, ulcerative colitis is more common in non-smokers.

5-Aminosalicylates

Intestinal inflammation may be reduced by 5-aminosalicylate (5-ASA), which is administered via modified release tablets to avoid absorption in the proximal intestine, and to deliver the drug to the ileum and colon. The mechanism of action of 5-ASA is unknown, although it may involve intracellular receptors such as PPAR-γ. 5-ASA is not substantially absorbed systemically, and may be active locally in the mucosa, where tissue concentrations can be quite high. The treatment with 5-ASA is generally well tolerated and without significant side effects. However, the efficacy of 5-ASA in treating active Crohn's disease, or in preventing relapses, is not high. In contrast, in ulcerative colitis, 5-ASA is moderately effective in inducing and maintaining remission.

Corticosteroids

The second line of treatment, particularly for moderately or severely active Crohn's disease, is to use corticosteroids. These reduce inflammation, and usually produce a dramatic improvement in the patient's symptoms. Relatively high doses are used for a short time, and the dose is reduced over a period of a few weeks.

In severe cases the steroids may be administered intravenously as hydrocortisone 100 mg four times daily. This is combined with a hydrocortisone enema preparation twice daily.

In moderate cases, oral prednisolone is used in a tapering dose. For example, 40 mg of prednisolone daily for 7 days, then 30 mg daily, then 20 mg, then 10 mg, and finally 5 mg per day for 7 days ('steroid tapering'). High doses of corticosteroids can produce severe side effects including changes in mood, disturbed sleep, weight gain, acneiform skin rash, steroid-induced diabetes mellitus in susceptible patients and, in the long term, osteoporosis. Patients should be warned about these potential side effects. To prevent osteoporosis, many clinicians prescribe calcium and vitamin D_3 supplements during steroid treatment.

Budesonide is an oral corticosteroid that is rapidly metabolised in the liver, and has minimal systemic side effects. This can be used for longer than prednisolone because of this safety advantage.

Treating the patient with corticosteroids is likely to induce remission from the Crohn's disease. However, the disease typically remits and then relapses, and multiple courses of tapering steroids may be needed. In these cases, a third line of therapy is needed.

Thiopurines

Immunomodulators such as the thiopurines azathioprine and mercaptopurine are currently third line agents.

They block DNA synthesis and interfere with the production of inflammatory leukocytes in the bone marrow. Thiopurines can cause life-threatening suppression of the bone marrow, as well as other side effects, and the treatment must be monitored by regularly checking the full blood count, liver function and monitoring the patient's clinical condition.

Methotrexate would not be offered to a female of reproductive age given the risk of foetal abnormalities if she were to become pregnant.

Corticosteroids and immunosuppressants are useful in treating ulcerative colitis and Crohn's disease.

Biological agents

A fourth line of medical treatment for Crohn's disease, particularly in patients who do not respond well to first, second and third line treatment, or who are intolerant of these treatments, is the use of antibodies to tumour necrosis factor α (anti-TNF-α).

The first of these therapeutic antibodies, infliximab, is a chimeric human–mouse protein, and is administered by intravenous infusion. It is often dramatically effective in inducing and maintaining remission. Antibodies to the antibody can develop, leading to reduced efficacy of subsequent infusions, and occasionally to allergic reactions. Newer agents, including the fully human anti-TNF antibody adalimumab, may circumvent these problems.

The treatment of Crohn's disease is evolving rapidly, and many experimental therapies may be available for the patient if conventional approaches are unattractive or ineffective. A top-down approach, using immunosuppressive agents and biological agents as a first line to allow mucosal healing early in a selective group of patients at the highest risk, is currently under investigation.

Surgery

Surgical resection of an affected segment of the bowel, for example the ileocaecal region in this case, may be indicated. This may offer a rapid and effective remedy for the patient.

The decision as to whether to opt for medical or surgical or combined treatment is best made by a multidisciplinary team, in consultation with the patient. Surgery does not, however, offer a cure as Crohn's disease can and does recur even after extensive resections. In this regard, it differs from ulcerative colitis, which is cured by the total removal of the colon (pan-proctocolectomy).

Emma responded rapidly to treatment with prednisolone and Pentasa. After tapering steroids, she continued to take Pentasa 1 g twice a day for a year. She then had a relapse, which responded poorly to treatment. Azathioprine was added to her treatment regimen. This seemed to be effective.

She has gained some weight, and after 3 months of iron supplementation her anaemia has been corrected. Her stools are more formed and there is no bleeding.

Outcome: what do you think happens next?

Eventually, about 80% of patients with Crohn's disease end up having some form of surgery for their disease.

Some patients require repeated surgery, and all medical and surgical attempts at inducing and maintaining remission are only partially effective in a minority of cases. Eventually about 20% of patients with ulcerative colitis undergo surgery for this condition at some point, and if the entire colon is removed, this is curative.

At any one time, 90% of treated patients with Crohn's disease remain in remission, and 10% experience relapses that require additional therapy. In the UK about 5% of patients require anti-TNF-α antibody treatment.

Overall, patients with Crohn's disease have a reduced life expectancy compared to healthy people. Patients with ulcerative colitis, in contrast, have a similar life expectancy to the general population.

CASE REVIEW

Chronic diarrhoea has many causes and the key is in a full history and examination.

Crohn's disease may affect young individuals who are ill for months before a diagnosis is reached. It can be familial, and can be more common in certain ethnic groups. Smoking can increase the risk.

Diagnosis is often established after exclusion of infection and other inflammatory processes. Stool examination, blood tests, endoscopic evaluation with biopsy and radiological studies provide a roadmap of disease extent and severity to guide therapy.

In the majority of cases the disease can be controlled by the careful use of available medical and surgical treatments, although an outright cure is not yet available. Perhaps this is because we do not fully understand the pathogenesis of the condition, and we do not know the cause.

KEY POINTS

- Coeliac disease is strongly associated with certain HLA haplotypes, and is strongly familial. In some parts of the world, such as western Ireland, the prevalence can be as high as 1:100.
- Inflammatory bowel disease can also run in families, and there is a strong hereditary predisposition. At least one gene has been associated with an increased risk of Crohn's disease – the *NOD2*, which mediates the interaction of our cells with bacterial products. People with IBD have a 15% chance of having at least one affected first degree relative
- A normal looking rectal mucosa at rigid sigmoidoscopy does not exclude IBD or colon cancer. However, the test may show an inflamed rectum, which can be interpreted as good evidence of ulcerative colitis if the history and examination support this diagnosis.
- Corticosteroids are powerful anti-inflammatory agents. They have profound systemic side effects that you must remember and warn patients about.

Case 10 A 51-year-old woman with acute nausea, vomiting and diarrhoea

Mrs Sharon Spue is a 51-year-old school teacher. She comes to the accident and emergency department with nausea, vomiting and loose stool. She describes a nagging lower abdominal discomfort. She looks dehydrated and unwell. You move her to a cubicle for further questioning and examination.

What features of the history are important?
Acute or chronic illness

- Duration of illness: how long has she been feeling unwell?
- Speed of onset: was it sudden or gradual?

Timing: what came first, the nausea and vomit, abdominal discomfort or loose stools? How has it evolved over time?

- An acute illness suggests an infective aetiology. A trigger can be searched for, but is not always found.

Nausea and vomiting

- What is the frequency of vomiting?
- What is the colour and consistency: is there altered food, gastric or bile-like fluid or faeculent material?
- Is there any blood or coffee-ground material?
- Vomiting is the mechanism to expel noxious stimuli or toxins. Repeated vomiting or retching can result in a tear in the oesophageal mucosa and thus bleeding.

Abdominal pain

- Describe the abdominal pain: location, radiation, intensity, frequency, nature of the pain, aggravating and relieving factors.
- Abdominal pain is usually the result of muscle spasms, distension of the intestine and mucosal response to inflammation.

Gastroenterology: Clinical Cases Uncovered, 1st edition.
© S. Keshav and E. Culver. Published 2011 by
Blackwell Publishing Ltd.

Bowel habit

Describe the stool colour, consistency and frequency. Are they watery? Is there any blood in the motions? Is there any mucus? Are there nocturnal symptoms or urgency? Is there incomplete evacuation of stool?

The Bristol stool chart can be shown to help patients identify their current stool type and help nursing staff to monitor the stool consistency and frequency whilst in hospital (see Fig. 9.1).

Associated features

- *Fever*: does she have hot sweats and chills? Fever may be present in bacterial, viral or amoebic infection and as part of a systemic response in inflammatory disease.
- *Meningism*: does she have a headache, photophobia or neck stiffness? A viral and bacterial meningitis may coexist.
- *Myalgia*: are her muscles weak and aching? Systemic features of fever, headache and myalgia are common in *Shigella*, *Campylobacter* and *Yersinia enterocolitica* infections.
- *Dehydration*: does she feel thirsty and dehydrated? Is she dizzy on standing due to postural hypotension?

Complications

- Haemolytic uraemic syndrome (HUS) may cause a purpuric rash.
- Erythema nodosum may occur in *Campylobacter* and *Yersinia* infections.
- Reiter's syndrome or reactive arthritis usually follows bacterial dysentery. The triad of arthralgia, conjunctivitis or uveitis and urethritis is classically associated with this. Ask about joint stiffness, aching and inflammation (arthritis), inflamed red and itchy eyes (conjunctivitis), pain in the eyes (uveitis), and discomfort and frequency in urination (urethritis).
- Guillain–Barré syndrome is an immune-mediated peripheral demyelination causing symmetrical weakness or numbness distally and ascending to involve the arms

and upper body. It occurs especially after *Campylobacter* infection. These patients need admission to hospital for monitoring of vital capacity, especially if there are symptoms of breathing difficulties. Treatment is with plasmapheresis.

Risk factors

The people most susceptible to infection include the elderly or very young, immunocompromised patients (with HIV/AIDS (acquired immune deficiency syndrome), organ transplant recipients, or on chemotherapy and immunosuppressive medications), those with hypogammaglobulinaemia, hyposplenism or a total gastrectomy.

Past medical and surgical history

• Do you have inflammatory bowel disease, an organ transplant or are known to be immunosuppressed?
• Have you had your spleen or stomach removed?

Medications

• Are you taking immunosuppressive medications such as steroids, chemotherapy or biological agents?
• Have you taken a course of antibiotics in the last few weeks/months? *Clostridium difficile* is associated with antibiotic use and can cause pseudomembranous colitis.
• Are you taking a protein pump inhibitor? Gastric acidity confers some protection against certain infections and the loss of this acidity can make people more susceptible.

Social history

• Have you been in contact with anyone who is unwell with similar symptoms? Have you been in close contact with someone in an institution? Nurseries, schools, hospitals and nursing homes allow rapid spread of gastroenteritis, particularly due to viruses such as rotavirus.
• Have you travelled abroad recently? Where did you go? Was anyone unwell there? Africa, the Far East and Latin America are hotspots for infection with various bacteria, viruses and protozoa.
• Have you eaten food that may have been prepared on a contaminated surface? Have you eaten any uncooked/undercooked meat or eggs or unpasteurised milk? Suspect food from take-aways, mass catering and conference dinners.
• Do you have good hand hygiene?

She tells you her symptoms began suddenly 48h ago. She felt nauseous then vomited. Her pain is in the upper abdomen and is crampy in nature. The loose stools developed a few hours later which are watery with no blood. She has passed stools every hour for the last 5h. She feels hot and sweaty and is aching all over. There are no other systemic symptoms.

She has had a hysterectomy but has no other medical problems. She is not taking any medications. She is a lifelong non-smoker and consumes little alcohol.

She went out for dinner with her husband two nights ago to a Chinese restaurant, but she ate the same food as him and he remains well. Her two children go to the local school and are both well. She last travelled to Africa 3 months ago, where she worked for 6 weeks as a teacher in a locally deprived school. She has been to the Lake District since for one weekend only. She took some antibiotics for cystitis 2 weeks ago, which has now resolved.

What features do you look for on examination?
General examination

• Look for evidence of the systemic inflammatory response syndrome (SIRS) or sepsis: hypothermia (especially in the elderly) or a fever of >37.5°C, pulse rate >100 beats/min, systolic blood pressure <90 mmHg, postural drop >20 mmHg.
• Look for clinical dehydration: dry mucous membranes, decreased skin turgor and low jugular venous pressure at a 45° angle.

Abdominal examination

• Is there abdominal tenderness, rebound or guarding, suggesting a toxic colon?
• Are the bowel sounds present and active suggestive of a functioning bowel?
• Are there any palpable masses, such as an appendiceal mass or diverticular abscess?

Digital rectal examination

In the presence of loose stools a DRE will confirm loose stool and ensure it is not overflow diarrhoea from impacted stool in the rectum; look for fresh blood and palpate for a rectal mass.

Specific findings

• Look at the eyes for evidence of conjunctivitis or uveitis.

- Look at the joints for signs of active inflammatory arthritis.
- Expose the patient and look at the skin for any hidden purpuric rashes.
- Do a neurological examination to look for evidence of ascending paralysis and exclude meningism in the presence of a headache.

> On examination she is tachycardic at 120 beats/min and pyrexial at 38.6°C. She is clinically dehydrated with dry mucus membranes and decreased skin turgor. On abdominal examination there is generalised tenderness with voluntary guarding but no rebound. Bowel sounds are present. The neurological exam is normal.

Differential diagnosis

This is an acute episode of nausea, vomiting, abdominal pain and loose stools. Her risk factors are a recent course of antibiotics, eating dinner in a restaurant and a previous travel history.

Possibilities include:
- Food poisoning.
- Viral gastroenteritis, such as Norwalk or rotavirus.
- Traveller's diarrhoea
- *Clostridium difficile* infection.
- Appendicitis should not be forgotten, although guarding and rebound are likely clinical findings on examination.

What investigations should you order to confirm your diagnosis?

Stool examination

A stool examination should be done for microscopy, cultures and sensitivity to look for bacterial, viral and amoebic causes of gastroenteritis. A separate request should be sent to look for parasites, ova and cysts. Three stool samples should also be sent for *Clostridium difficile*, as a single negative sample does not exclude the diagnosis.

Blood and leucocytes in the stool suggest an inflammatory cause of diarrhoea. Bacterial pathogens need stool culture. Viruses, such as rotavirus, can be detected by electron microscopy. Amoeba can be found by light microscopy. *Giardia* may be found on stool culture, but usually requires jejuneal aspiration and microscopy for confirmation.

Blood tests

Blood tests are needed to look for evidence of infection, inflammation and organ failure.

- A full blood count may show thrombocytopenia of HUS and an elevated white count (neutrophilia) is suggestive of infection. Coagulation studies may show evidence of disseminated intravascular coagulation of severe sepsis; the prothrombin time may be elevated in HUS.
- Urea and creatinine may be elevated due to renal failure from dehydration or HUS. Electrolytes may be abnormal; hypokalaemia and hypomagnesaemia can be due to diarrhoea, hypernatraemia to dehydration.
- Liver function tests may show a low albumin in systemic sepsis, an elevated isolated ALT if there is ischaemic liver injury and in conjunction with ALP in sepsis.
- Inflammatory markers such as C-reactive protein may be elevated.

Urine dipstick

This is done for blood and protein, which may indicate renal failure.

Abdominal X-ray

An abdominal X-ray should be taken if there is evidence of sepsis to look for mucosal oedema and exclude toxic megacolon.

Flexisigmoidoscopy

This may be required to look for macroscopic evidence of inflammatory or pseudomembranous colitis and to obtain a histological diagnosis if the symptoms do not settle with conservative medical management.

Whilst you are waiting for the results of stool specimens and blood tests, what treatment should you give her?

- She needs to be rehydrated. As she is in the accident and emergency department, she should have intravenous fluids via a cannula (1 L of saline 0.9% over 1 h). There is no previous cardiac history so volume replacement can be given quickly. In the community, dehydration can be treated with large volumes of oral fluid and rehydration sachets such as Dioralyte 500–3000 mL daily.
- It is likely she will be potassium depleted due to the diarrhoea, but if she has developed acute renal impairment the potassium may have risen so reserve potassium supplementation for when the blood tests are available.
- Antiemetics can be given for nausea, such as metoclopramide. There is a risk of dystonic reactions in younger patients and domperidone is an alternative.

- Antipyretics such as paracetamol should be given for pyrexia.
- Antispasmodics such as buscopan may be given for abdominal pain and cramps.
- Antibiotics should not be given blindly as she may have *Clostridium difficile* and the cause of her gastroenteritis is not known. Bacterial infections may benefit from empirical antibiotics such as ciprofloxacin 500 mg for 5 days if started early, limiting the duration of diarrhoea by 1–2 days at most. This depends on local resistance to antibiotics and the causative organism.

What other general advice do you give?

- She should be in isolated from other patients in a cubicle, and infection control measures, such as hand washing, gloves and aprons, should be used by medical personnel.
- Meticulous hand hygiene is important and she should use her own individual towel and wash her hands with soap and water.
- She should avoid constipating agents such as loperamide or lomitil as these prevent the toxins from leaving the gastrointestinal tract.

Her blood tests show an elevated white cell count at 17 × 10⁹/L and CRP at 56 mg/L. Her renal function is within normal range, although her potassium is low at 3.0 mmol/L. The remainder of her blood tests are normal.

An abdominal X-ray shows no evidence of mucosal oedema or toxic megacolon. Stool specimens were sent for bacterial culture and C. difficile exclusion.

What do you do now?

She should have further fluid resuscitation with potassium replacement (intravenous saline 0.9% with 40 mmol KCl). Once haemodynamically stable she should be discharged home with some oral rehydration sachets and advice to drink plenty of fluids, take regular paracetamol (1 g four times per day) for pyrexia and antiemetics as needed for nausea.

The symptoms may persist for up to a week. She should contact her general practitioner if they continue after this time or if she becomes more unwell. She should remain off work until the diarrhoea has settled.

The results of the stool cultures are called through to you from the microbiology department 48 h later. They are positive for Salmonella enteritidis. The specimens for C. difficile are negative.

Who do you need to inform of the result?

The patient's GP should be informed of the result of the stool specimens which may guide management in the future. Some patients can develop post-infective irritable bowel syndrome or the infection can trigger underlying inflammatory bowel disease.

Salmonella is a notifiable disease in the UK under the Public Health Regulations 1988. The Public Health Laboratory must be informed. Food handlers must be clear of symptoms for at least 48 h and have produced a negative stool sample before return to work.

Mrs Spue had an uncomplicated recovery and returned to work the following week. The Public Health Department was notified and the local Chinese restaurant was temporarily closed pending investigation.

Box 9.1 *Salmonella* enteritis

- *Salmonella* is a bacterium that causes one of the commonest forms of food poisoning worldwide. Numerous serotypes of *Salmonella* exist. *S. enteritidis* is the most common cause of *Salmonella* gastroenteritis. *S. typhi* and *S. paratyphi* can also cause systemic infection as described in typhoid fever.
- Pathogenicity is conferred due to the ability to invade intestinal mucosa and produce toxins.
- The source is usually of animal origin such as poultry, eggs and unpasteurised milk, but all foods can be contaminated. Organisms multiply rapidly in humid environments and cross-contamination occurs. Inadequate thawing of frozen food is a common source. It is spread by the faecal–oral route by poor hand hygiene.
- The incubation period is from 12 to 72 h.
- Symptoms include diarrhoea, which can be bloody, with fever and abdominal cramps. The illness tends to last 4–7 days and then recovery occurs.
- Signs of fever (temperature of 38–39°C) and dehydration are common. There is no typical rash of typhoid.
- Diagnosis is by culturing the organism from the stool. Full blood count shows an elevated white cell count. Agglutination tests, such as the Widal test, are not recommended as they are often false positive.
- Management consists of oral rehydration and hand washing to prevent spread of infection to others (faecal–oral route). Hospital admission may be needed in

the very young or elderly, immunosuppressed and in those with chronic gastrointestinal disease.

- Antibiotics may prolong the carrier stage and there are multiple antibiotic resistances. They may be used in the severely ill, especially immunocompromised patients.
- Sometimes antidiarrhoea or antispasmodic drugs may be required. Their use is controversial as prolongation of the transit time may prolong the disease.
- When diarrhoea has settled, the vast majority are not a risk to others and may return to work with no further testing.
- Mortality is about 0.4%. Most people recover uneventfully.
- Bacterial infection may rarely spread outside the gastrointestinal tract causing endocarditis, pneumonia or empyema, hepatic and splenic abscesses, meningitis, septic arthritis and osteomyelitis.

CASE REVIEW

Acute episodes of nausea and vomiting with diarrhoea and abdominal discomfort are usually infectious in origin. They often settle conservatively. It is important to be aware of the potential complications of gastroenteritis, depending on the organism involved and the underlying immune response of the individual. These include haemolytic uraemic syndrome and Guillain–Barré syndrome.

The diagnosis can be established by stool cultures and blood tests if the patient is systemically unwell, symptoms persist or there is other evidence of organ failure. Management concentrates on treating the dehydration and symptom control until the infective agent has gone. Certain groups of people require hospitalisation during this period for intravenous replacement of fluids and electrolytes.

KEY POINTS

- Gastroenteritis is caused by an infection of the gastrointestinal tract. It usually causes self-limiting illness although it can be responsible for widespread epidemics causing serious mortality.
- It can be caused by a number of bacteria, viruses, parasites and protozoa species. The organism is often not isolated.
- Certain infections are notifiable to the Public Health Department. The microbiology department should be able to advise.
- Typical symptoms are acute in onset and short in duration. These include abdominal pain, diarrhoea, nausea and vomiting and fever.
- Stool culture and microscopy are important in diagnosis. Blood and leucocytes in the stool identify inflammatory diarrhoea.
- Treatment is usually conservative with rehydration and electrolyte replacement in the community, although some people with systemic infection and susceptible individuals will need to be hospitalised.
- Potential complications of gastroenteritis include haemolytic uraemic syndrome, toxic megacolon and perforation, Guillain–Barré syndrome, seronegative arthropathy and post-infectious irritable bowel syndrome.

A 79-year-old woman with altered bowel habit and weight loss

Mrs Martha Bell is a 79-year-old woman who attends your outpatient clinic with her daughter. She tells you she is suffering from constipation and a vague abdominal discomfort. She has lost her appetite and her clothes have become looser over the last few months. She is otherwise well.

What are your main concerns? What other information do you need to know?

The main concern in an elderly patient with altered bowel habit and weight loss is malignancy. There are many other causes, however, so a full history and examination is essential.

Constipation

• Define constipated stool. The classic definition is stool passage less than every 3 days which may be hard or pellet-like. The definition of normal may vary for different people and it is important to establish what normal is for the individual.

• Define the length of time of constipation or altered bowel habit. It may have been present all her life, which is more suggestive of a functional or transit disorder. It may represent a change in bowel habit, for which a cause should be investigated.

Weight loss

• Establish the amount of weight lost over what time period. Has it been purposeful or non-intentional?

• Weight loss is one of the alarm symptoms that prompt the search for organic pathology, especially malignancy, malabsorptive and inflammatory processes.

Gastroenterology: Clinical Cases Uncovered, 1st edition.
© S. Keshav and E. Culver. Published 2011 by
Blackwell Publishing Ltd.

Abdominal discomfort

Describe the abdominal discomfort. Is it a superficial muscular ache that may be reproduced by movement, is it a deep-seated aching discomfort that is constant and may suggest sinister pathology, or is it related to the passage of stool?

Other symptoms

• *Rectal bleeding*: is there any fresh or altered rectal blood? Is this mixed in with the stool or separate on wiping/in the toilet pan? Is it constant or intermittent, associated with straining at stool? It is also an alarm symptom.

• *Nausea or vomiting*: does this sound obstructive in nature, occurring after eating and associated with bloating and abdominal distension?

• *Anaemia*: has she been excessively tired and fatigued? Does she get breathless on walking or had new angina symptoms?

She explains that she has felt constipated for the last year. Her bowel habit is regular, once per day, with hard, pellet-like stool. There is no excessive straining at stool and no rectal bleeding. Her abdominal discomfort is deep and constant. It is located around the epigastrum and does not radiate elsewhere. It has no relieving or aggravating factors.

She feels bloated most of the day. She does not have any nausea and never vomits. Her appetite has declined and she has probably lost about 6 kg in weight over the last 2 months (almost two dress sizes for her). She is happy with this. She feels tired and lethargic but puts this down to her age.

What other information do you need before planning investigations?
Past medical history

This is important to help decide on the best diagnostic tests (depending on anatomy) and may determine future treatment strategies.

- Previous malignancy, how it was treated and future management plans.
- Surgical history: prior gastrointestinal or gynaecological operations.
- Other medical history including cardiac and respiratory disease, especially if an operation may be needed in the future.

Medications

These may be the cause of current symptoms. The type of drug and timing of starting/finishing a medication is important.

- Constipating drugs, such as tricyclic antidepressants and opiates.
- Laxatives, which may mask the problem.
- Antiplatelet therapy or anticoagulants, which may need to be stopped before an investigative procedure.

Potential risk factors

- Smoking: does she smoke or has she ever smoked? If so, what is her pack-year history (number of years smoking 20 cigarettes per day)? Smoking increases the risk of many malignancies.
- Alcohol: history of consumption.
- Is there a family history of colorectal cancer? If so, which family members and what age at diagnosis? Has she ever been in a screening programme?

She suffers from ischaemic heart disease (recently diagnosed 6 months ago by her general practitioner), claudication on walking 200m and non-insulin dependent type 2 diabetes mellitus. She considers herself to be well. She lives alone and manages all activities around the house without assistance.

Her medications include aspirin, lisinopril, atorvastatin and metformin. She was recently started on iron supplements for anaemia. She has used lactulose as needed for constipated stool, usually once a month at most. She has no allergies. She takes no anticoagulants.

She is an ex-smoker of 20 years with a 30 pack-year history. There is a family history of diabetes and ischaemic heart disease but no colorectal cancer.

What is your differential diagnosis?

- *Colorectal cancer*: this is the main diagnosis to exclude in an elderly woman with a change of bowel habit and abdominal pain.
- *Hypothyroidism*: this can cause constipated stool, but is more likely to cause weight gain than loss.

- *Hypercalcaemia*: this can result in abdominal pain and constipation. The main causes for a high calcium level are related to either the parathyroid or malignancy.
- *Idiopathic constipation* (possibly age-related): the elderly population can suffer from age-related slowing of the bowels, most likely related to the level of exercise, dietary factors, amount of water consumed, as well as physiological changes.

What findings on the examination will confirm your suspicions?

- Look for signs of anaemia such as conjunctival pallor.
- Look for signs of weight loss, including loose skin and clothes that do not fit.
- Palpate for peripheral lymphadenopathy.
- Palpate for an abdominal fullness or mass in the colon.
- Palpate for organomegaly. A hard craggy liver suggests liver metastases.
- Digital rectal examination must be done to look for a rectal mass and may identify haemorrhoids, anal fissures and hard, pellet-like stool.
- Faecal occult blood (FOB) has a poor sensitivity in detecting colorectal cancer, and even if negative it would not change your investigation plan.

On examination she has conjunctival pallor. There is no lymphadenopathy. Her abdomen is soft and tender in the epigastrium with no obvious masses or organomegaly. There is nothing to find on rectal exam.

> **!RED FLAG**
>
> Change of bowel habit, abdominal pain, rectal bleeding or iron deficiency in older patients are alarm features to suggest malignancy.

What investigations do you choose?
Blood tests

- Full blood count and iron studies to look for iron-deficiency anaemia (although she is taking iron supplements which will misrepresent her iron stores).
- Urea, creatinine and electrolytes are important prior to deciding the type of bowel preparation for colonoscopy.
- Liver function results may suggest signs of metastatic disease, although they are a poor discriminator for this. An isolated elevated ALP may suggest bone involvement.

- Calcium, as hypercalcaemia can cause constipation and abdominal pain.
- Thyroid function, as hypothyroidism can lead to constipation and lethargy.

Colonoscopy

This is the best method to detect colorectal cancer. However, to decide if colonoscopy is appropriate, the presence of systemic disease, the administration of bowel preparation and the use of sedation should be considered.

The presence of co-morbidities such as cardiac or respiratory disease or organ failure puts the patient in a higher risk group for a procedure requiring bowel preparation and sedation. This can be avoidable.

Preparation given for colonoscopy depends on the presence of co-morbidities and renal function. Most units use Moviprep or Kleanprep with reduced risks of dehydration. Phosphate preparations have been associated with phosphate nephropathy and should be avoided in the elderly with renal disease who are at higher risk.

Sedation in the form of an opiate (fentanyl or pethidine) and a benzodiazepine (midazolam) is offered in most UK departments according to the British Society of Gastroenterology (BSG) safe sedation guidelines. An unsedated colonoscopy can be done in those who are intolerant or allergic to sedation and in those who request the procedure without it. However, this is associated with a longer time to completion and an increased risk of not completing the procedure to reach the caecum and thus potentially missing lesions. General anaesthetic is generally not given for diagnostic colonoscopy in adults in the UK. Propofol should not be used in the absence of anaesthetic support.

What are the other options instead of colonoscopy?

- CT colonography with oral gastrografin to opacify the stool.
- CT pneumocolon (virtual colonography).

When do you choose radiological investigation?

- If the patient was not fit for sedation or bowel preparation for colonoscopy. This again depends on co-morbidities and age.
- If the patient refused an invasive procedure. A patient has the right to consent to and withdraw consent from a procedure at any time.

If she had severe renal impairment, a CT colon with oral gastrografin preparation is less likely to cause serious side effects. However, bringing the patient into hospital overnight and rehydrating them pre- and post-colonoscopy is a viable alternative.

What if a lesion is found?

If a mass lesion is detected on imaging, an endoscopic examination would be needed to confirm radiological findings and obtain histology. A staging CT scan is also appropriate to look for the extent of disease and guide management.

> **KEY POINT**
>
> - Colonoscopy is currently the most sensitive and specific method to detect colorectal cancer, although there is a miss rate. The sensitivity of radiological techniques to detect colon lesions is improving. Imaging is a viable alternative to detect large lesions in patients who can not undergo or choose not to undergo endoscopic examination. This risks and benefits of this must be discussed with the patient.

Blood tests confirmed a microcytic anaemia with iron-deficiency pattern. She proceeded to CT colonography given her age and co-morbidities. This demonstrated thickening of a region in the ascending colon and scattered diverticula to the splenic flexure (Fig. 11.1).

She proceeded to have a colonoscopy, aware of the findings on the CT scan. She was admitted as an inpatient and given intravenous rehydration pre- and postoperatively. She tolerated the procedure well. The colonoscopy revealed a polypoid mass lesion causing partial obstruction in the ascending colon (see Plate 11.1). This looked malignant. The lesion was tattooed and biopsies were taken.

She was assessed by the colorectal nurse specialists the same day on the ward. She was then referred to the lower gastrointestinal multidisciplinary team. In the meantime, she returned home with an outpatient CT scan for staging organised and was to be seen in outpatients to discuss further management plans.

Staging CT of the abdomen, pelvis and chest revealed no significant lymphadenopathy or evidence of metastasis. There was no other pathology detected.

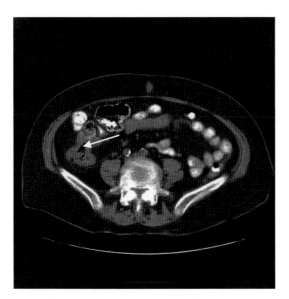

Fig. 11.1 CT colonography showing a thickened ascending colon (arrow) suggestive of a colonic malignancy. (Courtesy of the Gastroenterology Department, John Radcliffe Hospital.)

What are the management options?

These options should be discussed in a multidisciplinary team meeting with colorectal nurse specialists, colorectal surgeons, gastroenterologists, oncologists, colorectal radiologists and histopathologists. The options depend on the wishes of the patient, relevant co-morbidities, histopathology of the lesion including invasion, radiology assessment and evidence of metastases.

Surgery

Mrs Bell requires a preoperative assessment of risk factors prior to surgery.
• *Ischaemic heart disease.* Firstly, her anaemia should be corrected with iron supplements. Given the likely cause of this is the cancer, it may not return to normal until the cause has been removed. She will then need an exercise tolerance test and either appropriate anti-angina medication or angiography. Some patients require percutaneous intervention with stenting prior to an operation. Antiplatelet therapy then needs to be considered. An echocardiogram may be requested.
• *Diabetes control.* She has type 2 diabetes. Medication should be optimised and she may need insulin. This should be managed with the aid of a diabetic specialist nurse or doctor.

Chemotherapy

A course of postoperative adjuvant chemotherapy for 6 months would offer an approximate 5% benefit in 5-year survival. If she is keen to pursue this, discussion with the oncologist would be warranted. There are risks and complications of treatment.

Palliation of symptoms

This would not confer a survival benefit but would concentrate on support, medications and interventions as needed to improve quality of life. The palliative care team in hospital and the community palliative team in her local area would assist with this.

The case was re-discussed at the MDT meeting and surgical resection was deemed appropriate. She was assessed by the surgical team in clinic and discussed the risks and benefits of surgery. She was keen for an operation.

She underwent an exercise tolerance test and managed 3 min 25 s of the Bruce protocol, limited by dyspnoea. There was evidence of ST depression consistent with coronary artery disease. She was reviewed by the cardiologists and commenced on anti-anginal medication. This improved her symptoms. Echocardiogram confirmed good left ventricular function and no valvular disease.

Two weeks later, she underwent an extended right hemicolectomy. There were no complications. She remained in hospital for 5 days. Histology revealed a T4,N0,M0 moderately differentiated mucinous adenocarcinoma of the ascending colon (see Plate 11.2).

She was offered, but declined, adjuvant chemotherapy due to the potential risks and complications. She remains well 1 year later.

What about follow-up?

She requires a surveillance CT scan and colonoscopy 1 year postoperatively.

CASE REVIEW

A change of bowel habit, abdominal pain, rectal bleeding or iron deficiency in older patients should alert the clinician to consider a colorectal malignancy. Colonoscopy is the ideal investigation of choice. Radiological investigation of the bowel should be considered depending on age, frailty, co-morbidities and patient preference. The risks and benefits of each should be considered.

Management of colorectal cancer should be decided in a multidisciplinary team setting. This may include surgery, chemotherapy and palliative stenting of the colon for obstructive symptoms and/or medical management. Surveillance after initial management is in accordance with determined guidelines.

KEY POINTS

- Change of bowel habit, abdominal pain, rectal bleeding or iron deficiency in older patients should trigger the thought of colon cancer as the main differential.
- Colonoscopy is the optimal method to detect colon cancer.
- Radiological methods may be more appropriate in the elderly, frail or those with co-morbidity. These methods are becoming more sensitive and specific.
- Management is decided in a multidisciplinary team focusing on the best options for the patient and potential for cure versus risks associated with therapy.

Case 12 A 54-year-old man with rectal bleeding

Mr Palak Chandra is a 54-year-old mini-cab driver who attends your outpatient clinic because of persistent bleeding from the back passage. This has been a problem for the last few months. He has a friend who was recently diagnosed with colon cancer. He is very concerned that he may have cancer too. He has come to you for reassurance.

What are the important questions from the history that will help you to find a cause for his rectal bleeding?

Presenting complaint

• *Type of bleeding.* Is the blood bright red or dark or altered with clots? Is it mixed in with the stool or separate from it? Does it cover the lavatory after defecation and the toilet paper after wiping? This may help to determine the origin of blood loss; brighter, fresh red blood on wiping or in the pan is most likely related to anal disease (haemorrhoids, fissure, polyp or cancer); darker blood or blood mixed in with stool more often originates from higher in the colon.

• *Duration of bleeding.* Has the bleeding been present for days, weeks, months or years? Has it happened before? If so, how long ago and did it settle on its own?

• *Frequency of bleeding episodes.* Is it present every time he defecates or intermittently?

Other symptoms

• *Constipation.* Does he suffer from hard or pellet-like stool? Does he have any difficulty when defecating or strain when passing a stool? Has the bowel habit changed or is this longstanding? If there is a recent change in bowel habit, an obstructive mass should be excluded.

Straining at stool associated with bleeding suggests anal or rectal pathology.

• *Diarrhoea.* Is the stool loose with urgency of defection and nocturnal frequency? Inflammatory bowel disease, particularly ulcerative colitis, and some infective diarrhoea (shorter duration) may present with rectal bleeding, urgency and frequency. Radiation injury can also cause a radiation proctitis associated with bleeding, pain and urgency.

• *Perianal pain.* Is there a sudden onset of pain on defecation or is it constant? Pain on defecation suggests a protruding haemorrhoid or fissure.

• *Rectal fullness or a sensation of incomplete evacuation after defecation* (tenesmus). This may suggest a rectal lesion or a defecating disorder.

• *Palpable lumps.* Are there any visible or palpable haemorrhoids from his anus? Can they be pushed back in by himself or not? Are they painful?

• *Leakage.* Has he noticed any mucus or discharge leaking from the back passage? Does he suffer from perianal itch? What is his personal hygiene like?

• *Systemic symptoms* such as fever, lethargy or weight loss.

• *Extraintestinal manifestations of inflammatory bowel disease.* These include mouth ulceration, rashes, arthritis/arthralgia or eye inflammation.

Past medical history

• Does he have known inflammatory bowel disease?
• Has he had radiation treatment in the past?

Medications

• Is he taking any prescription or over-the-counter medications that may have caused altered bowel habit or bleeding?
• Is he taking warfarin or non-steroidal anti-inflammatory drugs?

Social history

• Does he smoke or drink alcohol?

Gastroenterology: Clinical Cases Uncovered, 1st edition.
© S. Keshav and E. Culver. Published 2011 by
Blackwell Publishing Ltd.

• What is his diet like? Does he consume sufficient dietary fibre and drink plenty of fluids?
• Has he travelled abroad recently? Could he have picked up an infection?
• What is his sexual orientation and is he sexually active?

Family history

• Is there any family history of colorectal or anal cancer? Which family members and at what age where they diagnosed?
• Is there any history of inflammatory bowel disease?

> *He tells you he sees bright red blood on the toilet paper after wiping and in the lavatory. The stool is coated in blood and he thinks it is also mixed in. He had his first episode 3 months ago and it has happened every week or so since. His stool has been loose but there is no urgency or nocturnal frequency. He has not noticed any lumps but feels generalised perianal discomfort and burning. His weight is stable and there are no other systemic symptoms.*
>
> *He has a past medical history of irritable bowel syndrome diagnosed by his general practitioner a few years earlier, suffering from episodic abdominal cramps and diarrhoea. He takes ibuprofen occasionally for a frozen shoulder.*
>
> *He is a smoker of 10 cigarettes per day, with a 20 pack-year history. He drinks 10 units of alcohol per week. His father had colon cancer aged 70 years. There is no other family history.*

What is your differential diagnosis at this stage?

The key features are rectal bleeding, both within and external to the stool, and his loose stool, which may be a component of his irritable bowel or associated with the bleeding. The differential diagnoses include:
• Haemorrhoids.
• Anal fissure.
• Proctitis.
• Polyp.
• Anal cancer.

Box 12.1 Causes of blood separate to the stool

• Haemorrhoids
• Anal fissure
• Drugs, such as anticoagulants (over-anticoagulated)

Box 12.2 Causes of blood mixed in with the stool

• Bacterial infection: *Salmonella, Campylobacter, Shigella, Escherichia coli* and *Clostridium difficile*
• Proctitis/colitis: radiation, inflammatory bowel disease (ulcerative or Crohn's colitis)
• Perianal or colorectal cancer
• Diverticular colitis and bleeding
• Ischaemic colitis
• Protozoal infection
• Schistosomiasis (rarely)

What would you look for on examination?

General examination

Examine for conjunctival pallor of anaemia and for evidence of nutritional deficiency such as koilonychia and angular stomatitis.

Abdominal examination

Examine for a palpable mass, especially in the left lower quadrant.

Digital rectal examination

DRE must be done in all patients with fresh rectal bleeding.
• *Inspection:* look for signs of perianal Crohn's disease such as fissures, skin tags or abscesses. Are there excoriations and broken skin from perianal itching? Are there external haemorrhoids?
• *Feel:* examine for anal tone by asking the patient to gently squeeze his anal passage and bear down on your gloved finger. Feel for internal haemorrhoids, anal fissures or an anal mass suggestive of a polyp or cancer. Is there fresh blood on your glove? There is no indication to do a faecal occult blood test in this setting.

Proctoscopy

Proctoscopy can reveal a distal rectal cancer and internal haemorrhoids.

Rigid sigmoidoscopy

This can visualise the rectal mucosa to identify an area of proctitis. A biopsy should be taken even if the mucosa is normal to identify Crohn's disease with rectal sparing or microscopic colitis.

KEY POINTS

- All patients must have a digital rectal examination in the context of rectal bleeding to exclude an anal tumour.
- Proctoscopy and/or rigid sigmoidoscopy are useful adjuncts in the outpatient clinic to identify distal rectal and anal lesions.

KEY POINT

- In those patients older than 40 years with rectal bleeding, or in patients with alarm symptoms, full colonic investigation should be considered. This can be endoscopic with or without radiology of the colon.

General and abdominal examinations were unremarkable. On rectal exam his perianal area was erythematous. There was good anal tone and no palpable masses or fissure.

Rigid sigmoidoscopy to 15cm showed normal healthy mucosa, which was biopsied. There were small internal haemorrhoids at 12 o'clock and 3 o'clock which were not thrombosed or prolapsed.

What investigations should you book?
Blood tests

These should include a full blood count to identify anaemia or thrombocytopenia, coagulation studies and C-reactive protein to look for an inflammatory cause. Given the history of loose stools, coeliac serology and thyroid function should be sent if not done previously.

Endoscopic tests

A serious cause of rectal bleeding should be excluded by colonic investigation. A flexible sigmoidoscopy should be done given the presence of fresh blood mixed in with the stool. This can be combined with a barium enema as the patient is aged over 40 years, to look for proximal lesions.

An alternative to the barium enema is a complete colonoscopy. This depends on resource availability and patient preference. If the stool is loose, a biopsy should be taken for microscopic colitis even if the mucosa appears normal.

Blood tests were normal. Flexible sigmoidoscopy showed diverticular disease of the sigmoid colon and confirmed internal haemorrhoids on retroversion of the scope. They were not thrombosed or actively bleeding. Barium enema also demonstrated some right-sided colonic diverticular disease. There were no colonic masses.

He returns to your gastroenterology clinic 2 weeks later to discuss the results.

What is the likely cause of his rectal bleeding and how would you explain this to him?

The likely cause of his fresh rectal bleeding is from his internal haemorrhoids that were identified on rectal exam and confirmed on sigmoidoscopy (Fig. 12.1). These are dilated rectal veins that usually develop due to straining at stool.

Diverticular disease was seen on sigmoidoscopy and barium enema (Fig. 12.2). Diverticula are outpouching of the large bowel wall that may become inflamed and bleed. The prevalence of colonic diverticula increases with age, present in 50% of the population aged over 50 years in developed countries. Over 90% of patients are asymptomatic. This risk is increased in males and in those taking NSAIDs.

It may be that the episodic abdominal cramps and diarrhoea he described over the last few years are due to a combination of irritable bowel and diverticulitis due to inflammation of the lining of the bowel around the diverticula. He can be reassured there is no evidence of cancer.

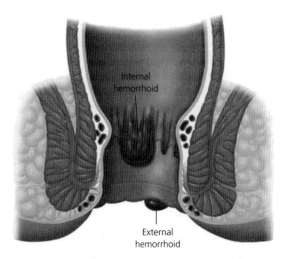

Fig. 12.1 Diagram of haemorrhoids. (From uptodate.com.)

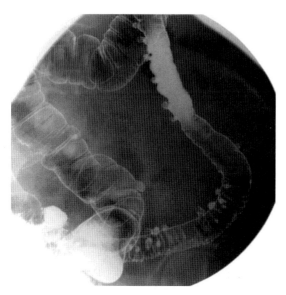

Fig. 12.2 Diverticular disease on barium enema. This barium study shows classic outpouching of the colonic wall. (From medicinet. com.)

On further questioning, Mr Chandra admits that he has suffered from constipated stool in the past and will spend a long time in the lavatory, straining at stool. This has been less of a problem in the last few months. He is reassured with the investigations and your explanation. He wants to know what options for treatment are available.

What are the management options?
Haemorrhoids

• A high fibre diet is advocated to reduce bleeding and defecation pain, particularly in the context of constipated stools.

• Laxatives such as lactulose and Movicol can be used if a high fibre diet is poorly tolerated or insufficient.

• Fluid intake should be adequate, at least 8 glasses of water/fluids per day.

• Topical preparations reduce burning and itching discomfort by local anaesthetic and anti-inflammatory effects, but may cause chronic perianal dermatitis if used in the long term. Mesalazine suppositories are well tolerated and can be effective.

• If external prolapse and thrombosis occurs, an ice pack relieves oedema, lidnocaine gel 1% is an anaesthetic agent for pain and lactulose 30 mL plus per day loosens stool.

• Conservative surgical intervention may be indicated for bleeding and persistent symptoms. These include rubber band ligation, infrared photocoagulation and injection sclerotherapy.

• Surgical therapy by external haemorrhoidectomy is only considered for large, permanently prolapsed haemorrhoids or following repetitive failed conservative treatments.

Diverticular disease

• Dietary fibre is again important in the context of constipation.

• Osmotic laxatives such as lactulose and Movicol can be used.

• Antispasmodics such as mebeverine 135 mg three times per day, peppermint oil 2 capsules three times per day and hyoscine 10–20 mg may help episodes of abdominal cramps.

Diverticulitis

This can be treated with oral fluid rehydration, analgesia and oral antibiotics, such as co-amoxiclav 625 mg three times per day and metronidazole 400 mg three times per day. Some patients, especially elderly and immunocompromised, may require hospital admission for intravenous fluids, antibiotics and analgesia. A CT scan of the abdomen and pelvis may be required to identify the presence of abscesses or fistula in complicated or refractory cases.

Diverticulosis

Surgery is indicated for complications of that do not settle with medical therapy. This includes recurrent infection, abscesses, perforation, fistulae, obstruction and major haemorrhage. It should be considered for localised disease after two episodes of diverticulitis as the recurrence is as high as 90%.

Mr Chandra increases his fibre and fluid intake accordingly and decides to try the mesalazine suppositories. His rectal bleeding settles down. He is discharged from the clinic to his general practitioner for follow-up.

Two months later he has a further flare of abdominal cramps, diarrhoea and fever. He goes to his local surgery and has some blood tests confirming elevated inflammatory markers. This is in keeping with diverticulitis. He takes a 10-day course of antibiotics and a period of bowel rest which resolves his symptoms.

CASE REVIEW

Rectal bleeding is an important symptom that requires investigation to exclude a serious cause. Investigations can be guided by the age of the patient, description of symptoms, presence of alarm symptoms and risk factors. A serious cause of rectal bleeding can be investigated by endoscopic examination of the bowel with or without radiological investigation. There may be more than one cause present.

Haemorrhoids can cause fresh rectal bleeding, prolapse and thrombosis. They are commonly associated with constipated bowel habit and straining at stool. They are usually managed conservatively with a high fibre diet and osmotic laxatives.

Colonic diverticular disease occurs frequently in middle-aged and elderly patients. It may cause episodic abdominal pain, diarrhoea and fever (diverticulitis). Recurrent diverticulosis may be more common in people presenting with a first attack at a young age, and in these patients earlier surgical intervention should be considered.

KEY POINTS

- Rectal bleeding can have many potential causes and should not be ignored.
- A serious cause must be excluded by endoscopic or radiological investigation if the patient is over the age of 40 years.
- Haemorrhoids are dilatations of the normal rectal submucosal venous plexus, which develop due to straining at stool. They can bleed, prolapse temporarily or permanently or become thrombosed.
- Symptoms include fresh rectal bleeding, a palpable lump from the anus, anal discharge and pruritis, and severe perianal pain if thrombosis occurs.
- Management involves increasing dietary fibre, laxatives and conservative surgical intervention if persistently symptomatic.
- The prevalence of colonic diverticula increases with age, present in 50% of the population aged over 50 years in developed countries.
- Over 90% of patients are asymptomatic.
- Common symptoms include colicky left iliac fossa pain relieved by defecation, bloating and flatulence, altered bowel habit and rectal bleeding.

PART 2: CASES

Mrs Irene Pale, a 66-year-old woman, comes to your clinic with her husband. She tells you her general practitioner took some blood tests after she went to see him. She was complaining of lethargy and breathlessness on exertion. She was told that she was anaemic and started on iron supplements. She has been taking these for the last 2 weeks. Her stool is now a dark green colour and she has been constipated since taking them. She feels otherwise well. She has a letter with her from the surgery detailing her blood test results: her haemoglobin was 7.8 g/dL, MCV 62 fL, ferritin 6 ng/mL and iron 3.6 µg/dL.

What do you want to know from the history?
Anaemia
• *Symptoms of anaemia:* fatigue, syncope, shortness of breath, chest pain. How long has she been symptomatic?
• *Evidence of bleeding:* gastrointestinal bleeding (fresh red blood in the stool, black tar-like melaena stool, coffee-ground vomit or haematemesis), post-menopausal bleeding in women, frank haematuria, recurrent epistaxis. How frequently and amount?

Associated symptoms
• Weight loss, suggestive of a carcinoma or malabsorption.
• Altered bowel habit. Diarrhoea may be suggestive of inflammatory bowel, celiac disease or colorectal malignancy.
• New or persistent dyspepsia, reflux or abdominal pain refractory to medications. Consider peptic ulceration or carcinoma.

Gastroenterology: Clinical Cases Uncovered, 1st edition.
© S. Keshav and E. Culver. Published 2011 by
Blackwell Publishing Ltd.

• New or progressive dysphagia or odonyophagia. Oesophageal ulceration is unlikely to cause anaemia, but consider oesophageal carcinoma.
• Bruising or bleeding easily, consider haematological disorders.
• Systemic features of an inflammatory condition such as mouth ulceration, arthralgia or rashes. Consider malabsorption and inflammatory bowel.

Reasons for anaemia
• Has she had any surgical operation to remove her stomach? Iron-deficiency anaemia is common in patients with partial or total gastrectomy, probably due to poor chelation and absorption of iron as a result of the loss of ascorbic acid and hydrochloric acid. These patients also have a two- to three-fold increased risk of gastric cancer after 20 years, and probably an increased risk of colon cancer.
• Is there a family history of colorectal cancer at a young age or inflammatory bowel disease?
• Is there a family history of a haematological disorder?
• Does she take any medications such as aspirin and NSAIDs?
• Does she eat red meat and other iron-containing foods? Is she a vegan or vegetarian?
• Has she donated blood recently?

She has been symptomatic for the last 3 months, thinking her exhaustion was due to the hyperactivity of her 2-year-old grandchild that she and her husband take care of twice a week. She denies any change in bowel habit, weight loss, systemic symptoms or post-menopausal bleeding.

She has a history of type 2 diabetes and hypertension, for which she takes metformin and ramipril. She also takes a single prophylactic aspirin per day, after reading an article in the Daily Mail newspaper about stroke prevention. She eats a varied diet including red meat. She has been a blood donor, last donating 1 year ago.

What features on the examination will you look for?
General examination
• Signs of iron deficiency, such as conjunctival pallor, cheilosis and koilonychias.
• Telangiectasia around the mouth and lips, found in hereditary haemorrhagic telangiectasia and Peutz–Jeghers syndrome.
• Mouth ulcers, which may be found in coeliac disease and inflammatory bowel disease.
• Bruises over the skin suggesting clotting or platelet abnormalities.
• Rash over the skin, especially over the buttocks, elbows or shoulders (dermatitis herpetiformis) of coeliac disease.

Abdominal examination
• Palpable abdominal mass, suggesting an inflammatory abscess or a tumour.
• Organomegaly: liver enlargement with a craggy edge if there are liver metastases, spleen enlargement in consumptive disorders.

Rectal examination
This is important to exclude rectal carcinoma. Faecal occult blood is of no benefit in the investigation of iron-deficiency anaemia as it is insensitive and non-specific.

> *On examination she is pale. There are no telangiectasia, mouth ulcers or signs of malabsorption. The abdomen is soft, non-tender with no palpable masses or organomegaly. Rectal exam reveals the presence of dark, iron-containing stool and no masses in the rectum.*

What are the most likely causes of iron-deficiency anaemia in this patient?
The differential diagnosis for iron-deficiency anaemia is broad. Although Mrs Pale denies suggestive symptoms of weight loss, altered bowel habit or reflux, these are generally unreliable. Carcinoma must be considered and excluded in all patients.

Differential diagnoses
• Drugs such as aspirin.
• Peptic ulcer.
• Coeliac disease.
• Colonic carcinoma.
• Dietary deficiency.
• Angiodysplasia.

Box 13.1 Causes of iron-deficiency anaemia

Common causes
• Drugs such as aspirin and non-steroidal anti-inflammatory drugs
• Colon carcinoma
• Gastric carcinoma
• Gastric ulceration
• Angiodysplasia
• Coeliac disease
• Partial or total gastrectomy
• *Helicobacter pylori* colonisation
• Inflammatory bowel disease

Less common causes
• Oesophagitis
• Oesophageal carcinoma
• Gastric antral vascular ectasia
• Small bowel tumours
• Mesenteric atrioventricular malformations
• Varicies from portal hypertension

Non gastrointestinal causes
• Renal cell carcinoma (haematuria)
• Haemoglobinopathies such as hereditary haemorrhagic telangiectasia
• Ovarian cancer
• Menstruation
• Blood donation

Which investigations will help you to find the cause of her anaemia?
Blood tests
• A full blood count will demonstrate a microcytic (MCV $<80\,fL$) and hypochromic (MCH $<27\,pg$) anaemia. This pattern may be due to iron deficiency, thalassaemia trait, sideroblastic anaemia or anaemia of chronic disease.
• A blood film may show target cells of severe iron deficiency, Howell–Jolly bodies of hyposplenism found in celiac disease or a mixed macrocytic/microcytic picture.
• Serum ferritin, iron and iron-binding capacity should be measured to confirm iron deficiency. Although serum ferritin is typically low ($<30\,pg/L$) in iron deficiency, it is an acute phase reactant so may be elevated with coexistent inflammatory disease, malignancy and liver disease. Low serum iron ($<10\,pmol/L$) with a high ($>70\,pmol/L$) or low ($<45\,pmol/L$) total iron-binding capacity suggests

iron deficiency and chronic disease, respectively. If these are normal, HbA2 should be measured for thalassaemia.

• Folate, vitamin B_{12} and albumin may demonstrate malabsorption.

• Renal function is important in anaemia of chronic disease and iron deficiency of renal cell carcinoma. Liver function and coagulation studies for evidence of portal hypertension and clotting abnormalities should be performed:

  • *Von Willebrand factor* (vWF) is a blood glycoprotein involved in haemostasis. It is deficient or defective in von Willebrand's disease and is involved in thrombotic thrombocytopenic purpura (TTP), Heyde's syndrome (aortic stenosis and angiodysplasia) and possibly in hemolytic uraemic syndrome.

• *Endomysial antibody* (EMA) or tissue transglutamase for coeliac disease. If coeliac serology is negative, small bowel biopsies should only be taken at endoscopy if there are other features that make coeliac disease more likely. If coeliac serology is positive, coeliac disease should be confirmed by distal duodenal biopsy.

Urinalysis

This should be done to detect microscopic haematuria, suggestive of a renal cell carcinoma. If blood is present, an intravenous urogram or CT of the renal system should be organised.

Endoscopy

Upper and lower gastrointestinal investigations should be considered in all post-menopausal female and all male patients where iron-deficiency anaemia has been confirmed. If there is significant co-morbidity or in frail and elderly patients, the appropriateness of investigations needs to be considered if it will not alter management. This should be discussed with the individual patient. Dual pathology occurs in 10–15% of patients, so patients should undergo both investigations, usually at the same session.

• *Upper GI endoscopy*: the presence of oesophagitis, erosions and peptic ulcer disease should not be accepted as the cause of anaemia until lower GI investigations have been done. Distal duodenal biopsies should be taken for coeliac disease. The CLO test for *Helicobacter pylori* can be done in the presence of active inflammation or ulceration.

• *Colonoscopy*: this allows visualisation of the lumen, assessment of the ability to biopsy, polyp removal, and can detect and treat angiodysplasia. It is associated with complications of sedation, bowel preparation, bleeding and perforation.

Imaging

Imaging may be more appropriate in patients who can not tolerate endoscopy to look for a mucosal lesion. If the patient can not tolerate an endoscopic procedure, it is unlikely they will be suitable for surgery, if needed.

• *Barium enema (double contrast)* with a sigmoidoscopy is an alternative to a full colonoscopy.

• *CT colon*: this does not necessitate bowel preparation and is more appropriate in elderly or frail patients.

• *Barium swallow or meal*: this allows an outline of the oesophageal and gastric compartments to identify large lesions or abnormalities.

Mrs Pale's blood tests confirm an iron-deficiency anaemia. Vitamin B_{12} and folate levels were normal. Coeliac serology was negative. Urinalysis did not demonstrate microscopic haematuria. Gastroscopy showed evidence of erosive gastritis with no ulceration. The CLO test was positive for Helicobacter pylori. Colonoscopy was unremarkable. Biopsies were normal.

What is the cause of her iron deficiency?

The gastroscopy demonstrated erosive gastritis whilst on aspirin therapy. She tested positive for *H. pylori* infection. Colonisation may impair iron uptake and increase iron loss thus leading to iron deficiency. There was no evidence of a colonic cause for anaemia.

What do you advise her to do?

The aim of treatment should be to restore her haemoglobin levels and red cell indices to normal, and to replenish iron stores. Treatment of an underlying cause should prevent further iron loss.

Treat the underlying cause

She should stop the aspirin therapy as she is taking this for 'prevention' of disease and it is causing more harm than benefit. If she had needed to take this medication, a protein pump inhibitor such as omeprazole should be co-prescribed.

  She should have a course of *H. pylori* eradication therapy (see Case 4), such as amoxicillin 1 g twice daily plus clarithromycin 500 mg twice daily plus omeprazole 20 mg twice daily. The omeprazole should be continued for a further 4 weeks at a dose of 20 mg daily to encourage healing of the gastric mucosa.

Correct anaemia and replenish iron

Iron supplementation with ferrous sulphate 200 mg twice daily should allow the haemoglobin to rise by 2 g/dL after 3–4 weeks. Other iron compounds such as ferrous fumarate and ferrous gluconate, or iron suspensions, may be tolerated better. Ascorbic acid (250–500 mg twice daily with the iron preparation) may enhance absorption.

Parenteral iron may be used when there is intolerance or non-compliance with oral preparations. Cosmofer or Ferrinject are preferred as they can be given as a single intravenous dose. Oral iron should be continued until 3 months after the iron deficiency has been corrected so that stores are replenished.

Blood transfusions should be reserved for patients with, or at risk of, cardiovascular instability due to their degree of anaemia. Transfusions should aim to restore haemoglobin to a safe level, but not necessarily normal values. Iron treatment should follow transfusion to replenish stores.

What follow-up should you organise?

The haemoglobin concentration and red cell indices should be monitored at 3-monthly intervals for 1 year then again after a further year. Additional oral iron should be given if the haemoglobin or ferritin levels fall below normal. Further investigation is only necessary if the haemoglobin can not be maintained.

She remains asymptomatic and has 3-monthly blood tests as recommended. After 9 months, her haemoglobin dropped to 11.1 g/dL and after a year her haemoglobin is 10.4 g/dL. Her iron indices are re-checked. Her ferritin is low at 15 ng/mL, iron levels are 5 ug/dL, and transferrin is within the normal range.

She is referred for further advice on management.

What do you do now?

It is important to retake the history for any new or missed symptoms. Repeat a full examination for new signs. Re-visit the previous investigations and ensure you have the results of all blood tests, endoscopy and biopsies done.

Asymptomatic symptoms

Further direct visualisation of the small bowel is probably not necessary unless her iron-deficiency anaemia becomes transfusion dependent.

Symptomatic symptoms

If she needed repeat transfusions or has overt gastrointestinal blood loss, repeat endoscopy and colonoscopy should be done by an experienced gastroenterologist.

• Capsule endoscopy is recommended to look for small bowel lesions and angiodysplasia. Young patients with recurrent iron deficiency are more likely to have a small bowel lesion (for example a gastrointestinal stromal tumour or carcinoid) and this should be searched for by capsule study or enteroscopy.

• Abdominal ultrasound should be done to look for portal hypertension.

• Mesenteric angiography may demonstrate vascular malformations or intestinal varices in transfusion-dependant anaemia.

• Diagnostic laparotomy with on-table endoscopy may be considered in recurrent bleeding.

She remained asymptomatic, was given further iron supplementation and had no further investigations. She remains well.

CASE REVIEW

Iron-deficiency anaemia should be confirmed by measurement of iron indices. A thorough history and examination should be done to identify possible causes of iron deficiency. Investigations should be directed by the clinical findings. Malignancy must always be excluded.

A coeliac screen is important in all patients with iron deficiency and can be done simply by serological testing. Upper endoscopy and colonoscopy should be done as the gold standard in all patients who are fit enough for the procedure to detect asymptomatic gastric and colonic carcinomas. Even if a benign cause is found at upper endoscopy, colonic investigation should be completed to exclude an asymptomatic malignancy. No cause is found in up to 15% of cases.

Treatment of the underlying cause is the most effective method of preventing further anaemia. Iron stores should be replenished.

Recurrent anaemia after sufficient iron replacement should be re-investigated, including re-taking a full history and doing a full examination. In young patients or in those that require transfusions, small bowel imaging is indicated. This may depend on the patient's preferences and co-morbidities.

KEY POINTS

- Iron-deficiency anaemia has a prevalence of 2–5% among adult men and post-menopausal women in the developed world and is a common cause of referral to gastroenterologists.
- Iron deficiency should be confirmed by a low serum ferritin, red cell microcytosis or hypochromia in the absence of chronic disease or haemoglobinopathies.
- Dual pathology occurs in 1–10% of patients, so upper and lower gastrointestinal investigations should be done.
- Menstrual blood loss is the commonest cause of iron-deficiency anaemia in pre-menopausal women.

- Blood loss from the gastrointestinal tract is the commonest cause in adult men and post-menopausal women.
- Asymptomatic colonic and gastric carcinoma and may present with iron-deficiency anaemia and must be excluded as a priority. Malabsorption causing iron-deficiency anaemia is most frequently from coeliac disease in the UK. However, iron-deficiency anaemia is often multifactorial.
- All patients should have iron supplementation both to correct anaemia and replenish body stores. Parenteral iron is appropriate if oral preparations are not tolerated.

Case 14 A 64-year-old man with abnormal liver function tests

Mr Jack Reynolds is a 64-year-old man who has recently been discharged from hospital after treatment for pneumonia. The discharge letter requested follow-up of 'abnormal liver function tests' that were discovered during the inpatient admission. He has come to see you to have this looked into further.

What questions should you ask him?
Presenting complaint

You want to know whether the 'abnormal liver function tests' may have preceded or occurred during the admission to hospital. This may be related to sepsis, drugs or an underlying liver or biliary pathology.

Ask him questions about his admission to hospital. Specifically, what were his symptoms prior to admission, the duration and severity of illness, antibiotics given and new medications (especially hepatotoxic ones) started by his GP or in the hospital.

Accompanying symptoms

Ask him about symptoms that may give you a clue about possible aetiology:

• Has he experienced jaundice, abdominal pain, fever, pruritus or a change in urine and stool colour? A history of jaundice associated with the sudden onset of severe right upper quadrant pain and shaking chills suggests choledocholithiasis and ascending cholangitis.

• Has he experienced jaundice before that resolved spontaneously? Consider Gilbert's syndrome as a cause

of hyperbilirubinaemia in the context of a concurrent illness.

• Does he have arthralgia, myalgia or a rash? A history of arthralgia and myalgia predating jaundice suggests viral or drug-related hepatitis.

• Has he lost his appetite and experienced weight loss? Malignancy must be considered, either as a primary or secondary involvement.

• Is there evidence of abdominal swelling of ascites or fluid retention? Does he get breathless on exertion or lying flat? This may occur in decompensated cirrhosis or congestive heart failure (transudate) or be in keeping with malignancy, or infective or inflammatory conditions (exudates).

Medical history

• Does he have a previous history of gallstone disease, liver disease or cardiac failure?

• Does he have a history of malignancy?

Medications

Has he been exposed to any chemicals, prescribed medication or over-the-counter medication that may be temporally related to the onset of liver function abnormalities? In addition, herbal preparations and illicit drug use must be considered.

Common causes of abnormal liver function tests (LFTs) include non-steroidal anti-inflammatory drugs, paracetamol, antibiotics, statins, antiepileptic drugs and antituberculous drugs. In particular consider antibiotics in this man with recent pneumonia.

Social history

• Risk factors for hepatitis B and C. Has he ever had a blood transfusion (when and where), a tattoo, used intravenous drugs or had high-risk sexual activity?

Gastroenterology: Clinical Cases Uncovered, 1st edition.
© S. Keshav and E. Culver. Published 2011 by
Blackwell Publishing Ltd.

• Risk factors for hepatitis A. Has he travelled to, or lived abroad in, an area with endemic hepatitis?
• Risk factors for hepatotoxins. Has he had occupational exposure? Has he been exposed to contaminated foods?
• Alcohol-related liver disease. What is his alcohol consumption on a weekly basis? Is the alcohol history reliable?

Family history
• Is there a family history of jaundice or liver disease?

Previous medical records
• What is the duration and pattern of liver function abnormalities?
• Has his liver function been investigated before in the past and if so, what tests have been done?

He explains that he was in hospital for just 5 days requiring intravenous antibiotics to treat his pneumonia and was put on oral tablets thereafter. He has been out of hospital for 2 weeks and feels much better with a residual cough only. He can not remember the name of the antibiotics but has a discharge letter with him. The letter tells you he was taking co-amoxiclav and clarithromycin for a total of 7 days, and used ibuprofen and paracetamol regularly for pleuritic pain.

He has a past history of type 2 diabetes, hypertension and hypothyroidism. He takes metformin, bendroflumethiazide and levothyroxine. He takes no over-the-counter medications or herbal treatments. He is a non-smoker and drinks a 'moderate' amount of alcohol, five bottles of beer a night. He has recently travelled to South India with his wife, staying in Kerala for a 2-week vacation. He has never had any known contact with hepatitis or been exposed to parenteral transfusions, drugs or tattoos. There is no family history of liver disease. His mother had thyroid disease and diabetes.

His liver function was checked over a year ago at his previous GP practice and he was not told of any abnormality in his liver tests then.

What do you look for on examination?
General examination
• Are there any stigmata of chronic liver disease?
• Are there signs suggestive of malignancy?
• Are there signs of longstanding disease, such as proximal muscle wasting?

Box 14.1 Stigmata of chronic liver disease

• Spider naevi, located above the nipple line (see Plate 14.1)
• Palmar erythema
• Digital clubbing
• Dupuytren's contractures
• Icteric sclera and skin
• Parotid gland enlargement
• Gynaecomastia
• Loss of axillary hair
• Caput medusae
• Abdominal ascites (portal hypertension)
• Splenomegaly (portal hypertension)
• Testicular atrophy

Box 14.2 Signs suggestive of malignancy

• Weight loss (loose skin folds or clothes)
• Craggy lymphadenopathy
• Virchow's node (left supraclavicular node) or periumbilical nodule suggestive of abdominal malignancy

---

Cardiac and respiratory examination
• Jugular venous pulse: is there jugular venous distension? This is a sign of right-sided heart failure, suggesting hepatic congestion.
• Pleural effusion (unilateral or bilateral): bilateral pleural effusions support cardiac failure. A right pleural effusion, in the absence of clinically apparent ascites, may be seen in advanced liver cirrhosis, malignancy or represent a para-pneumonic effusion.

Abdominal examination
• Feel for the size and consistency of the liver. A grossly enlarged nodular liver or an obvious abdominal mass suggests malignancy. An enlarged tender liver could be viral or alcoholic hepatitis. An enlarged liver may be an acutely congested secondary to right-sided heart failure. The liver may be pulsatile in severe tricuspid regurgitation.
• Feel for the size of the spleen (a palpable spleen is enlarged).
• Percuss for ascites. Is there a fluid wave or shifting dullness? Ascites in the presence of jaundice

suggests either cirrhosis or malignancy with peritoneal spread.

• Abdominal mass or tenderness. Severe right upper quadrant tenderness with respiratory arrest on inspiration (Murphy's sign) suggests cholecystitis or, occasionally, ascending cholangitis. A gallbladder or mass may be palpable.

> *On general examination he is overweight (BMI 29) with no stigmata of chronic liver disease. He has tanned skin but no scleral jaundice. On auscultation of his chest there are some inspiratory coarse crepitations at the right base with no clinical signs of effusion. Abdominal examination confirms a large distended abdomen which is soft and non-tender, with no palpable organomegaly or ascites.*

What is your differential diagnosis based on the information so far?

• Drug-induced (antibiotics, non-steroidal drugs, paracetamol) liver disease. The temporal relationship between medication and hepatotoxicity can be difficult to define but gradually resolves with removal of the offending agent.

• Sepsis-related pneumonia. Tests should normalise once the infection has resolved.

• Hepatic steatosis or steatohepatitis, based on co morbidities, BMI and physical examination.

• Alcohol-related liver disease. He consumes over 35 units/week of alcohol, which can lead to progressive liver damage.

• Haemochromatosis; He has bronzed skin (perhaps related to iron overload or his recent holiday in India).

• Viral hepatitis, based on his travel history.

• Autoimmune liver disease, based on his history of other autoimmune conditions such as diabetes and

thyroid disease and family history (although very rare in men).

How do you investigate this man further?

Liver chemistry (colloquially known as liver function tests or LFTs)

What was the initial abnormality in liver function and is it persistent? The liver chemistry should be repeated to determine a pattern.

The most commonly tested aspects of liver chemistry are:

• *Enzyme tests*:
  • Transaminases: serum aminotransferases (alanine aminotransferase (ALT) and aspartate aminotransferase (AST)).
  • Bile duct-expressed enzymes: alkaline phosphatase (ALP) and γ-glutamyl transferase (γ-GT).

• *Serum bilirubin*, which measures the liver's ability to detoxify metabolites and transport organic anions into bile.

• *Serum albumin*, which is a test of hepatic synthetic function

Additional critical information on hepatic function is obtained from the prothrombin time (PT), which depends on the synthesis of clotting factors in the liver, and is prolonged in liver disease, and in cases of vitamin K deficiency, which can be a consequence of biliary obstruction and consequent malabsorption of fat and fat-soluble vitamins.

Diseases causing hepatocellular injury typically cause a disproportionate elevation in serum ALT and AST compared with the ALP and γ-GT. An example is hepatitis.

Diseases causing biliary damage or cholestasis typically cause a disproportionate elevation in serum ALP and γ-GT compared with the AST and ALT. These patterns often overlap.

The serum bilirubin can be elevated in both hepatocellular and cholestatic conditions and therefore is not necessarily helpful in differentiating between the two.

The serum albumin and PT are useful to assess liver function. Low albumin suggests a chronic process such as cirrhosis or cancer. Normal albumin suggests a more acute process such as viral hepatitis or choledocholithiasis. Elevated PT indicates either vitamin K deficiency due to malabsorption or significant hepatocellular dysfunction. The failure of the PT to correct with parenteral administration of vitamin K indicates severe hepatocellular injury.

> **KEY POINT**
>
> • A complete history supported by an examination to look for signs of liver disease is the best method of determining the cause of abnormal liver function tests. The pattern of liver abnormalities and their fluctuation over time is important.

Urinalysis for bilirubin

The presence of bilirubin in the urine reflects direct hyperbilirubinaemia and therefore underlying hepatobiliary disease.

• Unconjugated bilirubin is tightly bound to albumin. It is not filtered by the glomerulus and is present in the urine unless there is underlying renal disease.

• Conjugated bilirubin may be found in the urine when the total serum bilirubin concentration is normal.

Abdominal ultrasound

An abdominal ultrasound (with Doppler flow if thrombosis of the hepatic or portal veins is in the differential) can identify abnormalities of the liver or spleen, the presence of ascites and lesions in the liver. Ultrasonography has a lower sensitivity than CT or MRI scanning for liver disease, but is less expensive and easily accessible.

Mr Reynolds' discharge letter referred to an elevated ALT of 120 IU/L as the predominant abnormality in liver function. He had not had inpatient investigation and repeat of the liver function tests was recommended 2 weeks post discharge.

His HbA$_{1C}$ was 9.6% suggesting poor diabetic control, his BP was 150/80 mmHg and his cholesterol was 6.7 mmol/L (predominantly elevated low density lipoprotein (LDL) cholesterol).

KEY POINT

• Key markers of liver function include bilirubin, ALT, ALP, γ-GT, albumin and prothrombin time. Repeating these tests can establish a pattern of abnormalities to direct further investigation.

What is the significance of his abnormal ALT?

An abnormal ALT is increasingly found in asymptomatic patients as part of screening tests. The serum ALT correlates with BMI and waist circumference, and so correlates with an increase in the obesity epidemic.

False-positive elevations in ALT can occur in those with a low pre-test probability of having liver disease. Normal test reference values are arbitrarily defined as those occurring within two standard deviations from the mean. As a result, 5% of healthy individuals who have a single screening test will have an abnormal result (2.5% will have an abnormally high result).

Individual patients can have baseline fluctuation in aminotransferases. Chronic (more than 6 months) persistent ALT elevations require further investigation.

How do you investigate an abnormal ALT?
Risk factors
Medications

The relationship between drug ingestion and toxicity is not always clear; patients may take multiple medications making the offending agent difficult to recognise, have concomitant diseases (such as alcoholism) that produce similar clinical/laboratory abnormalities, and may have a delay in the onset of hepatotoxicity. Features suggesting drug toxicity include lack of illness prior to ingesting the drug, clinical illness or biochemical abnormalities developing after beginning the drug, and improvement after the drug is withdrawn. The abnormalities will generally recur upon reintroduction of the offending substance, but re-challenge is generally not advised.

Alcohol abuse

The diagnosis of alcohol abuse can be difficult because many patients conceal this information. Several short questionnaires are of assistance (such as the CAGE questionnaire). Patterns of abnormalities supportive of alcohol abuse include an AST to ALT ratio of 2:1 or greater, and a two-fold elevation of the γ-GT in patients with an AST to ALT ratio greater than 2:1. It is unusual for the ALT to be greater than five-fold elevated. The ALT may even be normal in patients with severe alcoholic liver disease.

Hepatic causes of elevated ALT/AST
Viral hepatitis

This includes hepatitis A, B, C and E and cytomegalovirus (CMV) or Epstein–Barr virus (EBV) hepatitis.

• *Hepatitis B.* The risk is increased in patients with a history of parenteral exposure and travel to or residence in areas of high disease prevalence, such as South-East Asia, China and sub-Saharan Africa. Initial testing for patients suspected of having chronic hepatitis B is hepatitis B surface antigen (HBsAg), surface antibody (HBsAb) and core antibody (HBcAb).

Patients who are HBsAg and HBcAb positive are chronically infected. Additional testing in this group includes hepatitis B 'e' antigen (HBeAg) and 'e' antibody (HBeAb) and a hepatitis B virus (HBV) DNA. The presence of a positive HBV DNA in the presence or absence of HBeAg indicates viral replication. A positive HBV DNA and a negative HBeAg indicates a pre-core mutant. Both of these situations warrant further evaluation with a liver biopsy and possible treatment.

A positive HBsAg with a negative HBV DNA and a negative HBeAg suggests that the patient is a carrier of hepatitis B in a non-replicative state. The presence of a carrier state does not explain elevated aminotransferases and another cause needs to be found. A positive HBsAb and HBcAb suggests immunity to hepatitis B and another cause of aminotransferase elevation should be sought.

• *Hepatitis C.* The risk is increased in individuals with a history of parenteral exposure (blood transfusion, intravenous drug use, occupational), cocaine use, tattoos, body piercing and high risk sexual behaviour. The initial test for hepatitis C is the hepatitis C antibody (HCVAb).

A positive HCVAb in a patient with risk factors for the infection is sufficient to make the diagnosis, and a quantitative hepatitis C virus (HCV) RNA, HCV genotype and liver biopsy should be done to assess the patient's need and suitability for treatment. A positive HCVAb in a low risk patient should be verified with either a HCV recombinant immunoblast assay (RIBA) test or a qualitative polymerase chain reaction (PCR) test. A negative HCVAb in a patient with risk factors for hepatitis C should be verified with a qualitative PCR test.

Hereditary haemochromatosis (HHC)

Screening is by serum iron and total iron-binding capacity (TIBC), allowing the calculation of the transferrin saturation (serum iron/TIBC). An iron saturation of greater than 45% warrants serum ferritin evaluation. Ferritin is an acute phase reactant and therefore is less specific than the iron saturation. A serum ferritin concentration of >400 ng/mL in men and >300 ng/mL in women further supports the diagnosis of HHC.

Genetic testing (HFE genotype) has not replaced liver biopsy in the diagnosis of HHC. C282Y/C282Y and C282Y/H63D are responsible for 95% of genetic haemochromatosis. Not every patient who is homozygous for the HFE mutation has iron overload and not every patient with HHC has the identified HFE mutation. Thus, the biopsy may still be required to identify iron overload in some patients and is critical to determine the amount of fibrosis.

A liver biopsy should be performed if screening tests suggest iron overload to quantify hepatic iron and to assess the severity of liver injury. A hepatic iron index greater than 1.9 is consistent with homozygous HHC. Liver biopsy is not necessary for patients aged less than 40 years with genotypically defined haemochromatosis (C282Y homozygous) with normal liver function tests.

Patients with HHC and cirrhosis continue to have a high risk of developing hepatocellular carcinoma (HCC) even with depletion of body iron stores. These patients need to be identified and screened with AFP measurements and ultrasound evaluation for liver lesions as appropriate (usually 6 monthly if there is cirrhosis).

Box 14.3 Clinical features of hereditary haemochromatosis

• Skin pigmentation: bronzing
• Diabetes mellitus
• Arthropathy
• Fatigue
• Liver disease: jaundice and abdominal discomfort may occur
• Breathlessness due to cardiomegaly/cardiomyopathy
• Impotence

Hepatic steatosis (non-alcoholic fatty liver disease or NAFLD)

This can present with mild elevations of the serum aminotransferases, which are usually less than four-fold elevated.

The spectrum of NAFLD consists of four types:
• Type 1: fat alone.
• Type 2: fat + inflammation.
• Type 3: fat + ballooning degeneration.
• Type 4: fat + fibrosis and/or Mallory bodies.

Only types 3 and 4 have been definitively shown to progress to advanced liver disease and may be classified as non-alcoholic steatohepatitis (NASH).

Box 14.4 Primary causes of non-alcoholic fatty liver disease

• Increased insulin resistance syndrome
• Diabetes mellitus (type 2)
• Obesity
• Hyperlipidaemia
• Hypertension

Box 14.5 Secondary causes of non-alcoholic fatty liver disease

Drugs
- Corticosteroids
- Amiodarone
- Salicylates
- Nifedipine
- Tamoxifen
- Tetracycline
- Chloroquine
- Synth oestrogens
- Perhexiline

Surgical procedures
- Extensive small bowel resection
- Gastroplexy
- Jejunoileal bypass
- Biliopancreatic diversion

Miscellaneous causes
- Hepatitis C abetalipoproteinaemia
- Total parental nutrition with glucose
- Environmental toxins
- Small bowel diverticulosis
- Wilson's disease
- Malnutrition
- Inflammatory bowel disease
- HIV infection
- Weber–Christian disease

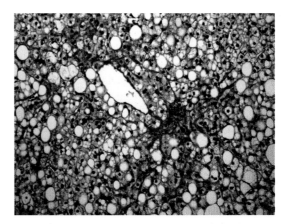

Fig. 14.1 Microvesicular steatosis seen in a liver biopsy in a patient with NAFLD.

mata of chronic liver disease, splenomegaly, cytopenia, abnormal iron studies, diabetes and/or significant obesity in an individual over the age of 45 years. There is no effective medical therapy for NASH.

Autoimmune hepatitis (AIH)

This is found predominantly in young to middle-aged women. The diagnosis is based upon the presence of elevated serum aminotransferases, the absence of other causes of chronic hepatitis and features (serological and pathological) suggestive of AIH. A useful screening test is the serum protein electrophoresis (over 80% of patients with AIH will have hypergammaglobulinaemia). Additional tests include antinuclear antibodies (ANAs), anti-smooth muscle antibodies (anti-SMAs) and liver–kidney microsomal antibodies (LKMAs).

Elevated γ-globulins and high titre of autoantibodies should prompt a liver biopsy to confirm the diagnosis of AIH. If the biopsy is consistent with chronic active hepatitis, patients should receive a trial of corticosteroids.

Wilson's disease

This is a genetic disorder of biliary copper excretion (Table 14.1), and may cause elevated aminotransferases

Non-alcoholic steatohepatitis

NASH is more common in women and is associated with obesity and type 2 diabetes mellitus. The ratio of AST to ALT is usually less than one. The presence of fatty infiltration of the liver can be seen radiologically by ultrasound, CT imaging or MRI. However, radiological imaging cannot identify inflammation.

The differentiation between steatosis and NASH requires a liver biopsy (Fig. 14.1). This should be done in the presence of the following features: peripheral stig-

Table 14.1 Prevalence of inherited liver diseases. (From Leggett *et al.*, 1990.)

Disease	Homozygote frequency	Gene frequency	Heterozygote frequency
Haemochromatosis	1:400	1:20	1:10
α_1-antitrypsin deficiency	1:1600	1:40	1:20
Cystic fibrosis	1:2500	1:50	1:25
Wilson's disease	1:30000	1:170	1:85

in asymptomatic patients. Patients usually present between the ages of 5 and 25 years, but case reports document patients from 3 to 80 years old.

The initial screening test is serum ceruloplasmin (reduced in approximately 85%). Patients should be examined by an ophthalmologist for Kayser–Fleischer rings. If the ceruloplasmin is normal and Kayser–Fleischer rings are absent, a 24 h urine collection for quantitative copper excretion can be done; a value of greater than 100 μg/day is suggestive of the diagnosis.

The diagnosis is usually confirmed by a liver biopsy for quantitative copper. Patients with Wilson's disease have liver copper levels of greater than 250 μg/g of dry weight.

Alpha-1 antitrypsin deficiency

In adults, α_1-antitrypsin deficiency should be suspected in patients who have a history of emphysema either at a young age or out of proportion to their smoking history. Decreased levels of α_1-antitrypsin can be detected either by direct measurement of serum concentrations or by the absence of the α_1 peak on serum protein electrophoresis.

Non-hepatic causes of elevated ALT/AST
Muscle disorders

Serum AST and ALT may both be elevated with muscle injury. Their ratio depends upon when they are assessed relative to the muscle injury. Consider subclinical inborn errors of muscle metabolism, polymyositis, seizures and heavy exercise such as long distance running. Determine the serum levels of creatinine kinase, lactate dehydrogenase (LDH) and aldolase (elevated at least to the same degree).

Thyroid disorders

Thyroid disorders can produce an elevated ALT/AST, although the mechanism is unclear. A TSH is a reasonable screening test for hypothyroidism while a full set of thyroid function tests should be checked if hyperthyroidism is suspected.

Coeliac disease

Elevated serum aminotransferases can occur in patients with undiagnosed coeliac disease. Liver tests return to normal when the patient is compliant with a gluten-free diet. Coeliac disease can be tested for by antibody screening (EMA, IgA antibody) and, definitively, by distal duodenal biopsies.

Adrenal insufficiency

Elevated ALT/AST levels (1.5–3 times the upper limits of normal) have been described in patients with adrenal insufficiency due to Addison's disease or secondary causes. Liver tests normalise with appropriate treatment.

Anorexia nervosa

This has been associated with aminotransferase elevation by mechanisms that are not well understood.

Mr Reynolds went on to have a full liver screen and abdominal ultrasound. The liver screen was negative for hepatitis and autoimmune disease. His immunoglobulins, ferritin and AFP were normal. An abdominal ultrasound showed evidence of fatty infiltration of the liver with a normal spleen and no free fluid.

Additional tests revealed a normal TSH, EMA and creatinine kinase level. He had an appropriate cortisol response to a synacthen test.

What is the most likely diagnosis and how would you manage this?

The most likely diagnosis is hepatic steatosis or NASH, based on the isolated abnormal ALT, normal liver screen, fatty liver on ultrasound and his co-morbidities.

He should be advised to reduce weight by reducing the consumption of fatty foods and overall calorie intake (this may be guided by a dietician) and increase his daily exercise (Fig. 14.2). He should reduce his alcohol consumption to within the recommended limits, and ideally

Define risk factors:	Goals:	Re-evaluate:
Evaluate BMI	Controlled weight loss	Repeat liver tests
Fasting glucose ⟶	Treat diabetes ⟶	Monitor weight and lipids
Fasting lipid profile	Treat hyperlipidaemia	US liver
Medications	Stop toxic meds and alcohol	Consider liver biopsy

Fig. 14.2 The management of NAFLD.

stop drinking all together given the contribution of alcohol to his liver disease.

He needs better control of his diabetes; consider gliclazide or a thioglitazone. He should control his blood pressure, with the addition of antihypertensive medication such as an angiotensin-converting enzyme (ACE) inhibitor. This medication is particularly important in the context of his diabetes, as an ACE inhibitor may help to control progression of disease and preserve his renal function. He should have a lipid profile taken, be given dietary advice for cholesterol reduction and may ultimately need a statin to lower the ALT level.

> *He stopped drinking alcohol, reduced the fat in his diet and started to walk every morning to collect the newspaper (15 min per day). He lost 4.5 kg over 3 months. His ALT fluctuated, but remained elevated between 80 and 110 IU/L over the next 6 months.*

What next? Do you continue to observe or proceed to liver biopsy?
When should you watch and wait?
Observation is probably appropriate in those in whom the ALT and AST are less than two-fold elevated and no chronic liver condition has been identified by non-invasive testing.

When should you consider liver biopsy?
A liver biopsy should be considered in those in whom the ALT and AST are persistently greater than two-fold elevated and the cause remains undefined. Although it is unlikely that the biopsy will provide a diagnosis or lead to changes in management, it reassures the patient and physician to know that there is no serious underlying disorder. At biopsy, the most frequent finding is non-alcoholic steatohepatitis or fatty liver (in two-thirds of cases). A biopsy should not be undertaken without due consideration of the risk : benefit ratio. The risk of significant bleeding, morbidity and mortality from percutaneous liver biopsy is 1 : 1000.

Patients who are at risk of progression to cirrhosis should be considered for biopsy.

Independent risk factors for fibrosis and/or cirrhosis (Day, 2002)
- Age >45 years.
- ALT more than two times normal.
- AST : ALT ratio >1.
- Obesity, particularly truncal.
- Type 2 diabetes or impaired glucose intolerance.
- Insulin resistance.
- Hyperlipidaemia (trigycerides >1.7).
- Hypertension.
- Iron overload.
- Hypertriglyceridaemia.

Box 14.6 Liver biopsy findings in abnormal liver function tests (Skelly et al., 2001)

- Normal: 6%
- Fibrosis: 26%
- Cirrhosis: 6%
- NASH: 34% (11% bridging fibrosis and 8% cirrhosis)
- Fatty liver: 32%
- Cryptogenic hepatitis: 9%
- Drug induced: 7.6%
- Alcoholic liver disease: 2.8%
- Autoimmune hepatitis: 1.9%
- Primary biliary cirrhosis: 1.4%
- Primary sclerosing cholangitis: 1.1%
- Granulomatous disease: 1.75%
- Haemochromatosis: 1%
- Amyloid: 0.3%
- Glycogen storage disease: 0.31%

> *He was referred for an ultrasound guided liver biopsy. There were no complications. He returned to clinic 2 weeks later. The liver biopsy confirmed fatty liver with no evidence of fibrosis or cirrhosis. Diet and exercise were reinforced. He was discharged back to your care.*

PART 2: CASES

CASE REVIEW

Abnormal liver function tests are may be identified incidentally on blood testing for other reasons. There are many liver-related and unrelated causes. The key is in the history to identify predisposing factors, and examination to support this.

Causes of abnormal liver function include medications, liver disease, cardiac failure, alcohol consumption, infection, malabsorption and many others. Investigations should be done to find the cause using the least invasive tests possible.

Non-alcoholic fatty liver disease is becoming increasingly prevalent in the Western world. Risk factors should be identified and treated. Goals include controlled weight loss, control of diabetes and hyperlipidaemia, and stopping alcohol and toxic medications. Liver biopsy may be needed in some patients to identify a progression to steatohepatitis, fibrosis and cirrhosis.

KEY POINTS

- Liver tests include enzyme tests (ALT, AST, ALP, γ-GT), serum bilirubin and measures of synthetic function (albumin and PT).
- A complete medical history is the most important part of the evaluation.
- The physical examination should focus upon findings suggesting the presence of liver disease.
- It is essential to determine the overall pattern of abnormal LFTs, which can be broadly divided into two categories: (1) patterns predominantly reflecting hepatocellular injury, and (2) patterns predominantly reflecting cholestasis.
- Many abnormal liver tests will return to normal spontaneously.
- Specific tests should be guided by the pre-test probability of the underlying liver disease, the pattern of abnormalities, and suggestive features obtained from the history and physical examination.
- The majority of patients in whom the diagnosis remains unclear after obtaining a history and laboratory testing will usually have alcoholic liver disease, steatosis or steatohepatitis.

A 45-year-old man with acute jaundice

PART 2: CASES

A 45-year-old radio producer, Jerrie Stroud, comes to your clinic with a 3-week history of yellow sclera and skin. This was noticed by his wife who encouraged him to seek help. She accompanies him today, but remains in the waiting room at his request.

What is this yellow discolouration and what are the possible causes?

Jaundice is a yellow discolouration of the tissues due to the accumulation of bilirubin. The circulating bilirubin should be in excess of 50 μmol/L for jaundice to be clinically apparent.

Jaundice can be classified into three main types. Prehepatic jaundice is predominately due to haemolysis. Hepatic jaundice is due to acute and chronic intrinsic liver disease. Cholestatic jaundice is due to intraheptaic cholestasis or post-hepatic biliary tract obstruction.

What features from the clinical history are important to define the cause of his jaundice?

The timing of jaundice and sequence of events is often helpful to distinguish between hepatic and cholestatic jaundice.

- Abdominal pain. Is this pain in the right upper quadrant, as a result of swelling and stretching of the fibrous liver capsule or preceding the impaction of a common bile duct gallstone? Is he pain-free? Insidious, painless jaundice may indicate a malignant process or bile duct stones in the elderly.
- Change in bowel habit. Is he passing fresh red blood mixed in with the stool (inflammatory bowel disease,

colorectal carcinoma), black tar-like melaena stool (upper GI bleed) or oily pale stool (chronic pancreatitis and malabsorption)? Is he constipated, which may predispose to encephalopathy?
- Confusion, slowness, personality change or disordered sleep pattern. These suggest encephalopathy.
- Easy bruising or bleeding. Could be due to thrombocytopenia and coagulopathy.
- Abdominal distension. This might represent ascites or a mass in the abdomen.
- Lower limb swelling. Bilateral pedal oedema is suggestive of a low albumin, cardiac failure or dependent oedema.
- Prodromal flu-like illness with fever, malaise, arthralgia and myalgia. This is typical of a viral hepatitis.
- Fever or rigors. Consider cholangitis or a liver abscess.
- Lost appetite and weight. This may indicate malignancy, malnutrition or chronic pancreatitis.
- Dark urine, pale stools and itching of cholestatic jaundice. This may be associated with nausea and vomiting.
- Pale, tired, lethargic and short of breath. This suggests anaemia.
- Haematuria. This may indicate haemolysis.

Past medical history

- Has he had previous episodes of jaundice as a child or in adulthood?
- Has he had previous biliary surgery? This may indicate an obstructive jaundice.
- Has he had a recent infection?

Medications

Drugs can cause prehepatic, hepatic and cholestatic jaundice. Enquire about prescribed drugs, over-the-counter drugs and herbal remedies, including teas and Chinese medicines. Ask about tablets and injections. Ask about overdose and the recent use of anaesthetic agents.

Common causes of drug-induced jaundice include paracetamol overdose, methotrexate, isoniazid, sodium

---

Gastroenterology: Clinical Cases Uncovered, 1st edition.
© S. Keshav and E. Culver. Published 2011 by
Blackwell Publishing Ltd.

Box 15.1 Causes of jaundice

Prehepatic (unconjugated bilirubin) jaundice

1 Congenital defects:
  • Gilbert's syndrome (common)
  • Criger–Najjar syndrome (rare)
2 Haemolysis:
  • Hereditary spherocytosis
  • Sickle cell disease
  • G6PD deficiency
  • Thalassaemia
  • Malaria
  • Autoimmune haemolysis
  • Hypersplenism
  • Incompatible blood transfusion

Hepatocellular jaundice

1 Acute hepatocellular disease:
  • Viral hepatitis (such as hepatitis A, B, C and E, EBV, CMV)
  • Infections (such as leptospirosis)
  • Liver abscess
  • Alcoholic hepatitis
  • Autoimmune hepatitis
  • Drug-induced (such as paracetamol)
  • Toxins (such as carbon tetrachloride)
  • Budd–Chiari syndrome
2 Chronic hepatocellular disease:
  • Chronic viral hepatitis
  • Chronic autoimmune hepatitis

  • Cirrhosis (e.g. due to alcohol)
  • Hepatic metastases
  • Hepatoma
  • Lymphoma
  • Wilson's disease
  • Haemochromatosis
  • Cardiac failure

Cholestatic (conjugated bilirubin) jaundice

1 Intrahepatic:
  • Drugs (such as chlorpromazine)
  • Primary biliary cirrhosis
  • Viral hepatitis
  • Pregnancy
2 Extrahepatic (obstructive):
  • Gallstones in the common bile duct
  • Benign stricture
  • Cholangitis
  • Sclerosing cholangitis (primary and secondary)
  • Cholangiocarcinoma
  • Pancreatic carcinoma
  • Chronic pancreatitis
  • Schistosomiasis infestation
  • Porta hepatis lymph nodes
  • Congenital biliary atresia
  • Parenteral nutrition

---

valproate, azathioprine, NSAIDs, co-amoxiclav, nitrofurantoin and allopurinol.

Social history

• Racial origin. Some conditions are more prevalent in certain ethnic groups.
• Occupation. Has there been industrial exposure, animal handling or ingestion of alcohol?
• Contact with jaundiced individuals, specifically exposure to hepatitis.
• Recent and past travel history, particularly to hepatitis-endemic areas or countries with a high rate of malaria.
• Sexual activity and hepatitis B exposure.
• Intravenous drug use or solvent abuse. Could he have shared needles with an infected individual?
• Tattoos. When and where were they done?
• Blood or plasma transfusions. When and where was this?
• Full alcohol history, including amount consumed, duration of excess exposure and features of dependence and addiction.

• Diet and oral intake of fluids and food.

Family history

Is there a family history of jaundice? Gilbert's syndrome is inherited as an autosomal dominant disorder.

He tells you he has been drinking alcohol to excess for the last 5 months due to stresses at work, up to one bottle of vodka per day, on a background of 5 years drinking 3 pints per day of real ale. He stopped drinking 5 days ago as he was feeling unwell. His wife noticed the yellow discolouration over the last few weeks.

He has no abdominal pain. He has a poor appetite and has lost 12.5 kg in weight in the last 6 months, mainly muscle mass. He feels weak and lethargic. He has not been eating well over the last few months as his alcohol intake increased. His bowels open normally twice per day with no blood.

He has a past medical history of asthma and anxiety. He takes inhalers as needed. He has never been on an antidepressant and denies any other medications. He is an ex-smoker with a 10 pack-year history. He travelled to Eastern Europe and India in the summer and was exposed to carbon tetrachloride. He had a hepatitis B vaccine prior to travelling. He has had no contact with individuals with hepatitis to his knowledge. There are no tattoos, blood transfusions or history of sexual promiscuity. He lives with his wife and has two healthy children. He works as a radio producer for a local radio station. He is severely needle phobic.

Examination
General examination
- *Vital signs*:
  - Fever may be present in patients with an abscess, cholangitis or hepatitis.
  - Tachycardia can be present in infection or acute hepatitis.
- *Skin and sclera*:
  - Evidence of clinical jaundice (the depth of jaundice is not a reliable indicator of causation).
  - Evidence of conjunctival pallor, indicating anaemia.
- *Asterixis* (liver flap): a liver flap, drowsiness and confusion are present in encephalopathy. This can be graded according to severity into four grades.
- *Signs of liver disease*: spider naevi, palmar erythema, leuconychia, clubbing, Duputren's contracture, loss of body hair, gynaecomastia, testicular atrophy, scratch marks, bruising and peripheral oedema.

Box 15.2 The West Haven criteria for grading encephalopathy

The severity of hepatic encephalopathy is graded with the West Haven criteria (Cash *et al.*, 2010):
- *Grade 1*: trivial lack of awareness; euphoria or anxiety; shortened attention span; impaired performance of addition or subtraction
- *Grade 2*: lethargy or apathy; minimal disorientation for time or place; subtle personality changes; in appropriate behaviour
- *Grade 3*: somnolence to semi-stupor, but responsive to verbal stimuli; confusion; gross disorientation
- *Grade 4*: coma (unresponsive to verbal or noxious stimuli)

Abdominal examination
- *Dilated periumbilical veins*: if the flow is towards the umbilicus, this indicates inferior vena cava obstruction. If the flow is away from the umbilicus, consider portal hypertension (caput medusae).
- *Abdominal swelling*: generalised abdominal swelling may indicate ascites. Percuss for a fluid thrill and shifting dullness to confirm a fluid–air level. Localised swelling may suggest a mass lesion or organomegaly.
- *Organomegaly*:
  - Hepatomegaly may be smooth, craggy or tender. Craggy enlargement suggests infiltration with malignancy. Tender enlargement suggests stretching of the capsule from hepatitis due to alcohol and viral causes most commonly.
  - Splenomegaly is a feature of portal hypertension, haemolysis and other haematological and infiltrative conditions.
  - A gallbladder mass, if present, suggests an enlarged, inflamed gallbladder or a carcinoma.
- *Arterial bruit over the liver*: this may be present in acute alcoholic hepatitis or hepatoma.

Box 15.3 Causes of generalised abdominal swelling: the five Fs

- Fat
- Fluid
- Faeces
- Flatus
- Fetus

Digital rectal examination
Do a DRE to assess stool colour and to feel for evidence of a rectal mass.

Neurological examination
Do a full neurological examination in patients with a history of alcohol excess. This may identify alcoholic peripheral neuropathy, cerebellar signs, features of Wernike's encephalopathy (confusion, ophthalmoplegia, ataxia, nystagmus) and Korsakoff's psychosis (confabulation).

On examination, he has a fever of 39.1°C, a pulse of 132 beats/min and a blood pressure of 145/90 mmHg. He is tremulous. There is no confusion or hepatic flap. His sclera are yellow. He has multiple spider naevi. There is hepatomegaly to 10cm below the costophrenic margin. The edge is smooth and tender. There is no ascites or peripheral oedema. Rectal examination is normal with dark brown stool on the glove.

What investigations do you want to order?
General investigations in all patients
Standard blood tests
• Full blood count for anaemia (malignancy and haemolysis), mean corpuscular volume (elevated in folate and B_{12} deficiency and in alcohol excess) and leucocytosis (in infection or haematological malignancy). Haematinics if anaemic.
• Urea and electrolytes, which may be elevated in hepatorenal syndrome and prerenal hypotensive renal failure.
• Liver function tests should include ALT, AST, ALP, γ-GT and albumin. Albumin may be low in liver disease or as the result of sepsis.
• Coagulation should be sent for a prolonged prothrombin time, a marker of synthetic liver function.
• C-reactive protein is elevated in inflammation and infection.

Urine sample
• Bilirubin (elevated in hepatic and cholestatic jaundice, absent in prehepatic causes).
• Urobilinogen (elevated in hepatic and some prehepatic causes, absent in cholestasis).

Septic screen
Given pyrexia, a full septic screen should be sent including blood cultures, urine for culture and sensitivity, a stool sample if there is diarrhoea, chest X-ray and an ascitic tap (if ascites is present).

Abdominal ultrasound with Doppler flow
This is useful to detect chronic scarring and hepatic size, vascular thrombosis, the presence of gallstones and dilated ducts of biliary obstruction, hepatic metastases and other lesions, splenomegaly, the pancreas, portal blood flow, lymphadenopathy and ascites. An abdominal ultrasound is not sensitive for discriminating cirrhosis, fibrosis and fatty change.

Chest X-ray
The presence of fever and liver dysfunction may be due to a chest infection.

Specific investigations
Haemolysis
• The reticulocyte count is elevated in haemolysis.
• Blood film for spherocytes.
• Coombs' test and serum haptoglobins.
• Ham's test for paroxysmal nocturnal haemoglobinuria.

Hepatocellular jaundice
• Paracetamol level if drug toxicity is suspected.
• Viral antibodies for hepatitis A, B, C and E (if from an endemic area), CMV and EBV.
• Autoimmune screen for anti-smooth muscle antibody, antinuclear antibody and anti-mitochondrial antibody for autoimmune hepatitis and immunoglobulins (IgG, IgA, IgM).
• Serum iron, total iron-binding capacity and ferritin. Ferritin is non-specifically elevated as an acute phase reactant in inflammatory and infective processes, and in high alcohol consumption. It is elevated in haemochromatosis (often over 1000 ng/mL) with transferring saturations of over 50%. Do a HFE gene test to confirm.
• Serum copper and ceruloplasmin are both reduced in Wilson's disease. If low do a 24 h urinary copper excretion.
• Serum α_1-antrtrypsin is low in α_1-antitrypsin deficiency.
• Serum for atypical infections such as leptospirosis; complement fixation test for leptospiropsis.
• Alpha-fetoprotein (AFP) is a marker for hepatocellular carcinoma.

Cholestatic jaundice
• Abdominal ultrasound to detect gallstones and dilated bile ducts.
• Endoscopic ultrasound or magnetic resonance cholangiopancreatography (MRCP) may detect gallstones in a dilated common bile duct and exclude a tumour.
• If a gallstone is in a dilated duct with obstructive jaundice, ascending cholangitis or recurrent pancreatitis, this should be removed urgently by endoscopic retrograde cholangiopancreatography (ERCP). A percutanous approach is used if this is not technically feasible.

His blood tests revealed a low sodium of 127 mmol/L, a low potassium of 2.9 mmol/L and a low phosphate of 0.44 mmol/L. He had normal renal function. His CRP was elevated at 56 mg/L. His haemoglobin was low at 11.1 g/dL and MCV was elevated at 102 fL. The liver function was abnormal: bilirubin 358 μmol/L, ALT 47 U/L, ALP 430 U/L, γ-GT 284 IU/L and albumin 36 g/L. He was folate deficient. His ferritin was elevated at 1772 ng/mL.

His chest X-ray was unremarkable. The septic screen was negative.

Abdominal ultrasound with Doppler showed an enlarged liver at 23 cm. The liver parenchyma was diffusely homogeneous but granular and echogenic, suggesting marked fatty change. There were no focal liver lesions. The spleen was homogeneous but bulky at 15 cm. The portal vein was mildly dilated at 13 mm at the porta hepatis but flow was hepatopetal. The gallbladder, ducts, pancreas and kidneys were normal.

The liver screen demonstrated an elevated ferritin with a negative HFE genotype. The AFP was normal. The autoimmune and hepatitis screen was negative. He was EBV IgG positive, indicating prior infection. Immunoglobulins showed an elevated IgG and IgA.

What are the causes of liver inflammation (hepatitis) and acute liver disease?

Rapidly progressive damage to the liver causes acute liver disease. This damage is usually caused by one of, or a combination of, the following.

Drugs and toxins

• Alcohol interferes with energy metabolism causing fatty liver, and causes inflammation and thus alcoholic hepatitis. Progressive alcohol consumption can lead to cirrhosis.
• Paracetamol overdose can cause massive hepatic necrosis.
• Hepatotoxic drugs.

Viral infection

• Hepatitis A, B, C and E cause inflammation that may be self-limiting but can progress to chronic hepatitis and cirrhosis.
• Cytomegalovirus and Epstein–Barr virus.

Immune damage

Autoimmune hepatitis is characterised by self-reactivity against the liver. It typically affects women who have high circulating autoantibodies.

Vascular damage

• Budd–Chiari syndrome is caused by hepatic vein thrombosis resulting in hepatic congestion. It is associated with thrombophilia.
• Veno-occlusive disease.

Biliary obstruction

• Ascending cholangitis due to gallstone disease results in bacterial infection of the biliary tree and liver.

Tumour infiltration

• Hepatocellular carcinoma or metastatic disease.

What is the most likely cause for this man's jaundice?

The most likely cause for this man's jaundice is alcoholic hepatitis. Acute hepatitis has characteristic signs of jaundice, fever, signs of alcohol withdrawal, tender hepatomegaly and biochemical liver changes of hepatitis or cholestasis. It is often precipitated by a heavy binge of alcohol. Hepatic failure can occur.

Alcohol-induced liver damage causes typical Mallory bodies, formed from precipitated intracellular proteins. In alcoholic hepatitis, neutrophils and other inflammatory cells infiltrate the parenchyma and portal tracts. The amount of alcohol consumed is not directly correlated with amount of damage.

How should you manage him?

He needs supportive management. He should be treated for vitamin deficiency with Pabrinex intravenously and started on an alcohol withdrawal protocol to prevent seizures and delirium tremens. He requires nutritional assessment and high calorie supplement drinks. This should be done after replacing electrolytes intravenously or orally, as he is at risk of refeeding syndrome (hypophosphataemia).

If anxiety and depression are factors in his alcoholic dependency then he should see a specialist whilst an inpatient. He may be started on antidepressant or anti-anxiety medications.

When do you consider steroids?

The indication for steroids in alcoholic hepatitis depends on its severity. Most patients do not require a liver biopsy, although this is the gold standard to determine inflammation. The Glasgow alcoholic hepatitis score (GAHS) has been shown to be more accurate than the modified Maddrey's discriminant function (mDF) in the prediction of outcome from alcoholic hepatitis, and guides corticosteroid use.

Glasgow alcoholic hepatitis score

A GAHS of greater than or equal to 9 predicts poor prognosis and is an indication for steroids (Table 15.1).

Table 15.1 Calculating the GAHS.

Criteria	Points		
	1	**2**	**3**
Age	<50	>50	
WBC (×10⁹/L)	<15	>15	
Urea (mmol/L)	<5	>5	
INR	<1.5	1.5-2.5	>2.5
Bilirubin (μmol/L)	<125	125-250	>250

Maddrey's discriminant function

A mDF of greater than or equal to 32 suggests a poor prognosis in severe alcoholic hepatitis and steroids should be given. The mDF can be calculated using the following formula:

$$\{4.6 \times [\text{actual PT} - \text{control PT (seconds)}] + [\text{bilirubin (mg/dL or mol/L)}]\}/17$$

He was treated for alcoholic hepatitis. He did not initially meet the criteria for steroids: his GAHS was 8 and Maddrey score was 38. He was given intravenous thiamine, electrolytes were replaced and he was placed on an alcohol withdrawal protocol. He ate regular meals, snacks and supplements including Ensure plus. His electrolytes were monitored daily for refeeding syndrome.

Prednisolone 40 mg daily was started on day 3 of admission as his bilirubin remained high. He showed a good response within a few days: bilirubin 268 μmol/L, renal function normal and electrolytes normalised.

He was discharged after 7 days admission with outpatient follow-up in 4 weeks. He remained well and was started on Seroxat for depression. His biochemistry improved.

CASE REVIEW

Jaundice is a yellow discolouration of the tissues due to the accumulation of bilirubin. The causes can be divided into prehepatic, hepatic and post-hepatic. Investigations are done to define the cause of jaundice and detect complications associated with it. These include blood tests, urinalysis and abdominal imaging. Management depends on correcting the underlying cause.

This man presented with features of alcoholic hepatitis. He was jaundiced, feverish and had tender hepatomegaly. Treatment was mainly supportive with nutrition, electrolyte and vitamin replacement. Steroids were given for evidence of severe inflammation, determined by using the Glasgow alcoholic hepatitis score. The main goal is long-term abstinence from alcohol. Acute alcoholic hepatitis can progress to hepatic failure and decompensated liver disease.

KEY POINTS

- Jaundice may be due to prehepatic, hepatocelullar or cholestatic causes or a combination.
- History and examination to determine the likely cause will guide further investigations.
- Hepatitis can be the result of drugs, viral infections, immune and vascular damage, biliary obstruction and tumour infiltration.
- Alcoholic hepatitis can progress to hepatic cirrhosis and failure.
- Steroid treatment is determined by the level of liver inflammation, guided by a scoring system designed to assess various marker and to determine prognosis. The risk of steroids lies in causing or exacerbating underlying infection.

A 53-year-old woman with jaundice and abnormal liver tests

A 53-year-old woman, Irene Rice, first came to your clinic 2 years ago with a 6-month history of malaise, anorexia and general arthralgia and a 1-month history of jaundice. Past medical history was of autoimmune thyroiditis and diabetes.

Blood tests confirmed an elevated ALT of 250 U/L and a low albumin of 29 g/L. Serum IgG was elevated. ANA and anti-smooth muscle antibody were positive. Liver biopsy confirmed autoimmune chronic hepatitis. Histology showed a mononuclear infiltrate of the portal and periportal areas, plasma cells and fibrosis. Iron and copper stains were negative.

She had treatment with corticosteroids, monitoring the response with serial ALT measurements. Her hepatitis recurred on the discontinuation of steroids and she was started on azathioprine as a steroid-sparing agent. Her last ALT was 100 U/L.

She has returned to the clinic with a history of abdominal distension and ankle swelling over the last few weeks. She feels generally tired and lethargic.

What questions do you want to ask her?

This woman has chronic autoimmune hepatitis. She is not known to be cirrhotic. She has developed ascites and pedal oedema. You must decide if she has developed clinical features of cirrhosis.

Ascites

• What is the timing of onset and progression of the abdominal distension and pedal oedema? Is it an acute and rapid onset or has it been accumulating over time?
• Does she suffer from shortness of breath at rest or on exertion? The ascites may splint the diaphragm making breathing difficult if tense and of large volume.

Gastroenterology: Clinical Cases Uncovered, 1st edition.
© S. Keshav and E. Culver. Published 2011 by
Blackwell Publishing Ltd.

• Does she describe orthopnoea or paroxysmal nocturnal dyspnoea, characteristic in cardiac failure?
• Does she have generalised or localised abdominal discomfort or pain? Think of spontaneous bacterial peritonitis.

Decompensated liver disease

Ask about symptoms suggestive of liver disease:
• Does she have a tendency to bruise easily, suggesting a coagulopathy or thrombocytopenia?
• Is she suffering from mood and sleep disturbances, which may be a marker of encephalopathy? Is she having coordination or balance difficulties?
• Has she become jaundiced and/or itchy from bilirubin?
• Has she noticed muscle wasting and weakness, a feature of malnutrition in liver disease?
• Has she lost her appetite or any weight?
  Ask about risk factors for decompensation:
• Has she had a change in her bowel habit? Is she constipated?
• Has she started any new medications, such as sedatives, analgesics or diuretics?
• Has she started drinking alcohol to excess?
• Has she had a recent infection of the chest, urine or skin?
• Consider new malignancy, particularly hepatocellular carcinoma.

Portal hypertension

• Has she developed varicies and are these bleeding?
• Does she have black melaena stool, fresh rectal blood or haematemesis?

What features are you looking for on examination?
Signs of chronic liver disease and decompensation

This includes jaundice, ascites, peripheral oedema, asterixis and constructional apraxia, loss of muscle bulk, cutaneous signs, splenomegaly and hepatomegaly.

Digital rectal examination

This should be done to identify melaena stool.

She tells you she has a poor appetite, and has lost weight and muscle mass. She bruises easily. She is drinking alcohol, two glasses of wine per night but not to excess. She has cutaneous signs of liver disease, ascites and peripheral oedema on examination. There is no melaena stool on rectal examination.

What are the causes of liver cirrhosis?

Longstanding liver damage eventually leads to fibrosis, scarring and cirrhosis. There are many different causes of liver cirrhosis. In some, there are multiple causes that accelerate damage further. Defining the exact cause will guide management and therapeutic options.

Box 16.1 Causes of cirrhosis

- Alcohol, one of the most common causes in the Western world
- Chronic viral hepatitis, hepatitis B and C
- Autoimmune hepatitis
- Primary biliary cirrhosis, affecting women more frequently than men
- Haemochromatosis
- Non-alcoholic fatty liver (NASH)
- Alpha-1 antitrypsin deficiency
- Primary sclerosing cholangitis
- Secondary biliary: strictures, sclerosing cholangitis, atresia, cystic fibrosis
- Cardiac, such as chronic right heart failure
- Budd–Chiari syndrome
- Wilson's disease
- Cryptogenic

KEY POINT

- The main causes of liver cirrhosis in the Western world are alcohol, non-alcoholic steatohepatitis and chronic viral hepatitis.

What are the features of decompensated liver cirrhosis?

Hepatic decompensation usually occurs in an individual with chronic liver disease. There is usually a reversible component, so the cause should be identified and aggressive management instituted.

Features of hepatic decompensation include:
- Jaundice and associated pruritis of the skin.
- Encephalopathy, causing mood and sleep disturbances, a characteristic flapping tremor of the hands and constructional apraxia (tested by asking the patient to draw a five-pointed star or joining the dots).
- Abdominal ascites and peripheral oedema.
- Coagulopathy and bleeding.
- Susceptibility to infections such as spontaneous bacterial peritonitis, caused by the translocation of bacteria from the intestinal lumen into protein-rich ascitic fluid.

Box 16.2 Causes of hepatic decompensation

- Infection from the urinary tract or chest, or spontaneous bacterial peritonitis
- Drug-induced, such as diuretics causing dehydration and electrolyte disturbance, sedative and opiates
- Intestinal bleeding from varices or peptic ulceration
- Constipation due to hyperammonia from amino acid catabolism and intestinal bacterial overload, causing encephalopathy
- Alcohol abuse with coexistent alcoholic hepatitis
- Development of hepatocellular carcinoma
- Progressive liver damage

What investigations should be done for decompensated liver disease?

Blood tests

All of these tests may be normal despite advanced cirrhosis:
- Full blood count (leucopenia and thrombocytopenia of severe liver disease, macrocytic anaemia of alcohol excess or vitamin B_{12}/folate deficiency).
- Urea, creatinine and electrolytes (deranged in prerenal failure, hepatorenal syndrome or isolated elevated urea suggestive of a gastrointestinal bleed).
- Liver function (raised liver enzymes, raised bilirubin and low albumin).
- Coagulation (elevated prothrombin time as a maker of synthetic liver function)

Liver screen

A full liver screen may identify a cause of cirrhosis and should be guided by the history and examination:

- Viral hepatitis screen (hepatitis A, B, C and E, CMV, EBV).
- Autoimmune screen (antinuclear antibody, anti-smooth muscle antibody, anti-mitochondrial antibody, anti-liver–kidney microsomial antibody).
- Immunoglobulins (IgG, IgA, IgM).
- Serum ferritin (and HFE gene if ferritin is over 1000 ng/mL).
- AFP for hepatocellular carcinoma detection.
- Serum ceruloplasmin and copper (and 24 h urinary copper for Wilson's disaese).
- Alpha-1 antitrypsin (if history issuggestive of α_1-antitrypsin deficiency, for example evidence of basal emphysema at a young age).

Septic screen

Urine microscopy and culture, blood cultures, sputum culture and chest X-ray should be done to identify a source of infection.

Ascitic tap

An urgent differential white blood cell count (WBC) should be done to detect a neutrophilia of spontaneous bacterial peritonitis (neutrophil count over 250%).

Abdominal ultrasound with Doppler

This detects an abnormal liver texture and size, the presence of hepatic lesions representing HCC, and splenomegaly due to portal hypertension. Doppler studies are conducted to identify portal and hepatic vein flow, which are diminished or absent in Budd–Chiari and other veno-occlusive diseases.

Computerised tomography

This is more sensitive in detecting hepatic lesions and can identify portosystemic vascular shunts. Triple phase CT scanning of the liver is the investigation of choice to identify hepatocellular carcinoma in a cirrhotic liver.

Liver biopsy

A live biopsy is used to identify a cause or confirm a diagnosis. This is often delayed until after acute decompensation. Coagulation should be normalised (INR less than 3) with vitamin K and fresh frozen plasma products prior to percutaneous approach, given the risk of haemorrhage. A transjugular approach in the presence of ascites or irreversible coagulopathy is preferred.

It classically shows fibrosis and regenerative hepatocyte nodules (Fig. 16.1). Special immunohistochemical stains are used.

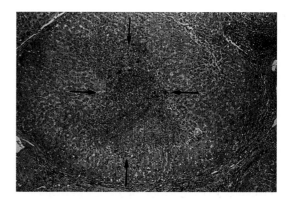

Fig. 16.1 Central regenerative nodule with surrounding fibrosis on liver biopsy.

Endoscopy

This is done to identify signs of portal hypertension with oesophageal and/or gastric varices and portal hypertensive gastropathy.

Primary prophylaxis to prevent bleeding of oesophageal varices is with β-blockers such as propranolol. Nitrates can be considered in those who are intolerant of β-blockade. After an episode of variceal bleeding, either oesophageal banding and/or propranolol are given to reduce portal pressure. Measurement of hepatic portal wedge pressure can be done in specialist liver centres. Surveillance endoscopy and repeat banding should be done depending on the size and intervention to the oesophageal varices.

Repeat blood tests showed a coagulopathy (PT 18s) and low albumin (22 g/L). An ascitic tap confirmed that her ascites was a transudate. There were no organisms on Gram stain. There were only 10 polymorphs in the cell differential.

She is not constipated, dehydrated or in renal failure. There are no new medications. She denies excess alcohol. There is no obvious factor causing the decompensation.

What are the aims of treatment?

Liver cirrhosis is largely irreversible. The main aims of treatment are palliation of symptoms, preventing further liver damage, delaying complications and avoiding liver failure. If decompensation occurs, identify and treat the provoking factor.

Palliation of symptoms

• Malnutrition and weight loss should be combated by giving regular, high calorie meals (watch for the risk of refeeding syndrome) or food supplements. Protein-rich foods are important to help build muscle. Thiamine intravenously should be given to malnourished patients and alcoholics with deficiency.

• Ascites and pedal oedema can be treated with salt restriction (no added salt diet), fluid restriction and diuretics such as spironolactone.

• If jaundice occurs, pruritis can be treated with sedating antihistamines (such as piriton) and oral bile-binding resins (such as cholestyramine) to reduce the enterohepatic circulation.

• Encephalopathy is treated by correcting identifiable causes. Stimulant laxatives such as lactulose are sufficient to reduce intestinal bacterial load. Enema therapy should be started if the patient is intolerant of lactulose, the oral route is not available or there has been no effect despite high doses.

• Correction of electrolytes, rehydration and discontinuation of sedatives and opioid analgesics may be sufficient to correct encephalopathy.

• Spontaneous bacterial peritonitis is treated by antibiotics and human albumin solution. Intravenous cephalosporins are given until an organism is identified.

• If there is evidence of active bleeding, fluid resuscitation and blood products must be given prior to endoscopic therapy. If there is severe bleeding from varices, a Sengstaken–Blakemore tube can be inserted and the gastric balloon inflated to cause a tamponade and stop the bleeding. Varices should be banded and ulcers should be injected if actively bleeding or if there are stigmata of recent haemorrhage. Antibiotic cover should be given after a variceal bleed as there could be translocation of bacteria through the intestinal wall. A protein pump inhibitor is started once varices have been banded.

KEY POINT

• The aims of treatment are palliation of symptoms, preventing further liver damage, delaying complications and avoiding liver failure. If decompensation occurs, identify causal factors and treat them.

Specific treatments

Specific treatments are available for some forms of liver disease (Table 16.1).

Liver transplantation is an option in some forms of cirrhosis. Orthotic liver transplant, where the original liver is replaced by a donor organ, can give an 85% 5-year survival postoperatively, depending on the underlying liver disease. Unfortunately, disease may recur in the transplanted liver, rejection may occur and immunosuppressive side effects can be devastating.

Table 16.1 Specific treatments for different types of liver disease.

Cause of liver cirrhosis	Specific treatment options
Chronic hepatitis B and C	Antiviral medication: • interferon and ribavirin in hepatitis C • oral nucleoside analogues in hepatitis B
Alcohol	Abstinence from alcohol (for at least 6 months if transplantation is considered)
Autoimmune disease	Corticosteroids Immunosuppressives
PBC and PSC	Ursodeoxycholic acid
Haemochromatosis	Venesection
Wilson's disease	Penicillamine

CASE REVIEW

Liver cirrhosis is characterised by the replacement of healthy liver tissue by fibrosis, scar tissue and regenerative nodules leading to loss of liver function. There are many causes. The most frequent in the Western world are alcohol, fatty liver disease (NASH) and chronic viral hepatitis.

Decompensation of liver disease can present with jaundice, encephalopathy, ascites and peripheral oedema, coagulopathy and susceptibility to infections. The causes of decompensation include gastrointestinal bleeding, infection, malignancy, drugs, dehydration and constipation. Management is aimed at reversing and treating these causes. Ultimately, liver transplantation is the final goal, although timing is crucial.

This woman had a history of chronic autoimmune hepatitis. She had a history of other autoimmune disorders. Despite steroid treatment, she developed chronic liver disease and hepatic decompensation. This was likely the natural progression of her liver disease. She responded to supportive management of her symptoms. Liver transplantation may be an option for her in the future.

KEY POINTS

- Liver cirrhosis is the loss of normal hepatic architecture due to fibrosis with nodular regeneration.
- It implies irreversible liver disease, although because of the large excess reserve capacity of the liver, evidence of liver disease may be unapparent. This is compensated liver disease.
- Chronic liver disease can decompensate due to a variety of causes including infection, intestinal haemorrhage, drugs, constipation, alcohol abuse, tumour development and progression of underlying liver disease.
- Investigations should be directed at determining the underlying cause of this decompensation.
- Management of the acute episode involves identifying and treating the cause of decompensation and supportive management.

PART 2: CASES

A 53-year-old man with abdominal swelling

Mike Higgs, a 53-year-old lorry driver, was referred to your gastroenterology clinic by his GP. He has a history of generalised abdominal distension and weight gain. The GP detected what he thought was 'shifting dullness' on examination of his abdomen, indicative of fluid. He has asked you for further assessment.

What are the possible causes of generalised abdominal swelling?

There are five main causes of generalised abdominal swelling. They are often referred to as the 'five Fs':

- Fat.
- Fluid.
- Faeces.
- Flatus.
- Fetus.

This man has been referred with fluid in his abdomen (ascites). What questions do you want to ask in the history?

Ascites is the accumulation of excess free fluid in the peritoneal cavity.

Abdominal swelling

- Length of time the swelling has been present and speed of onset? Sudden onset may be due to rapid decompensation of cirrhosis, malignancy, thrombosis or Budd–Chiari syndrome.

Abdominal pain

- Describe the features of the pain.
- Is there an associated fever or chills? Consider spontaneous bacterial peritonitis in patients with painful ascites.

Gastroenterology: Clinical Cases Uncovered, 1st edition.
© S. Keshav and E. Culver. Published 2011 by Blackwell Publishing Ltd.

- Is there a palpable mass or lump? Consider peritoneal metastases from an abdominal primary. Assess for localised masses or organomegaly.

Peripheral oedema

- Does he have ankle swelling or sacral oedema? This may be due to hypoalbuminaemia due to cirrhosis, nephritic syndrome or congestive cardiac failure.
- Is he short of breath? This may be due to diaphragmatic splinting or cardiac failure with pleural effusions or dilated cardiomyopathy.
- Does he suffer from orthopnoea or paroxysmal nocturnal dyspnoea? This is suggestive of congestive cardiac failure.

Risk factors for ascites
Liver cirrhosis

- Alcohol consumption. How much alcohol, in units, does he take on a daily basis? What is the duration of this intake? Does he binge drink or is this constant? Remember individuals often underestimate their alcohol consumption and may even lie about alcohol intake due to embarrassment or denial.
- Exposure to hepatitis. Has he had tattoos, intravenous drug use or blood transfusions? What is his sexual history? Has he travelled to endemic areas?
- Prior history of jaundice.
- Family history of liver disease, such as haemochromatosis or Wilson's disease.
- Was there emphysema at a young age? Consider α_1-antitrypsin deficiency.
- Autoimmune conditions. Does he suffer from other autoimmune condition such as type 1 diabetes or autoimmune thyroid disease, which may increase the risk of autoimmune liver disease?

Malignancy

- Smoking history: this results in an increased risk of many cancers.

- History of abdominal or pelvic malignancy.
- History of other malignancy that may have metasta-sised with peritoneal infiltration, for example prostate, testicular or haematological malignancy.
- Exposure to asbestos, a risk factor for mesothelioma.

Cardiac failure

- History of ischaemic heart disease, hypertension, periph-eral vascular disease or atherosclerosis.
- Consider dilated cardiomyopathy caused by ischaemia, alcohol excess, iron deposition or thyroid disease.

Tuberculosis

- Exposure to tuberculosis by travel to developing coun-tries or infected contacts.
- Family history of tuberculosis.
- Childhood vaccinations (BCG) against tuberculosis.
- Immunosuppression by medication or other disease process.

Pancreatitis

- Pancreatic inflammation resulting in ascites.

Thrombotic factors

- Clotting abnormalities which may predispose to Budd–Chiari disease or portal vein thrombosis.

What do you look for on examination?
General examination

- Assess haemodynamics in terms of blood pressure, pulse rate and fluid balance.
- Look for conjunctival pallor of anaemia.
- Look for icteric sclera, liver flaps and/or signs of chronic liver disease.
- Palpate for lymphadenopathy, which may be present in malignancy, lymphoma and tuberculosis.

Cardiovascular examination

- Look for an elevated jugular venous pressure (JVP) at a 45° angle, suggestive of cardiac failure.
- Look for a prominent V wave of tricuspid regur-gitation, with pulsatile hepatomegaly and right heart failure.
- Look for an elevated JVP on inspiration (Kussmaul's sign) in a pericardial effusion.
- Palpate for a displaced apex beat from cardiomegaly, due to dilated cardiomyopathy or cardiac failure.
- Palpate for peripheral pedal and/or sacral oedema. This occurs in cirrhosis, cardiac failure, malabsorption,

nephrotic syndrome and obstructed lymphatic flow due to intra-abdominal or pelvic tumours.
- Listen for heart sounds. These may be muffled with a pericardial effusion. A third heart sound may be audible in cardiac failure.
- Listen for murmurs. A tricuspid pansystolic murmur may be present in tricuspid regurgitation. If present, palpate for a pulsatile enlarged liver.
- Listen for a pericardial friction rub or knock in pericarditis.
- Listen to the chest for bilateral fine inspiratory crepita-tions of pulmonary oedema.
- Percuss the chest for dullness of a pleural effusion.

Abdominal examination

- Look for signs of chronic liver disease. These include spider naevi, palmar erythema, finger clubbing, jaundice, loss of body hair, gynaecomastia and caput medusae.
- Palpate for hepatomegaly and splenomegaly in portal hypertension and hepatic and haematological malignancies.
- Assess for ascites; shifting dullness and fluid thrill are classic signs.

Digital rectal examination

- A rectal exam is done to palpate a rectal carcinoma.
- In women, a vaginal examination may identify a pelvic adnexal mass.

Mr Higgs explains the abdominal distension has developed over the last few months. He noticed ankle swelling prior to this. He feels breathless on exertion but denies any orthopnoea or paroxysmal nocturnal dyspnoea. He has not noticed jaundice.

Past medical history is of hypertension, for which he takes bendroflumethiazide, amlodipine and ramipril, and chronic obstructive airways disease. He drinks alcohol, usually two home measures of whiskey per night but denies drinking to excess. He smokes 40 cigarettes per day. He has never injected drugs but has had a previous blood transfusion 30 years ago after a fractured femur and has multiple tattoos on his arms.

Examination reveals an elevated jugular pressure, normal heart sounds and a clear chest. There are no stigmata of chronic liver disease. He has shifting dullness but no demonstrable fluid thrill. There is no palpable organomegaly. He has pitting bilateral pedal oedema to his knees. The rectal examination is normal.

Which general investigations are important to help identify a cause?

Investigations should be directed at finding the underlying cause of the ascites guided by the history and examination.

Box 17.1 Causes of ascites

Hepatic
- Cirrhosis
- Hepatocellular carcinoma or metastases

Cardiac
- Cardiac failure
- Constrictive pericarditis
- Tricuspid incompetence

Renal
- Nephrotic syndrome

Malignant
- Abdominal or pelvic tumour
- Carcinomatosis
- Primary mesothelioma
- Pseudomyxoma peritonei

Venous obstruction
- Veno-occlusive disease
- Budd–Chiari syndrome
- Hepatic portal vein obstruction
- Inferior vena cava obstruction

Gastrointestinal
- Pancreatitis
- Malabsorption
- Bile ascites

Peritonitis
- Tuberculosis
- Spontaneous bacterial

General investigations
Urine dipstick

This is performed to test for protein in the nephrotic syndrome; if it is strongly positive, send a 24 h urine collection to confirm. A protein content of above 3.5 g is diagnostic.

Blood tests

- Full blood count for anaemia and differential white cell count in malignancy.

- Urea and creatinine may be elevated in renal failure due to a hepatorenal syndrome, hypovolaemia and intrinsic renal disease. Electrolytes can be abnormal in cirrhosis, cardiac failure and renal disease.
- Liver function may be abnormal in liver disease. Albumin is low in cirrhosis.
- Coagulopathy of liver cirrhosis.

Electrocardiogram

This is used to detect evidence of left or right ventricular strain or ischaemia in cardiac disease.

Chest X-ray

A CXR is performed to detect signs of cardiac failure such as cardiomegaly, pulmonary oedema with 'bat-wing' upper venous diversion and Kerley B lines. There may be evidence of pleural effusions – bilateral due to cardiac failure, unilateral in malignancy or if related to the ascites. A mass in the lung is suggestive of carcinoma or metastases. Calcified nodules are found in tuberculosis.

Abdominal ultrasound

This will confirm the presence of ascites. It can show a coarse echo texture or fatty deposits in liver cirrhosis. The liver may be enlarged or shrunken with liver lesions suggestive of hepatocellular carcinoma or metastases. Splenomegaly can be identified. Dilated collateral veins may be seen in hepatic or portal venous obstruction. Other intra-abdominal pathology may be detected.

Doppler ultrasound

This is indicated to detect thrombosis of the hepatic or portal veins as the cause of the ascites.

Ascitic tap

The commonest site for an ascitic tap is approximately 15 cm lateral to the umbilicus, done in the left or right lower abdominal quadrant, with care being taken to avoid enlarged organs. For diagnostic purposes, 10–20 mL of ascitic fluid should be withdrawn and sent for biochemistry, microbiology and cytological examination.

Diagnosis

- *Appearance*: the appearance of the ascitic fluid may give a clue as to the cause (Table 17.1). Straw-coloured is the most common. Milky white fluid (chylous) is due to obstruction of the lymphatic ducts. Haemorrhagic fluid occurs in malignancy, tuberculosis and trauma. Bile-stained fluid suggests bile peritonitis.

Table 17.1 Possible causes of ascites based on the appearance of the ascitic fluid.

Colour of fluid	Possible causes
Straw/yellow	Liver cirrhosis, cardiac failure, nephritic syndrome
Milky white	Lymphatic ducts obstructed
Blood-stained	Malignancy, tuberculosis, trauma
Bile-stained	Bile peritonitis

• *Biochemical analysis*: this is done for protein content, glucose, amylase, bilirubin and triglyceride levels. The protein level helps to classify the fluid as a transudate (less than 25 g/L) or an exudate (greater than 25 g/dL). It is not as simple as this, however, and the serum ascites–albumin gradient (SA-AG) should be calculated to categorise ascites, with 97% accuracy:

$$\text{SA-AG} = (\text{serum albumin concentration}) - (\text{ascitic fluid albumin concentration})$$

A gradient of >11 g/L occurs in cirrhosis, cardiac failure and nephrotic syndrome. A gradient of <11 g/L occurs in malignancy, pancreatitis and tuberculosis.

Glucose is low in bacterial infection. Amylase is high in pancreatic ascites. Triglyceride is elevated in chylous ascites. Bilirubin is elevated in bilious ascites.

• *Cytology*: this is important to determine the differential WCC for classification of bacterial peritonitis (neutrophil count >250 cells/mm^3 or WCC >500 cells/mm^3) or tuberculosis peritonitis (lymphocytosis). Gram and Ziehl–Neelsen staining with cultures are rarely helpful. Blood culture bottles detect a greater yield for bacterial infection.

• *Pathology*: pathology and cytology samples are sent to look for malignant cells.

Complications of ascitic taps

These occur in up to 1% of patients (abdominal haematomas) but are rarely serious. More serious complications such as haemoperitoneum or bowel perforation are rare (1 in 1000 procedures).

His blood tests showed normal full blood count, liver function and coagulation. His urea was elevated at 7.2 mmol/L with a normal creatinine and electrolytes.

Urinalysis did not show an excess of protein. An electrocardiogram showed evidence of P-pulmonale and left ventricular hypertrophy. A chest X-ray showed an enlarged heart with normal lung markings and no effusions.

Abdominal ultrasound confirmed the presence of ascites with no organomegaly or abdominal masses. Ascitic fluid was an exudate with an ascitic protein content of 29 g/dL. The SA-AG was >11 g/L.

What specific investigations can be done to confirm the suspected cause?

• *Echocardiogram*: to look for left and right ventricular dysfunction, evidence of a pericardial effusion and colour Doppler flow of tricuspid regurgitation.

• *Liver screen*: to determine the cause of cirrhosis, guided by risk factors from the history. A full liver screen includes viral serology (hepatitis A, B, C and E, EBV, CMV), autoimmune screen (antinuclear antibody, anti-smooth muscle antibody, anti-mitochondrial antibody) immunoglobulins and biochemistry (AFP, ferritin, α1-antrypsin level, caeruloplasmin).

• *Liver biopsy*: to determine or confirm the cause of liver cirrhosis.

• *Renal biopsy*: to determine the cause of the nephritic syndrome.

• *Portal venography*: to confirm veno-occlusive disease and Budd–Chiari syndrome.

An echocardiogram confirmed normal left ventricular function and normal flow through the valves. There was significant right ventricular dilatation and diastolic dysfunction.

What is the explanation for this man's ascites?

The most likely cause is right heart failure, due to chronic obstructive airways disease (COPD).

How do you treat the ascites?

Treatment should be of the underlying cause of ascites. The ascitic fluid can be managed by the use of diuretics and/or abdominal large volume paracentesis. Refractory ascites is peritoneal fluid that is difficult to remove or recurrent despite repeated attempts to treat it. It can be resistant to diuretics or refractory to them because of diuretic-induced complications.

- In *left cardiac failure*, optimise the heart function by cardiac medications (ACE inhibitors, calcium channel blockers and β-blockers) and use frusemide (furosemide) as the first line diuretic.
- In *right heart failure*, offload the right heart by optimising ventilation with treatment of the COPD. He needs to stop smoking and use inhaled medications, such as steroid inhalers and tiotropium, as guided by the respiratory team.
- In *liver failure*, salt restriction (low salt diet) and fluid restriction to 1500 mL/day are important. Spironolactone

is used as the first line diuretic, increasing every 3–5 days in a logarithmic fashion if ascites is resistant, whist monitoring the renal function, fluid balance and weight. Large volume abdominal paracentesis can be done for diuretic-resistant or refractory ascites.

A LeVeen (peritoneovenous) shunt or transjugular intrahepatic portal-systemic shunt (TIPSS) can be inserted, with risk of encephalopathy and shunt blockage as the main complications. Liver transplantation should be considered at an early stage; criteria for considering transplant depend on the underlying cause.

CASE REVIEW

Ascites, the presence of fluid in the peritoneal cavity, is a cause of generalised abdominal swelling. It can be detected by examining for shifting dullness or a fluid thrill. The causes can be divided into those producing a transudate (such as nephritic syndrome, liver cirrhosis, cardiac failure) or exudate (such as tuberculosis, malignancy). This can be worked out by calculating the serum ascites–albumin gradient.

Investigation of ascites includes blood tests and imaging of the abdomen, chest and heart. This will be guided by the history and examination findings. Treatments include fluid restriction, no added salt diet, diuretics and paracentesis. Shunts and transplantation are reserved for cases refractory to these measures.

This man in this case presented with gradual onset abdominal distension, weight gain, ankle swelling and shortness of breath on exertion. Examination confirmed an elevated jugular venous pressure, shifting dullness of ascites and peripheral pitting oedema. There was no evidence of liver disease. Investigations suggested a cardiac cause with left ventricular hypertrophy on his electrocardiogram consistent with his hypertension, and p pulmonale consistent with right heart disease. an echocardiogram confirmed right heart and diastolic dysfunction. He was treated by optimising the preload and afterload to the heart and given diuretics.

KEY POINTS

- Generalised abdominal swelling may be attributed to one of the 'five Fs – fat, faeces, flatus, fluid and fetus.
- Ascites is the accumulation of excess free peritoneal fluid. It has many causes, including liver cirrhosis.

- Investigations are guided by the history and examination to determine a cause of ascites.
- An ascitic tap is crucial to define if the fluid is a transudate or exudate, and to detect spontaneous bacterial peritonitis in patients with liver disease.

A 36-year-old man who drinks alcohol

AndrewWilliams, a 36-year-old man, is brought to accident and emergency by the paramedics, accompanied by his partner. She tells you he is a 'drinker' and that he has been off alcohol for the last 48h. Over the last few hours he has been anxious and sweaty. She found him having a fit on the living room floor, shaking his limbs. She called an ambulance. He is now awake and appears agitated.

What do you want to know from his history?

This sounds like an alcohol-related withdrawal seizure. You should confirm this by taking a history of his 'fit', documenting an alcohol history and excluding other organic causes of his seizure. He may not be able to give an accurate account of events. His partner may give a valuable collateral history.

The 'fit'

- Was there any aura or altered sensation before the event?
- Did he loose consciousness?
- Was there any tongue biting or urinary incontinence?
- Did he come around quickly or more gradually (postictal period)?
- Did he feel exhausted or tired afterwards?
- Ask the partner to describe his activity and limb movements.
- Has he had a seizure before, and was this linked to alcohol use?

Alcohol consumption

Most physicians know and employ the CAGE questioning technique as a screening tool for alcohol misuse. A single positive response to the CAGE questions is considered suggestive of an alcohol problem. Two or more posi-

tive responses indicate the presence of an alcohol problem with a sensitivity and specificity of approximately 90%.

- How much alcohol does he consume on a daily basis (in units)? An alcohol unit is 10 mL or 8 g of absolute alcohol. This equates approximately to half a pint of beer (285 mL), one glass of fortified wine (50 mL), one single measure of spirits (25 mL) and one glass of average strength wine (125 mL). The recommended weekly alcohol allowance for women is 14 units per week and f or men 21 units per week. Individuals frequently underestimate their consumption. This underestimation may be attributed to denial, one of the hallmarks of the disease.
- The type and strength (%) of alcohol? This influences the toxicity of alcohol.
- Drinking alone or in company? Drinking alone is more indicative of an alcohol dependence or problem.
- How long has he been drinking this amount? Did he drink more or less in the past?
- Explore any events or reasons for him drinking heavily. These may be personal and better explored by an alcohol councillor, if available.
- When did he last drink any alcohol? This is important when dealing with alcohol withdrawal seizures and the possibility of delirium tremens.
- Withdrawal symptoms that occur when not drinking regularly, such as being agitated or anxious, sweaty, tremulous or confused.

Gastroenterology: Clinical Cases Uncovered, 1st edition.
© S. Keshav and E. Culver. Published 2011 by
Blackwell Publishing Ltd.

Box 18.1 The CAGE questionnaire

- C: Have you ever felt you should **C**ut down on your drinking?
- A: Have people **A**nnoyed you by criticising your drinking?
- G: Have you ever felt **G**uilty about your drinking
- E: Have you ever had a drink first thing in the morning (**E**ye-opener) to steady your nerves or to get rid of a hangover

He tells you he has little recollection of the fit but feels exhausted now. He usually drinks up to 0.5 L of vodka each night with the occasional beer at a weekend, and usually drinks with friends but always at his home or theirs. He has drunk heavily like this for months. He has been feeling unwell for the last few days and had reduced his alcohol intake quickly. He had his last drink 26 h ago.

He has had two fits before and was fully investigated to exclude epilepsy by brain scan and other tests. His partner confirms he was drinking alcohol at this time. He refuses to comment on this.

His partner gives an account of the episode. He was fidgety and agitated. Then suddenly he went rigid and dropped to the floor. His arms and legs shook for seconds and then stopped. She is unsure if he hit his head but there is no bruising. His tongue was bleeding after the event.

What other information do you want to know?

Symptoms of alcohol-related harm

Ask about other symptoms of alcohol-induced physical or psychological injury.

Gastrointestinal

• Has he been retching or vomiting up any fresh red blood? This may suggest a superficial oesophageal tear (Mallory–Weiss tear) or ulceration.
• Does he suffer from reflux or heartburn? He may have alcohol-induced gastric erosions and inflammation.
• Does he have swallowing difficulties and are these progressive? There is an increased risk of oesophageal carcinoma with alcohol consumption.
• Does he have unintentional weight loss? Is he eating any nutritional foods? Does he have an appetite? Patients with alcohol dependence may source their calories from alcohol and either feel too nauseous to eat or have a reduced appetite. This may lead to loss of muscle mass and fat deposition over time.
• Does he suffer from abdominal or back pain or altered bowel habit? This is suggestive of pancreatic inflammation and insufficiency.
• Has he been jaundiced or developed abdominal distension and peripheral fluid retention? Look for features of liver disease.

Cardiac

• Does he have palpitations? If so, describe them. Arrhythmias are provoked by alcohol.

• Does he get breathlessness or have chest pain on exertion? This may suggest development of alcoholic dilated cardiomyopathy.

Neurological

• Does he have problems with his balance (ataxia), vision, memory and recall? Cerebellar symptoms, Wernicke's encephalopathy and Korsakoff's psychosis must be detected and treated.
• Does he suffer sensory disturbance in his feet and lower limbs. An alcoholic peripheral neuropathy can present early in these patients. Alternative causes such as diabetes and drug-induced ones should be looked for and excluded.
• Does he have hallucinations or periods of amnesia as a result of alcohol?

Musculoskeletal

• Is he prone to accidents and injury? Does he fracture bones easily? Be aware of osteoporosis in those with high alcohol consumption.
• Does he complain of muscular pain or weakness?

Endocrine

• Is he suffering from impotence?
• Does he have testicular atrophy or male breast tissue? These are features of liver disease.

Past medical history

• Explore other organic causes for seizures as organic disease and alcohol misuse can coexist. Consider diabetes.
• Does he have a history of depression, anxiety or a psychiatric disorder?

Medications

Does he take any antidepressant, anti-anxiety or other prescribed medications that may interact with his alcohol or lower the seizure threshold?

Social history

• Obtain information on prior alcohol detoxifications, concomitant use of other substances, date of first use, and time interval from last use. Does he smoke? Does he take illegal substances? Does he inject drugs? Consider risk factors for hepatitis and HIV.
• Find out his employment status and the responsibilities in his job, such as driving, handling equipment and caring for dependants.

• Find out his social situation; who does he live with, what is his social support network? Does he have difficulties with interpersonal relationships and social situations?

He tells you he suffers from severe reflux and heartburn most days but has no swallowing difficulties. He vomits occasionally with no blood. He has lost weight but is not eating as he has no appetite. He is off balance when he walks and needs to hold on to furniture to steady himself. This has been the case for the last few weeks.

He has no medical history and takes no medications or illicit drugs. He lives with his partner although they fight a lot. He is unemployed and has been for over a year.

What are you looking for on examination?

Look for signs of alcohol misuse and alcohol-related disease.

General examination

• Blood glucose: measure his blood glucose (BM test) for hypoglycaemia.
• Vital signs: pulse for tachyarrhythmias and blood pressure for hyper- or hypotension.
• Signs of withdrawal: agitated, tremulous or sweaty.
• Signs of alcoholic hepatitis: febrile, tremulous, tender liver.
• Signs of neglect: unkempt and untidy clothes, hair, basic hygiene.
• Inspect for evidence of traumatic injury.

Directed examination

• Stigmata of chronic liver disease: cutaneous spider naevi, telangiectasia, jaundice, ascites and hepatosplenomegaly.
• Neurological exam for ataxia, nystagmus, ophthalmoplegia, peripheral neuropathy and muscular weakness.

He is shaky and tremulous. He appears malnourished and in a state of neglect with dirty fingernails, unwashed hair and unshaven beard. There are no stigmata of chronic liver disease.

On neurological examination he has ataxia, nystagmus to lateral gaze and a 6th cranial nerve palsy. He uses the bed and chair to steady himself on standing.

He has had a withdrawal seizure. What do you do now?

He requires early treatment to prevent further seizures. An immediate dose of fast acting benzodiazepine, such as lorazepam, will reduce the likelihood of further seizures.

Delirium tremens occurs in less than 5% of people withdrawing from alcohol, usually after 72h of stopping alcohol. It is characterised by a coarse tremor, agitation, profound confusion, delusions and hallucinations, fever and tachycardia. Hyperpyrexia, ketoacidosis and profound circulatory collapse may develop. It is a medical emergency and is easier to prevent than treat.

Oral lorazepam is the first line treatment. Parenteral lorazepam, haloperidol or olanzapine can be given if this is refused or not tolerated.

He has neurological signs on examination. What should you do now?

He has symptoms and signs suggestive of Wernicke's encephalopathy. This characteristically involves symptomatic confusion and signs of nystagmus, ocular palsy and ataxia. It is a medical emergency and reversible with intravenous thiamine. Korsakoff's psychosis can also develop over time causing short-term memory loss and confabulation.

He should be admitted for intravenous thiamine and alcohol detoxification.

• Intravenous Pabrinex is given daily, three doses per day for 5 days minimum. This is converted to oral thiamine 300mg daily thereafter.
• Detoxification using long-acting benzodiazepines such as chlordiazepoxide should be started in the emergency department and prescribed on a daily reducing regimen to avoid accumulation and oversedation. Reduction is tailored individually and guided by symptoms.
• Agitation should be controlled with extra benzodiazepines as needed or haloperidol if this is unsuccessful.
• Lorazepam or intravenous diazepam can be given if seizures occur.
• Dehydration should be corrected with oral fluids, avoiding overhydration and rapid correction of sodium.
• Electrolytes should be replaced, particularly potassium as hypokalaemia is common.
• Nutrition should be encouraged including supplements and high calorie drinks. Refeeding syndrome should be considered in those malnourished due to alcohol. Phosphate depletion is one of the most important markers of this.

> **KEY POINT**
>
> - Wernicke's encephalopathy must be considered early in those with harmful or hazardous drinking, malnutrition or decompensated liver disease. Clinical features include global confusion, eye muscle weakness and ataxia. Thiamine (parenteral) should be given in those patients at risk or in those exhibiting features.

He is confused about why he had a 'fit'. What do you tell him?

The most likely cause for his seizure was alcohol withdrawal. Approximately 40% of those who misuse alcohol develop alcohol withdrawal syndrome.

Most people with withdrawal manifest minor symptoms between 6 to 8h after abrupt changes in alcohol intake. Theses include generalised hyperactivity, anxiety, tremor, sweating, nausea, retching, tachycardia, hypertension and mild pyrexia. The symptoms peak at 20h. They often resolve by 50h. Seizures manifest in the first 24–48h after abrupt withdrawal of alcohol. Auditory and visual hallucinations may also occur and last for up to 6 days. Treatment with a benzodiazepine or carbamezapine should treat the symptoms of acute alcohol withdrawal. A symptom-triggered regimen should follow on from this, with regular assessment and monitoring for symptoms.

He asks you if he is an 'alcoholic' or an 'addict'. How do you define this?

Alcohol dependence or addiction is a syndrome characterised by the presence of three or more of the following:

- A strong desire or compulsion to drink.
- Difficulty controlling the onset and termination of drinking or the level of alcohol use.
- A physiological withdrawal state on cessation of alcohol or its use to avoid withdrawal symptoms.
- Increasing tolerance to alcohol so that more is needed in order to achieve similar effects to those produced originally by smaller amounts.
- Progressive neglect of other interests.
- Persisting use of alcohol despite clear evidence and an awareness of the nature and extent of the harm it is causing.

An alcoholic can be defined as an individual that is experiencing alcohol-related harm, either physically or psychologically. Predisposition to harm comes from the availability and cost of alcohol, advertising campaigns, cultural factors, and parental and peer group influences.

This patient has experienced an alcohol-related seizure and has compulsion to drink, withdrawal on cessation, neglect for other things and persistent drinking despite the consequences. He fulfils these criteria.

> **Box 18.2 Alcohol-related physical harm**
>
> **Gastrointestinal**
> - Oesophagitis, gastro-oesophageal reflux and ulceration
> - Mallory–Weiss tear from vomiting and retching
> - Oesophageal carcinoma
> - Gastritis erosions (acute and chronic)
> - Pancreatitis (acute and chronic)
> - Pancreatic exocrine insufficiency from chronic pancreatitis (may need enzyme supplementation if there is steatorrhoea or poor nutrition)
> - Malabsorption
> - Liver damage: fatty change, hepatitis (may need steroids), cirrhosis (may need transplantation)
> - Acute alcohol poisoning
>
> **Other systems**
> - Accidents and injury
> - Cardiovascular: arrhythmia, cardiomyopathy, coronary hearty disease, hypertension, cerebrovascular accidents
> - Nervous system: Wernicke's encephalopathy, Korsakoff's psychosis, cerebellar degeneration, central pontine myelinolysis, alcoholic dementia, peripheral neuropathy, withdrawal seizures
> - Skeletal muscle: acute rhabdomyolysis, chronic myopathy
> - Bone: osteoporosis
> - Skin disorders: spider naevi, linear telangiectasia
> - Malignancy, including mouth, larynx, pharynx, oesophagus, breast
> - Hypoglycaemia
> - Aspiration pneumonia
> - Infertility
> - Fetal damage

> **Box 18.3 Alcohol-related social and psychological harm**
>
> - Interpersonal relationships damaged
> - Employment-related problems
> - Criminal behaviour
> - Social disintegration

- Depression and anxiety symptoms
- Psychotic illness
- Alcoholic hallucinosis
- Amnesia
- Morbid jealousy

KEY POINT

- Alcohol abuse is associated with physical, psychological and social harm.

Which investigations will you do whilst he is an inpatient?
Blood tests
• Full blood count for macrocytosis and thrombocytopenia. If macrocytic, B_{12} and folate levels should be sent.
• Urea, creatinine and electrolytes may show a low urea, potassium, magnesium, sodium and phosphate. These should be replaced prior to feeding.
• Liver function tests for evidence of fatty change or hepatitis. Remember, liver tests can be normal in the presence of severe cirrhosis and not all liver dysfunction in patients with alcohol misuse is necessarily due to the alcohol.
• Coagulation for signs of hepatic synthetic function.

Electrocardiogram
Look for evidence of arrhythmias or left ventricular hypertrophy of hypertension.

Chest X-ray
Look for dilated cardiomyopathy and evidence of aspiration after a seizure, especially if the patient is vomiting and not protecting his airway.

Abdominal ultrasound
This should be done in the presence of abnormal liver tests or signs of liver disease. It can show a fatty liver, enlarged liver, small cirrhotic liver or evidence of portal hypertension with splenomegaly. Ultrasound may not detect abnormalities despite the presence of liver disease.

Upper GI endoscopy
This should be done if there is cirrhosis, acute overt upper GI bleeding or iron-deficiency anaemia. It may identify varices, oesophagitis, gastric erosions or a Mallory–Weiss tear.

He is on his fourth day of detoxification and is feeling better, but still a little shaky and unsteady on his feet. He can now stand slowly unaided and uses a single stick to support him to walk. The physiotherapist feels this will improve with time. He is motivated to get better. He wants to go home with his remaining medication. He promises you he will not drink again. He is not in touch with an alcohol support service.

Should you discharge him?
Inpatient detoxification is time consuming but should be completed for patients in acute alcohol withdrawal with withdrawal seizures, delirium tremens or at high risk of these. Benzodiazepines given on prescription can be sold, abused or taken with alcohol, which may have serious consequences. Detoxification can be done in the community but only under the supervision of a community specialist nurse. Offer advice about sudden reduction in alcohol intake and information about local support services.

Inpatient detoxification gives the individual time to understand how alcohol has affected him and make the appropriate changes on discharge to the community. An alcohol liaison service should be available for further input and regular contact on discharge. He should be put in touch with specialist services, such as alcohol treatment units, community-based services and Alcoholics Anonymous.

In patients under the age of 16, offer admission to hospital for physical and psychosocial assessment in addition to medically assisted alcohol withdrawal.

He completed his 7-day course of detoxification and was transferred to a rehabilitation unit.

PART 2: CASES

CASE REVIEW

Continued harmful drinking can result in alcohol dependence and tolerance, with a risk of alcohol withdrawal on abrupt cessation of drinking. It may cause both physical and psychosocial damage.

Alcohol withdrawal may be managed in the community by specialist support agencies, specialist nurses or in conjunction with the general practitioner. Alcohol withdrawal is managed in hospital if there are complications such as withdrawal seizures and delirium tremens, the presence of organ damage or failure such as liver disease, pancreatitis or electrolyte disturbances, and in those patients under the age of 16 who also need both physical and psychological assessment. A symptoms-triggered regimen involves tailoring the treatment to the individual's symptoms and signs of withdrawal.

This young man had features of alcohol dependence and alcohol-related harm. He presented to the emergency department with an alcohol withdrawal seizure. He had neurological features of Wernicke's encephalopathy that required urgent medical treatment with intravenous thiamine. Inpatient alcohol detoxification was completed and he was discharged to a rehabilitation centre for ongoing input.

KEY POINTS

- Alcohol abuse is a pattern of drinking associated with the development of alcohol-related harm.
- Alcohol-related harm can be physical and psychological.
- Withdrawal is characterised by tremor, agitation, insomnia and diaphoresis. Seizures may develop within 24–72 h after the abrupt discontinuation of alcohol.
- Delerium tremens begins after 3–5 days, characterised by disorientation, fever and visual hallucinations. It is a medical emergency and should be treated as on an inpatient basis.

- Wernicke's encephalopathy is defined by confusion, ataxia, nystagmus and opthalmoplegia or ocular palsies. It requires emergency treatment as an inpatient with intravenous thiamine.
- Detoxification with long-acting benzodiazepines is best done in the community under the guidance of a clinical nurse specialist or specialist centre. If this service is unavailable or the patient has other medical complications, inpatient admission is advisable.

A 79-year-old man with right upper quadrant colicky abdominal discomfort

Mr Stone is a 79-year-old retired pharmaceutical representative. He comes to the outpatient clinic with a 3-month history of intermittent right upper quadrant abdominal discomfort, loss of appetite and general lethargy. He thinks it may be due to gallstones. He has come for further investigation.

What are the likely causes of right upper quadrant pain or discomfort?

Pain or discomfort in the right upper quadrant may be due to:

- Gallbladder and gallstone disease.
- Hepatobiliary disease.
- Pancreatic disease.
- Peptic ulcer disease.
- Right colon disease.
- Right kidney disease.
- Referred pain from the chest or heart.
- Abdominal wall pain.

What important features in the history will help to narrow your differential diagnosis?

Abdominal pain

- Describe the abdominal pain: character, location, radiation, intensity, frequency, duration, aggravating and relieving factors, and associated symptoms.
- Gallstone related pain is typically colicky and frequent, lasting seconds to minutes. The pain may be aggravated by fatty meals, which stimulate cholecystokinin release and gallbladder contraction.

Associated features

- Loss of appetite? Loss of weight? This may occur in systemic disease, inflammatory conditions, malignancy and if there is prolonged anorexia.
- Nausea and vomiting. Most of the above causes can lead to nausea and vomiting. Even severe pain can stimulate a feeling of nausea.
- Jaundiced and/or itching. This is due to an accumulation of bilirubin and bile salts, respectively.
- Pale stools. This is due to absent bile pigment in the intestine.
- Oily stools that are smelly and difficult to flush (steatorrhoea) may occur in pancreatic insufficiency.
- Dark orange urine. This is due to excretion of conjugated bilirubin.
- Fever or rigors. This may occur in bacterial infection of a dilated biliary system.
- Heartburn or reflux may be a feature, alongside dyspepsia, of peptic ulcer disease.
- Flatulence and bloating can occur in bacterial overgrowth, malabsorption, gallstone disease and functional disorders.
- Urinary symptoms. These are often present in renal tract and urinary system pathology.
- Respiratory symptoms such as a cough, wheeze, sputum and breathlessness, suggesting chest disease.
- Cardiac symptoms such as palpitations, chest pain, orthopnoea and syncope, suggesting cardiac disease.

His abdominal pain is in the right upper quadrant. It is colicky, in acute recurrent episodes lasting 60s, usually for a few days at a time. He is then pain free for a few weeks. He is intolerant of fatty foods and describes excessive flatulence. There is no change in his bowel habit and no urinary symptoms. He has not been feverish.

Gastroenterology: Clinical Cases Uncovered, 1st edition.
© S. Keshav and E. Culver. Published 2011 by
Blackwell Publishing Ltd.

The history of presenting complaint is suggestive of gallstones. What other information do you need to establish?

Medical background
• Does he have any conditions that predispose to gallstones?

Black pigment stones
• Does he have chronic haemolysis from a prosthetic valve, sickle cell or spherocytosis?
• Does he have a biliary infection?

Brown pigment stones
• Does he suffer from sclerosing cholangitis?

Cholesterol stones
• Has he had a pervious resection of the terminal ileum for cancer or inflammatory bowel disease?
• Is he obese or have a diet lacking in fibre?
• Does he have cirrhosis of the liver?

Medications
Use of the oral contraceptive pill may increase the risk of gallstones.

Family history
Predisposition to gallstones may run in families, although the genetic basis is not well understood.

He has had primary immune thrombocytopenia, diverticular disease and duodenal ulcer. He also has essential hypertension and type 2 diabetes mellitus. His medications are ranitidine 150 mg bd, omeprazole 20 mg od, amlodipine 10 mg od and mebeverine 135 mg tds. He is an ex-smoker of 30 years with a 20 pack-year history. He drinks up to a bottle of wine and a nip of whiskey per night. He has a healthy diet. There is no family history.

What features are you interested in on examination?

General examination
• Does he have evidence of pyrexia, tachycardia or hypotension suggestive of systemic sepsis?
• Does he have jaundiced skin or sclera? Are there any scratch marks or excoriations?
• Are there xanthalasma of the eyelids or xanthomas in the palmar creases or tendons?

Abdominal examination
• Does he have right upper quadrant tenderness? Is there rebound tenderness or local peritonism?
• Is there a palpable, inflamed and tender gallbladder or liver?

On examination, he is clinically well. He is not jaundiced. There is tenderness to deep palpation in the right upper quadrant with active bowel sounds. There is no palpable organomegaly.

What investigations do you want to do?
Tests should be directed at identifying the presence of gallstones and their consequences.

Bloods tests
These may be normal despite the presence of gallstones, chronic cholecystitis and, in the elderly, even in the presence of cholangitis.
• Liver chemistry and the prothrombin time as a measure of hepatic synthetic function are the most important tests. A raised conjugated bilirubin, ALP and γ-GT suggest common bile duct (CBD) stones. An elevated ALT may be seen in acute biliary obstruction. Coagulopathy may be present due to malabsorption of fats and fat-soluble vitamins including vitamin K, which is necessary for the maturation of certain clotting factors.
• A full blood count may show a leucocytosis in acute cholecystitis and cholangitis. Thrombocytopenia is probable in this man with idiopathic thrombocytopenia. Platelets may also be raised in inflammation or may fall in acute sepsis.
• Elevated CRP can be seen in acute cholecystitis and cholangitis.

Ultrasound scan
This should be done to detect gallstones in the gallbladder. These may not be seen due to gas, unusual anatomy or small size. The scan may show dilated bile ducts from obstruction, gallbladder inflammation with a thickened wall, or a dilated pancreatic duct and pancreatic inflammation.

Abdominal X-ray
This may show calcified gallstones. It is not done routinely in most patients unless looking for obstruction, mucosal oedema or a toxic megacolon.

Magnetic resonance cholangiopancreatography

MRCP is a sensitive and specific method of detecting bile duct dilatation and gallstones in the biliary system. It also allows for detection of other lesions such as pancreatic head tumours or cholangiocarcinoma, where the symptoms can mimic those caused by gallstones.

Endoscopic retrograde cholangiopancreatography

ERCP can also be used to detect gallstones and the biliary and pancreatic ducts, although the risk of potential complications, such as pancreatitis, bleeding, perforation and sedation effects, means that it is much less favoured.

ERCP allows the endoscopist to potentially remove gallstones that are obstructing the bile ducts or pancreatic duct (Fig. 19.1). Therefore it remains a good combined diagnostic and therapeutic procedure.

> *His blood tests confirmed normal liver function. Amylase was normal.*
>
> *The abdominal ultrasound showed a fatty liver and an 11 mm gallbladder calculus, with sludge in the gallbladder. The gallbladder was contracted and small. The gallbladder wall and common bile duct were normal.*

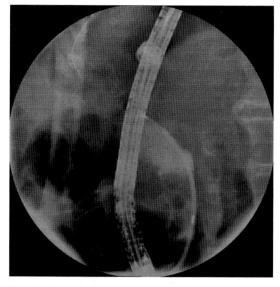

Fig. 19.1 ERCP showing multifaceted gallstones in the distal common bile duct. A plastic stent is being inserted. (Courtesy of the Gastroenterology Department, John Radcliffe Hospital.)

You have the results of his investigations. What do you tell him?

The ultrasound shows the presence of gallstones and biliary sludge in the gallbladder. Up to 15% of the normal population have gallstones, which become more common with increasing age. Most gallstones stay in the fundus of the gallbladder and do not cause any symptoms. It is likely that one of his gallstones has become stuck in the cystic duct, a passage between the gallbladder and the common bile duct, which is causing his symptoms.

He probably has chronic cholecystitis with recurrent episodes of biliary colic. Dyspepsia aggravated by eating fatty meals is a typical symptom of gallstone-associated disease.

What treatment do you offer him?

Surgical intervention by elective laparoscopic or open cholecystectomy (removal of the gallbladder) is indicated for acute and chronic cholecystitis. Laparoscopic techniques are preferred to shorten the hospital stay, reduce postoperative pain and increase speed of returning to work.

Rare complications include biliary leak, stricture of the bile duct and retained stones. Post-cholecystectomy syndrome, which is associated with ongoing pain in the right upper quadrant, may occur in as many as 10% of those undergoing cholecystectomy.

> *He talks to a general surgeon about the risks of the procedure and goes away to think about the operation.*
>
> *Two months later he returns with shaking episodes and hot flushes. He describes nausea, vomiting, severe right upper abdominal pain and loss of appetite with 6 kg weight loss. On examination he is pyrexial, clinically jaundiced and tender in the right upper quadrant with no signs of peritonism.*

What has happened?

He has developed a complication of gallstone disease. Gallstones may pass into the bile ducts and cause transient or persistent obstruction, which carries a risk of infection in the obstructed duct system. A stone in the cystic duct obstructing the gallbladder can cause cholecystitis. An impacted stone in the common bile duct, intra- and extrahepatic ducts can cause ascending cholangitis. Pancreatitis may be due to a stone obstructing the ampulla of Vater or the common bile duct causing pancreatic obstruction and inflammation.

PART 2: CASES

Box 19.1 Consequences of gallstones

- *Acute cholecystitis* caused by a gallstone in the cystic duct or acalculus disease due to trauma or polyarteritis. It presents with persistent right upper abdominal pain, fever and raised inflammatory markers
- *Chronic cholecystitis* causing intermittent biliary colic, fat intolerance, dyspepsia and other non-specific symptoms
- *CBD stones* can cause transient or persistent obstruction. They may pass spontaneously and can cause jaundice and abdominal pain
- *Cholangitis* is an ascending infection in the biliary tree due to obstruction of the main bile ducts. The most common cause is an impacted CBD stone. Features include abdominal pain, jaundice and fever (Charcot's triad)
- *Mirizzi's syndrome* is due to a stone in the cystic duct causing compression of the hepatic duct and resulting in obstructive jaundice
- *Pancreatitis* can be caused by a gallstone blocking the pancreatic duct
- *Empyema of the gallbladder* can cause gangrene and is the result of recurrent and persistent infection. It presents with a pattern of sepsis. Perforation and peritonitis can occur
- *Biliary fistula* can form from a chronically inflamed gallbladder. A gallstone ileus can occur due to impaction of the stone at the ileocaecal valve
- *Carcinoma of the gallbladder or bile ducts* (cholangiocarcinoma) presents with jaundice abdominal pain and weight loss

---

What investigations are needed now?

These tests should confirm a consequence of gallstone disease and look for other possible causes including carcinoma.

- *Repeat blood tests* including full blood count, liver function, coagulation and C-reactive protein.
- *Abdominal ultrasound scan* to look for dilated ducts and a CBD stone, and for gallbladder wall thickening and inflammation.
- *MRCP* to identify dilated ducts and a CBD stone or obstructing mass.
- *Endoscopic ultrasound* is used in some specialised centres to visualise gallstones in the biliary tree.
- *CT scans* are used in other centres to look for a dilated duct which is not visualised on ultrasound. They are less sensitive than MRCP at detecting gallstone.

Blood tests showed an elevated bilirubin of 33 μmol/L, ALP 211 U/L, γ-GT 350 IU/L, ALT 220 U/L and albumin 27 g/L. His prothrombin time was prolonged at 16 s. His inflammatory markers were elevated, with a CRP of 45 mg/L and WCC of 14.2 × 10⁹/L. His platelets were 18 × 10⁹/L.

An MRCP demonstrated dilatation of the CBD to 9 mm and a well-defined oval signal void (calculus) in the lower common bile duct. There were multiple calculi in a normal gallbladder.

What is the treatment?

He has bacterial cholangitis due to a distal CBD stone. Mortality can be as high as 10%.

General management

He should be given intravenous fluids, analgesia and broad-spectrum antibiotics. Blood cultures should be taken to identify an organism and target antibiotic cover. A third generation cephalosporin or ciprofloxacin with metronidazole to provide cover against enteric Gram-negative organisms and anaerobes are reasonable choices for empirical treatment. Vitamin K is given parenterally to correct vitamin K deficiency and reverse clotting abnormalities prior to drainage.

Endoscopic retrograde cholangiopancreatography

Urgent drainage is required by ERCP. This provides contrast-enhanced images of the biliary tree in real time. Stones can be removed endoscopically by basket or balloon trawl and allowed to pass spontaneously after sphincterotomy. Stents may be inserted.

Percutaneous transhepatic cholangiography

This is indicated in the presence of dilated ducts when ERCP is not technically possible.

Surgical intervention

Emergency surgery in bacterial cholangitis has a high mortality. Early elective laparoscopic or open cholecystectomy should be done after ERCP and sphincterotomy done to remove the source of the stones. Perioperative cholangiography is advocated by some to confirm clearance of the bile duct, even after sphincterotomy.

He was admitted to the hospital and treated with intravenous fluids and intravenous tazocin (according to local antibiotic guidelines). He received three doses of vitamin K for coagulopathy and was given 60mg of prednisolone for 72h as advised by the haematologists for his idiopathic thrombocytopenia.

Urgent ERCP demonstrated a 1cm lower CBD stone and proximal CBD dilatation. A biliary sphincterotomy and balloon trawl was done to remove the stone. His symptoms settled quickly and his biochemical abnormalities resolved over the next few days.

Two months later he had an uncomplicated laparoscopic cholecystectomy.

CASE REVIEW

Right upper quadrant pain has many causes. This may be due to disease of organs in the direct anatomical area or due to disease in other organs with pain referred from elsewhere.

Gallstone disease is asymptomatic in the majority (up to 80%) of patients. Complications include cholecystitis, cholangitis, pancreatitis, empyema, fistula and cancer. The presence of complicated disease necessitates more urgent treatment.

This patient had features consistent with chronic cholecystitis. He developed ascending cholangitis. MRCP confirmed a common bile duct stone with dilated proximal ducts. He required urgent drainage by ERCP and sphincterotomy and proceeded to elective outpatient cholecystectomy with no further complications.

KEY POINTS

- Gallstones affect up to 20% of the population in the Western world and the incidence increases with age.
- Gallstones are asymptomatic in over 80% of patients and ARE detected incidentally on imaging for other reasons.
- Gallstones are only treated if symptomatic.
- Gallstones are easily detected by abdominal ultrasound scan, and are poorly visible on X-ray and CT scan because they are typically rich in fat.
- MRCP is a good way to delineate the biliary tree and any stones non-invasively.
- ERCP allows the endoscopist to treat gallstone disease by removing stones, although it carries a risk of causing pancreatitis and ascending cholangitis.
- Gallstones can cause severe symptoms, including acute and chronic cholecystitis, ascending cholangitis, acute and chronic pancreatitis and multisystem failure.
- If there is acute cholangitis or recurrent pancreatitis, gallstones can be effectively removed by ERCP.
- Symptomatic gallstones disease should be treated by cholecystectomy, which should ideally be performed electively.

PART 2: CASES

Case 20 A 19-year-old man with acute abdominal pain

A 19-year-old man, Ian Grove, presents to the emergency department with severe central abdominal pain with nausea and vomiting. He is rolling around in agony with tears in his eyes. He has never experienced pain like this before.

What is the first thing you want to do?

Ask him if he has any allergies or takes any regular pain medications. Prescribe him a small amount of fast-acting opioid analgesia, such as pethidine or morphine. This will make him more comfortable, enable him to answer your questions and examine him.

What do you want to know about his abdominal pain?

Abdominal pain

There are 10 main features you want to address when asking a patient to describe abdominal pain:

- Character: dull ache, colicky spasms, deep or superficial.
- Location.
- Radiation: to back, loins, groin, chest, shoulder tip or other area of the abdomen.
- Onset: sudden or gradual.
- Progression: is it becoming more severe and intense or constant?
- Intensity: grading scale from 1 to 10, with 10 the worst pain imaginable.
- Frequency: this can be the number of times in a day/week/month/year.
- Duration: when was it first noticed? This may be a prior episode.

- Aggravating and relieving factors: related to posture, eating meals, worsened by movement, inspiration or coughing, better on lying still.
- Associated symptoms.

Associated gastrointestinal symptoms

- Does he have heartburn or reflux? Think peptic ulcer.
- Is there associated nausea and vomiting? Did this precede the pain? What is its frequency and character? Is there haematemesis? Think gallstones, appendicitis and pancreatitis.
- Has he lost his appetite? Is there any weight loss? He may have an inflammatory condition, such as Crohn's disease with a stricture and obstructive symptoms. He is young and unlikely to have a malignant process.
- Has he had a change in bowel habit? Is there rectal bleeding or melaena? Are there oily stools that are smelly and difficult to flush (steatorrhoea)? Think peptic ulcer and pancreatitis, respectively.
- Does he feel feverish or has he had a rigor? Has he become jaundiced? Is he itching? Think of cholecystitis and cholangitis.

Systemic enquiry

Ask questions to identify evidence of multisystem disease, referred pain or additional pathology.

- Does he have any respiratory symptoms such as a cough, wheeze, sputum and breathlessness? Consider basal pneumonia and pleurisy.
- Does he have cardiac symptoms such as palpitations, chest pain, orthopnoea or syncope? Consider cardiac ischaemia, mesenteric ischaemia or pericarditis causing pain.
- Does he have neurological symptoms such as weakness, paraesthesia, spinal pain, gait disturbance or incontinence? Consider spinal lesions or prolapse with radiation of pain.
- Does he have any urological symptoms of frequency, urgency, loin pain or haematuria? Is he in urinary retention? Pain may radiate from renal calculi.

Gastroenterology: Clinical Cases Uncovered, 1st edition.
© S. Keshav and E. Culver. Published 2011 by Blackwell Publishing Ltd.

• Dose he have a rash? Consider herpes zoster even in the absence of a rash if the pain is dermatomal in distribution.
• Does he have a hernia or testicular problem? Could he have torsion of his testes?
• Has he had a prodromal viral illness? Consider viral or bacterial pancreatitis.

Past history

• Has he had recent surgery? Adhesions could cause intestinal obstruction.
• Has he had recent traumatic injury? Consider delayed splenic rupture.
• Has he had a recent viral infection? Consider pancreatitis due to mumps.
• Does he have a history of gallstone disease or peptic ulcer?

Medications

• Does he take any regular analgesics for pain? Opioid addiction should not be assumed but always considered in the context of prior seeking for opioid drugs.
• Does he take other medications either prescribed or over-the-counter? For example, a side effect of thiopurines (azathioprine, mercaptopurine) is pancreatitis.

Social history

• Does he drink alcohol, and how much? Does alcohol influence the pain? Consider pancreatitis.
• Does he smoke or is he a recent ex-smoker? This is relevant in inflammatory bowel disease.

Family history

• Are there any abdominal complaints that could be inherited? For example, hereditary pancreatitis.

He tells you the pain started suddenly in the central upper abdomen yesterday and has become progressively worse. It is constant and dull. It makes him feel sick and he has vomited food and bilious fluid three to four times. He has loose stools, opening his bowels three times today. He did not look to see if there was blood. He feels warm but does not describe a fever or rigors.

He has no previous medical problems and takes no regular medications. He does not smoke and only drinks at weekends with his friends. He denies binge drinking. He is studying to be a vet and is in his third term at university. There is no family history.

Examination
General examination

• *Vital signs*: determine his temperature, pulse, blood pressure, respiratory rate and oxygen saturations to look for haemodynamic compromise.
• *Glasgow coma score*: determine level of consciousness (beware because opiate analgesia can cause drowsiness and constricted pinpoint pupils).
• *Scleral icterus*: jaundice may be accompanied by excoriations or scratch marks from itching.
• *Cervical lymphadenopathy*: suggestive of mesenteric adenitis.

Abdominal examination

• Bluish discolouration around the umbilicus (Cullen's sign) or reddish-brown discolouration along the flanks (Grey Turner's sign) from retroperitoneal blood in severe necrotising pancreatitis (see Plate 20.1).
• Scars, distension or visible peristalsis. Consider adhesions if there has been prior surgery.
• Abdominal tenderness, rebound and guarding. Are there signs of peritonism?
• Palpable masses or organomegaly, for example an appendiceal abscess or inflamed gallbladder.
• Bowel sounds may be hyperactive in obstruction and quiet in peritonitis.
• Hernia orifices should be examined for an obstructed hernia.

Digital rectal examination

Tender rectal examination may occur in appendicitis, depending on the position of the inflamed appendix.

Testes examination

A testes exam should be done to exclude torsion.

Systemic examination

• Chest exam: are there chest crepitations indicative of a pneumonia or acute respiratory distress syndrome (ARDS)? Is there a clinical pleural effusion?
• Cardiac exam: pericarditic rub or heart murmur?
• Neurological exam: focal neurology or spinal tenderness with a sensory level?
• Renal angles: loin tenderness?
• Skin exam: rash with vesicles from herpes zoster? Widespread purpuric rash from disseminated intravascular coagulation (DIC)?

He looks unwell on examination. His blood pressure is 80/40 mmHg, pulse is 120 beats/min and he has a low grade pyrexia of 37.5°C. His abdomen is tender in the epigastrium and central abdomen with voluntary guarding and hypoactive bowel sounds. He is not peritonitic. Chest sounds are vesicular bilaterally and heart sounds are normal with no rubs or murmurs. There is no musculoskeletal tenderness or focal neurology. His testes are normal. There is no tenderness on DRE.

KEY POINTS

- A careful abdominal pain history is crucial in narrowing the range of differential causes.
- Referred pain from non-abdominal sites should be considered in the differential.
- Never forget the testes and hernia orifices in assessment of abdominal pain.

What is your differential diagnosis?

The differential diagnosis of acute abdominal pain is vast. He is a young man, only 19 years old, and describes an epigastric, dull, constant ache with associated nausea, vomiting and change of bowel habit. Differential diagnoses include:

- Peptic ulcer.
- Gastritis.
- Acute pancreatitis.
- Gallstones.
- Renal stones.
- Mesenteric adenitis.
- Intestinal obstruction.
- Cholecystitis.
- Addison's crisis.
- Sickle cell crisis.
- Acute intermittent porphyria.

What investigations are appropriate?

There are some general investigations that should be done for all causes of abdominal pain and more specific ones depending on the likely cause.

General investigations
Blood tests

- Full blood count should be taken for evidence of anaemia (inflammatory bowel disease, peptic ulcer) and leucocytosis (inflammatory or infective disease).
- C-reactive protein is elevated in many inflammatory and infective conditions.

- Urea, creatinine and electrolytes may be affected by dehydration, vomiting and diarrhoea.
- Liver function may be abnormal in cholangitis, hepatitis and sepsis of any source.
- Coagulation may be impaired, especially in sepsis with DIC.
- Serum amylase and/or lipase may be markedly raised in acute pancreatitis and minimally elevated in small intestinal obstruction, mesenteric ischaemia, infarcted bowel, perforated peptic ulcer or renal insufficiency.
- Calcium and albumin levels to detect hypercalcaemia, which may cause abdominal pain.
- Blood glucose for pancreatic endocrine dysfunction and in diabetic ketoacidosis.

Urine

Dipstick may show blood and protein in pyelonephritis. A midstream urine specimen should be sent for culture.

Electrocardiogram

This will identify an arrhythmia or ischaemia.

Arterial blood gas

- Metabolic acidosis in sepsis, infarcted bowel and diabetic ketoacidosis. Lactate may be raised.
- Hypoxia may occur in chest pathology.

Chest X-ray

A CXR will look for evidence of air under the diaphragm from a perforated viscus. This will also identify consolidation or an effusion.

Abdominal X-ray

This is used to look for dilated loops of bowel in obstruction, mucosal oedema of an inflamed colon, local ileus (sentinel loop) in pancreatitis or appendicitis. Calculi in the renal system and gallbladder may be seen. Pancreatic calcification may be seen in chronic pancreatitis.

Abdominal ultrasound

This is used to identify a localised abscess, free fluid in the abdomen, gallstone disease and dilated ducts, gallbladder empyema, pancreatic inflammation and oedema.

Specific investigations

- Calcium, cholesterol and triglycerides. These levels are important in the aetiology of pancreatitis (hypercalcaemia, hyperlipidaemia) or complications of pancreatitis (hypocalcaemia).

- Sickling test. This should be done for sickle cell disease.
- Short Synacthen test. This should be done to exclude Addison's disease. A random cortisol is not sufficient to make the diagnosis.
- Urinary porphobilogens. Consider for acute intermittent porphyria.
- CT abdomen. This may be done to look for abdominal catastrophe, infarcted bowel or a perforated viscus. It may show evidence of pancreatic inflammation, oedema and necrosis or complications such as pseudocysts or fluid collections.
- Upper gastrointestinal endoscopy. It should be done if peptic ulcer disease is suspected.
- Small bowel enema or MRI enterocolysis ± colonoscopy. These should be done to detect small bowel and colonic Crohn's disease or lymphoma.

Mr Grove's blood tests show a grossly elevated amylase at 2000 U/dL. His liver function and coagulation are normal. His calcium level is normal. Abdominal X-ray and chest X-rays are normal. There is no evidence of free air.

An abdominal ultrasound was booked to look for evidence of gallstones or pancreatic inflammation or cysts. There are no stones. There is fat standing around a poorly visualised pancreas.

What is the most likely diagnosis?

Acute pancreatitis is diagnosed from classic clinical features of severe constant abdominal pain, which may radiate to the back in half of patients, with nausea, vomiting and elevated pancreatic enzymes. Pancreatic enzymes are released that autodigest duct tissue, causing damage and possible necrosis. It is a multisystem disorder.

What are the causes of acute pancreatitis?

According to the British Society of Gastroenterology guidelines the aetiology of acute pancreatitis should be determined in at least 80% of cases (no more than 20% should be classified as idiopathic). Alcohol exposure and biliary tract disease cause most cases.

Box 20.1 Causes of acute pancreatitis

- Gallstones: the most important cause in most developed countries is a small stone passing into the bile duct and becoming lodged at the sphincter of Oddi

- Alcohol: this usually affects habitual drinkers although it may develop in those with a binging habit. Alcoholics are usually admitted with an acute exacerbation of chronic pancreatitis
- Post-ERCP pancreatitis: prospective studies have shown the risk is at least 5%. The risk is increased with an inexperienced endoscopist, sphincter of Oddi dysfunction or manometry on the sphincter
- Trauma: pancreatic injury occurs more often in penetrating injuries (e.g. from knives, bullets) than in blunt abdominal trauma (e.g. from steering wheels, bicycles)
- Drugs: these cause a mild pancreatitis. Examples include azathioprine, 6-mercaptopurine, sulfonamides, tetracycline, sodium valproate, methyldopa, oestrogens, frusemide (furosemide), 5-aminosalicylic acid compounds, corticosteroids and octreotide
- Infection: several infections can cause pancreatitis. Viral causes include mumps, EBV, coxsackie virus, echovirus, varicella-zoster and measles. Bacterial causes include *Mycoplasma pneumoniae*, *Salmonella*, *Campylobacter* and *Mycobacterium tuberculosis*
- Autoimmune pancreatitis: IgG4 levels are measured and raised. Typical imaging and histological features and response to steroids help to confirm diagnosis
- Hereditary: this is due to mutations in PRSSI, CFTR or SPINK-1
- Hypercalcaemia: causes include hyperparathyroidism, excessive doses of vitamin D, familial hypocalciuric hypercalcaemia and total parenteral nutrition
- Hypertriglyceridaemia: clinically significant pancreatitis occurs with a serum triglyceride level of over 20 mmol/L. It is associated with type I and type V hyperlipidaemia
- Malignancy obstructing the pancreatic ductal system
- Developmental abnormalities of the pancreas: pancreas divisium and annular pancreas
- Vascular abnormalities: vasculitis can predispose to pancreatic ischaemia, especially in those with polyarteritis nodosa and systemic lupus erythematosus
- Idiopathic: occult microlithiasis is probably responsible for most cases of idiopathic acute pancreatitis

What specific investigations should be ordered?

Tests are ordered to determine the cause and severity of acute pancreatitis.

- *Blood tests* include pancreatic enzymes in plasma, liver function tests, fasting plasma lipids and fasting plasma calcium.

• *Imaging* includes ultrasound of the gallbladder to identify gallstones, MRCP or CT-enhanced imaging (helical or multislice with pancreas protocol) to look for evidence of pancreatic inflammation, tumour and complications of pancreatitis.

What are the severity markers of acute pancreatitis?

The Glasgow system is a simple prognostic system that uses the data collected during the first 48 h following an admission for pancreatitis (Table 20.1). There is a minimum score of 0 and maximum score of 8. Severe pancreatitis is likely with a score equal or greater than 3.

Patients with persisting organ failure and new organ failure, and in those with persisting pain and signs of sepsis after a week of admission, will require evaluation by dynamic contrast-enhanced CT. CT evidence of necrosis correlates well with the risk of other local and systemic complications.

Table 20.1 Glasgow scoring system for pancreatitis.

Parameter	Finding at any time during initial 48 h	Points
Age	>55 years	1
	≤55 years	0
Serum albumin	<3.2 g/dL	1
	≥3.2 g/dL	0
Prterial PO_2 on room air	<60 mmHg	1
	≥60 mmHg	0
Serum calcium	<8 mg/dL	1
	≥8 mg/dL	0
Blood glucose	>180 mg/dL	1
	≤180 mg/dL	0
Serum LDH	>600 U/L	1
	≤600 U/L	0
Serum urea nitrogen	>45 mg/dL	1
	≤45 mg/dL	0
WBC count	>15 000 cells/μL	1
	≤15 000 cells/μL	0

What are the treatment options for acute pancreatitis?

The management of acute pancreatitis is mainly supportive. The aim is to provide aggressive supportive care, to decrease inflammation, to limit infection or superinfection, and to identify and treat complications as appropriate.

• Oxygenation (to maintain saturations of over 95%).

• Aggressive prompt fluid resuscitation to treat haemodynamic instability and prevent potential systemic complications.

• Fluid balance and urine output should be measured. A central venous catheter should be inserted in high-risk individuals. Urinary catheterisation to monitor urine output may be necessary.

• He should remain nil by mouth initially, to allow inflammation to settle.

• Feeding should be introduced enterally as the patient's anorexia and pain resolves, starting on a low fat diet.

• Analgesics are administered for pain relief.

• Antibiotics are generally not indicated, although in the presence of fever and evidence of systemic sepsis which may suggest necrosis, broad-spectrum antibiotics are often given. There is no consensus in the type of antibiotic used or duration of use. Intravenous co-amoxiclav and metronidazole are often prescribed.

• High dependency care should be offered to all patients with severe acute pancreatitis. They should be managed in a high dependency unit with full monitoring and systems support. Within hours to days a number of complications may develop. These include shock, pulmonary failure, renal failure, gastrointestinal bleeding and multiorgan system failure. Infection of necrosis is the most serious local complication of acute pancreatitis and is associated with a high mortality rate of up to 40%.

• Therapeutic ERCP with sphincterotomy should be performed urgently if an ultrasound shows evidence of gallstones and if the cause of pancreatitis is believed to be biliary, in patients who have severe pancreatitis, and if there is cholangitis, jaundice or a dilated common bile duct.

• Cholecystectomy should be performed during the same hospital admission if gallstone pancreatitis is thought to be the cause. This is the ideal, although some units refer for urgent outpatient cholecystectomy.

• Surgical treatment is not needed for most patients with acute pancreatitis. Those with infected necrosis will require intervention to completely debride all cavities containing necrotic material. The choice of surgical technique for necrosectomy, and subsequent postoperative management, depends on individual features and locally available expertise.

Mr Grove was admitted to hospital. He had a severity score of 1 in the first 48 h. He received oxygen, intravenous fluids and antibiotics. His pain settled over the first 72 h and his amylase gradually decreased. On day 5 he was discharged pain free.

He re-presented 4 weeks later with severe upper abdominal pain with an associated rise in amylase level.

What may have happened?

He recovered well from his acute pancreatitis and had a low severity score on the Glasgow criteria. He has presented again with features of acute pancreatitis or a possible complication, such as a pancreatic pseudocyst (Table 20.2).

What tests should be done for recurrent acute idiopathic pancreatitis?

• Repeat abdominal ultrasound to detect gallstones missed on the initial scan.

• Viral antibody titres for viral infections.
• IgG4 for autoimmune pancreatitis in those with no other risk factors.
• Autoantibodies for vasculitis.
• Pancreatic function tests to exclude chronic pancreatitis.
• Genetic analysis in those with a family history or in those that present at a young age.
• Consider an endoscopic ultrasound, ERCP with bile and pancreatic cytology, and sphincter of Oddi manometry in those with a possible biliary source.

What is chronic pancreatitis?

Chronic pancreatitis is the result of recurrent pancreatic inflammation. This can cause endocrine and exocrine deficiency. Abdominal pain may be severe and constant due to damage of sensory nerves and scarring and obstruction of the duct.

Malabsorption develops due to pancreatic enzyme deficiency and diabetes mellitus due to insulin insufficiency. Treatment includes oral pancreatic supplements, insulin if diabetic and analgesia.

Table 20.2 Complications of pancreatitis.

Complications	Description
Pseudocysts	These are collections of pancreatic fluid enclosed by a wall of granulation tissue
	Features include abdominal pain and persistent elevated serum amylase, usually 4 weeks after the acute episode. They may be palpable as an abdominal mass. They are detected by ultrasound or CT scanning
	Treatment involves analgesia and nutritional support
	They usually resolve spontaneously if less than 6 cm. If they continue to grow and are associated with obstructive jaundice or persistent pain then drainage is indicated by endoscopic, percutaneous or surgical means
Acute fluid collections	These occur early in the course of acute pancreatitis
	They are detected by imaging studies
	They require no specific therapy as they lack a defined wall and usually regress spontaneously
Intra-abdominal infections	Fluid collections or pancreatic necrosis can become infected within the first 3 weeks
Pancreatic abscess	This is a circumscribed intra-abdominal collection of pus, within or in proximity to the pancreas. It may arise from localised necrosis, with subsequent liquefaction that becomes infected. It may develop in the first 3–6 weeks
Pancreatic necrosis	This is a non-viable area of pancreatic parenchyma that is often associated with peripancreatic fat necrosis. It is diagnosed on dynamic spiral CT scans. Distinguishing between infected and sterile pancreatic necrosis is difficult
	Sterile pancreatic necrosis is treated with aggressive medical management. Infected pancreatic necrosis requires surgical debridement or percutaneous drainage

PART 2: CASES

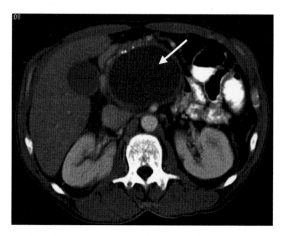

Fig. 20.1 CT abdomen showing a large pancreatic pseudocyst. (Courtesy of the Gastroenterology Department, John Radcliffe Hospital.)

He had a repeat abdominal ultrasound which showed multiple, small, fluid-filled pseudocysts (maximum diameter 4 cm) around the pancreatic tail. There were no gallstones or biliary dilatation. A CT abdomen confirmed the pseudocysts and demonstrated an oedematous pancreas (Fig. 20.1).

He had a full screen for recurrent pancreatitis with negative results. He eventually returned to the clinic for genetic screening and was found to be SPINK-1 positive. He was diagnosed with hereditary pancreatitis. There is no definite treatment for this. He has a 40% risk of developing pancreatic carcinoma by the age of 70 years.

CASE REVIEW

Acute abdominal pain has a wide list of differential causes. Often, the key to finding the cause is in a careful abdominal pain history and abdominal examination. This should include an examination of the hernia, testes and a digital rectal exam. A systemic search for causes of referred pain is also important. This can be complemented by blood tests and imaging.

This young man had severe central and upper abdominal pain with nausea, vomiting and altered bowel habit. Investigations confirmed an elevated amylase level consistent with acute pancreatitis. Gallstones and alcohol are the most common causes.

Patients with pancreatitis require assessment into the initial severity, evidence or organ failure and complications. Calculation of the Glasgow score on admission helps to predict prognosis. Treatment is predominately supportive and directed at reversal of an underlying cause if found. Recurrent episodes should encourage a repeat exclusion of the common causes and a screen for atypical causes in an effort to limit complications and preserve pancreatic function.

KEY POINTS

- Acute abdominal pain has many causes: gastrointestinal, hepatobiliary, urological, gynaecological, vascular, retroperitoneal, musculoskeletal, referred pain and medical causes.
- Symptoms and signs will guide further investigations.
- Acute pancreatitis is diagnosed by classic abdominal pain, nausea and vomiting and markedly elevated pancreatic enzymes.

- Where doubt exists, pancreatic imaging by contrast-enhanced CT scan provides good evidence for the presence or absence of pancreatitis. In the presence of persisting organ failure, signs of sepsis or deterioration in clinical status, a CT scan should also be done.
- Complications of pancreatitis can develop weeks after the initial infection.

Miss Jackie Potts, a 35-year-old woman, was admitted to the medical assessment unit. You are the physician on call. She had been reviewed by a locum general practitioner at home that morning after 'collapsing' to the floor. Over the last few weeks she has become progressively weak and unable to stand. When the GP arrived, her friend was with her. Her blood sugar (BM test) was 2.mmol/L. He gave her some Glucogel glucose solution and arranged for emergency admission to the hospital. He has never met her before.

You are the first to see her in the medical assessment unit. She looks thin and weak. What questions will you ask?
Presenting complaint
Obtain the details of her collapse. Was there a prodrome? Has it happened before? Did she hit her head or loose consciousness? Was there any seizure activity or post-ictal period? Did she definitely collapse? If so, do you think her collapse was the result of the low glucose level or could there be another cause and this was just an incidental finding?

Low glucose
• Was she sweaty, hungry or tremulous (autonomic features of hypoglycaemia)?
• Was she drowsy, agitated or did she have a seizure (neuroglycopenic features of hypoglycaemia)?
• When was the last time she ate? Is this fasting or post-prandial hypoglycaemia?
• If this is due to fasting, does she have diabetes? Is she taking sulphonureas or insulin? Has she taken someone else's insulin? Has she been on a recent alcohol binge without eating?

Gastroenterology: Clinical Cases Uncovered, 1st edition.
© S. Keshav and E. Culver. Published 2011 by
Blackwell Publishing Ltd.

• Does she suffer from liver disease or Addison's disease?
• Is she starving herself? Is she known to have a psychiatric condition or eating disorder?

She tells you she has felt progressively weaker over the last few weeks and called her friend for help with the shopping. When her friend arrived, she felt tired and a little light-headed. She could barely stand and the GP was informed. There was no actual collapse. She did not hit her head or loose consciousness.

Further questioning reveals a 10-year history of anorexia nervosa. She has had five prior admissions to the centre for adult eating disorders with significant psychopathology relative to body image. She feels her life isn't worth living. Her brother has recently relapsed with myeloma and she has subsequently slipped backwards with regards to eating and weight. She feels ashamed of this but is reluctant for help.

What other information do you want to know?
Symptoms of malnutrition and vitamin/mineral deficiencies (Table 21.1)
• Does she feel listless and lethargic? Malnutrition and anaemia as well as other systemic illnesses can cause this non-specific symptom.
• Does she have paraesthesia, focal weakness and balance or coordination difficulties?
• Does she have problems with her memory or recall?
• Does she have any new rashes or skin complaints? Are her gums bleeding?
• Is she experiencing altered bowel habit or abdominal discomfort?
• Is she menstruating? When was the last time she had a normal menstrual period? Anorexia and malnutrition can cause secondary ovarian failure and amenorrhoea.
• Symptoms of anaemia. Does she have chest pains or breathlessness on exertion?

Table 21.1 Clinical features of mineral and vitamin deficiency.

Deficiency	Clinical features
Mineral deficiency	
Iron (ferritin <15 μg/L)	Glossitis, cheiliosis, koilonychias and anaemia (microcytic)
Calcium (corrected <2.2 mmol/L)	Chvostek's sign (jaw), Trousseau's sign (arm) tetany
	Weakness, proximal myopathy and perioral paraesthesia
Magnesium (<0.7 mmol/L)	Myopathy
Phosphate (<0.8 mmol/L)	Proximal myopathy
Copper (red cell superoxide dismutase activity)	Osteoporosis, anaemia (hypochromic) and low white cell count
Zinc (<6 μmol/L)	Crusty red rash, anorexia, depression, diarrhoea and candidaisis
Selenium (glutathione peroxidase activity)	Cardiac failure
Vitamin deficiency	
Vitamin C (ascorbic acid)	Poor wound healing, gum hyperplasia and bleeding, and perifollicular haemorrhages
Folate (<120 ng/L)	Anaemia (macrocytic)
Vitamin B_{12} (<150 ng/L)	Painful neuropathy, ataxia, poor proprioception and anaemia (macrocytic)
Thiamine B_1 (red cell transketolase)	Ophthalmoplegia, ataxia, neuropathy, confusion, psychosis and cardiac failure
Riboflavin B_2 (red cell glutathione reductase)	Angular stomatitis, fissures in the lips, ataxia, apathy and anaemia (normochromic)
Pyridoxine B_6 (aminotransferase activity)	Neuropathy and anaemia (sideroblastic)
Nicotinamide (urine metabolities)	Dermatitis, diarrhoea and memory impairment/dementia

Past medical history
- Does she have any other medical co-morbidity?
- Does she suffer from depression or psychiatric illness?

Medications
- Does she abuse laxatives, diuretics or antiobesity pills?
- Does she take over-the-counter 'slimming tablets'?

Social history
- Does she drink alcohol or smoke cigarettes?
- Is she employed?
- What is her social support network like? Does she have family and friends who she can trust and support her?

She feels tired and lethargic all the time. She never goes out to visit friends as she has no energy. She has difficulties with balance but considers this due to her weakness. She has difficulty combing her hair and rising from a chair.

Her medical history is of osteoporosis and depression. There is no history of deliberate self-harm or suicidal intent. Medications include alendronate once weekly, Adcal-D₃, citalopram, folate supplementation, domperidone and Movicol.

She lives with her husband, but they have no children. She has not been able to conceive. She is a non smoker and consumes little alcohol. She has not worked for years and claims disability allowance.

What do you look for on examination?
General examination
- Firstly, calculate her body mass index (BMI). The BMI, skin-fold thickness and muscle mass are low in anorexia and malnutrition.
- Document her vital signs for evidence of hypotension, tachycardia or bradycardia and temperature regulation.
- Document the blood glucose and chart this at hourly intervals (given the admission glucose level was low).
- Look for evidence of dehydration.
- Look at and in her mouth. Does she have angular stomatitis, mucosal fissures, glossitis, oral *Candida*, gum hyperplasia and bleeding?
- Look at her skin. Does she have dermatitis, perifollicular haemorrhages or a crusty erythematous rash?
- Look at the nails for evidence of koilonychia.

Specific examination

• *Neurological examination.* Look for peripheral neuropathy, ophthalmoplegia, poor proprioception, ataxia or other focal abnormality.

• *Musculoskeletal examination.* Examine for proximal myopathy by standing from seated with arms folded across the chest, or raising the arms to the back of the head.

• *Cardiac examination.* Look for evidence of cardiac failure. Peripheral oedema may be present due to protein–energy malnutrition (Kwashiorkor).

> On examination she is drowsy, dehydrated and cachexic. She is hypothermic with a core body temperature of 32.8°C. She is bradycardic at 50 beats/min and hypotensive with a pressure of 90/52 mmHg.
>
> She weighs 29.4 kg with a BMI of 11.1. She has mucosal fissures and angular stomatitis. There is a proximal myopathy involving the arms and legs bilaterally. There is no muscle wasting or focal neurology. Respiratory, cardiovascular and abdominal exams are otherwise unremarkable.

What is anorexia nervosa?

Anorexia nervosa is an illness in which individuals maintain a low body weight by dieting, vomiting or excessively exercising. The illness is caused by an anxiety about their body shape and weight. This originates from a fear of being fat or from wanting to be thin. They often see themselves differently to other people and challenge the idea that they should gain weight. They use their ability to be thin as positive reinforcement and a sense of achievement to increase confidence and self-esteem.

Anorexia can cause severe physical and emotional problems because of the effects of starvation on the body. This can lead to loss of muscle strength, reduced bone strength, loss of menstrual periods, sexual disinterest and infertility. The illness can affect relationships with family and friends. It can damage progress in education and employment opportunities.

People who suspect they might have an eating disorder may find it difficult or embarrassing to admit to the problem, seek help and talk about their symptoms to family, friends or health care professionals. They may fear they will be criticised or treated unsympathetically.

What investigations would you like to do for this woman in the medical assessment unit?

Urine dipstick

Urind dipstick test for glucose, ketones (starvation), protein and blood (renal disease).

Blood tests

• Full blood count and haematinics. This should include iron studies, B_{12} and folate levels. Look for evidence of anaemia, marrow suppression and vitamin deficiency.

• Urea, creatinine, liver function and coagulation should be taken for evidence of single or multiple organ failure.

• Electrolytes such as potassium and sodium (routine), magnesium, calcium and phosphate should be checked for low levels that require replacement. These should be corrected prior to feeding being commenced in anyone who is malnourished.

• Random glucose to look for hypoglycaemia.

• Venous bicarbonate should be checked for evidence of metabolic acidosis or alkalosis.

Electrocardiogram

Perform an ECG to measure the corrected QT interval, given the risk of arrhythmias.

> Blood tests show a random glucose of 5.3 mmol/L (after glucose solution). Electrolytes are low: sodium (124 mmol/L), potassium (3.2 mmol/L), phosphate (0.2 mmol/L), magnesium (0.5 mmol/L) and calcium corrected (2.2 mmol/L).
>
> Biochemistry shows a high urea (15.8 mmol/L), normal creatinine (80 μmol/L) and high bilirubin (45 μmol/L), ALT (373 U/L) and ALP (311 U/L), and normal albumin (41 g/L).
>
> Haematology reveals a haemoglobin of 15.6 g/dL, MCV 88 fL and platelets 38 × 10^9/L. Prothrombin time is prolonged at 17.4 s.
>
> On venous gas she had a normal acid–base balance and normal lactate. The ECG shows sinus bradcardia with a normal QT interval. Urine dipstick reveals a trace of protein and blood.

What should you do now?

She has symptoms, signs and blood tests suggestive of severe malnutrition and metabolic compromise. She needs admission into the hospital for intensive treatment.

Does she need sectioning under the Mental Health Act or will she agree to treatment?

If you become so physically ill that there is a serious and immediate risk that you might die, you could be fed against your will. This happens very rarely and will take place only as a last resort. You will be told about your legal rights under the Mental Health Act 1983.

What does treatment involve?

Her management requires a multidisciplinary approach from psychiatrists, gastroenterologists, dieticians, physiotherapists and allied health professionals.
• The first aim is to replace the electrolyte imbalance, vitamins and minerals to allow for gradual feeding.
• The second aim is to increase her weight, usually by 0.5–1 kg a week by nasogastric feeding.
• In addition, psychological treatment should be provided. This is best done by a specialist team from the eating disorders unit. The aims of psychological treatment are to reduce the risk of harm, to encourage weight gain and healthy eating, to reduce other symptoms related to the eating disorder, and to help psychological recovery.

She was willing to have treatment, although reluctant, and did not require a mental health section. She was admitted to the gastroenterology ward under agreement of the lead consultant gastroenterologist. The consultant psychiatrist was actively involved in her care.

She was started on intravenous vitamins (Pabrinex for 72 h) and multivitamins. Intravenous glucose was given to treat hypoglycaemia. She was rehydrated with saline. Electrolytes were replaced intravenously. Refeeding was implemented according to a designed protocol by the dietician at a rate of 5 kcal/kg of feed via a fine bore nasogastric feeding tube.

What are the complications of severe anorexia?

• Haemodynamic instability (blood pressure <80/50, P <40).
• Severe electrolyte imbalance.
• Renal failure.
• Persistent hypoglycaemia, blood glucose <2.5.
• Myelosuppression with platelets $<100 \times 10^9$/L and WCC $<1 \times 10^9$/L.
• QT prolongation on ECG >450 ms.
• Refeeding syndrome once feeding commences.

What is refeeding syndrome and who is at risk?

Refeeding syndrome is the potentially fatal shifts in fluid and electrolytes that may occur in malnourished patients receiving artificial feeding. The hallmark biochemical feature of refeeding is hypophosphataemia.

At-risk groups include the following:
• Those with a BMI <16.
• Unintentional weight loss >15% in the past 3–6 months.
• Starvation (or poor nutritional intake) >10 days.
• Chronic alcoholics.
• Low levels of potassium, magnesium or phosphate prior to feeding.

Box 21.1 Refeeding syndrome

Severe fluid and electrolyte shifts and metabolic implications in malnourished patients undergoing refeeding:
• Hypophosphataemia
• Hypokalaemia
• Hypomagnesaemia
• Altered glucose metabolism
• Fluid balance abnormalities
• Vitamin deficiency

What is the treatment for this?

Provide metabolic and nutritional support during the period of risk (usually 7–10 days). Electrolytes should be replaced:
• Low phosphate <0.3 mmol/L: Addiphos 40 mmol in 500 mL NaCl over 6 h.
• Low potassium <2.5 mmol/L: Sando-K 2 tablets tds or IV fluids with 40 mmol KCl.
• Low magnesium <0.5 mmol/L: IV 50% $MgSO_4$ 24 mmol in 500 mL NaCl over 6–12 h.
• Low calcium: IV calcium gluconate.
• Thiamine: IV Pabrinex (1 pair ampoules) at least 30 min before feed starts and for 72 h after. Thereafter oral thiamine can be administered as needed.
• Low glucose: PO glucose tablets or IV dextrose.

When all biochemistry is normal, feeding can commence. Feeding should start at 5 kcal/kg in those with severe risk, and 20 kcal/kg for those with moderate risk, for the first 24 h then increase gradually over the first week. The dietician (and nutritional team in some hospitals) is responsible for regulating the feeding regimen.

Cardiac monitoring should be done in high-risk patients. Electrolyte levels should be measured daily for the first 3 days until electrolyte levels have stabilised, then three times a week for the next 2 weeks. The fluid balance should be carefully monitored.

> *She developed refeeding syndrome requiring intravenous supplementation with magnesium, phosphate and potassium. She needed daily bloods for electrolytes, close monitoring of fluid balance and gradual nasogastric feeding coordinated by the dietician.*

What was the cause of her abnormal liver function and thrombocytopenia?

Multiple organ failure can develop in malnutrition. Liver dysfunction and failure were primarily due to malnutrition. Coagulopathy was due to vitamin K deficiency, requiring intravenous vitamin K for 3 days. Thrombocytopenia was due to bone marrow failure consistent with malnutrition. These all corrected with feeding and increased weight.

Where should she be discharged to?

Continuous psychiatric support is essential after hospital admission to treat profound metabolic disturbance. She should go to an eating disorders unit for ongoing care.

> *She was discharged for ongoing nutrition to a centre for adult eating disorders 4 weeks after admission. Her weight on discharge was 39.4 kg. She received inpatient psychiatric review and outpatient follow-up. She continued on daily meal plans.*

PART 2: CASES

CASE REVIEW

Anorexia nervosa may present at any age of life, but is most commonly identified in teenagers and young adults. It must not be forgotten in later life. Patients may display symptoms and signs suggestive of vitamin and mineral deficiencies, organ failure and psychological anxiety and distress.

Complications of severe anorexia include haemodynamic instability, electrolyte imbalance, renal failure, persistent hypoglycaemia, myelosuppression, arrhythmias and refeeding syndrome once feeding commences.

Treatment should be done in a multidisciplinary setting. It concentrates on replacing electrolytes, vitamins and minerals, gradual nutritional supplementation to promote weight gain by nasogastric feeding, and extensive psychological input.

It is essential that all members of the team strive towards one goal and that only the dietician regulates food intake. Anorexic patients can be very manipulative in an attempt to stop feeding and gain self-control.

KEY POINTS

- Compared to other psychiatric illnesses anorexia nervosa carries a high risk of mortality.
- Clinical features are those of severe malnutrition, vitamin and mineral deficiencies.
- Severe anorexia leads to hypoglycaemia, electrolyte disturbances and multiple organ failure.
- Management of inpatients with severe anorexia nervosa requires a multidisciplinary team approach.

- Psychiatric assessment and appraisal is essential for all patients.
- Refeeding syndrome with metabolic disturbance is an important complication that can occur in malnourished patients when feeding re-commences.
- Electrolytes and fluid balance must be monitored carefully.

Case 22 # A 48-year-old man with an increased body mass index

Mr Harry Butcher has just joined your general practice. He moved from Northampton 2 months ago and is working as a butcher in the central village. He filled in a questionnaire given to him by the reception staff and has made an appointment to see you for a routine medical examination.

The form tells you he is 48 years old and has no known medical problems. He admits to the smoking cigarettes, up to five per day, and drinking a 'moderate' amount of alcohol with no estimated units given. He takes no medication. You work out his BMI, which is 36. He is sitting in the waiting room and is the next patient to be called.

You decide to address the issue of his weight. What questions should be asked?

His perception of his weight
• Does he consider himself overweight?
• Has his weight changed recently, or has it crept up gradually? Is there a reason for this?
• Has he ever tried any measures to reduce weight in the past or is he currently doing so?

Impact of his body habitus
• Does he complain of symptoms related to his weight? Consider fatigue, poor sleep and snoring, difficulty with breathing on exertion, arthralgia and arthritis, dyspepsia or heartburn.

Past medical history
• Does he suffer from any co-morbid conditions? Does he have cardiac, respiratory, endocrine, gastrointestinal, hepatic or rheumatological disease? Consider type 2 diabetes mellitus, hypertension, coronary artery disease,

vascular disease, osteoarthritis, dyslipidaemia and sleep apnoea.
• Are there any psychological problems such as depression?

Medications
• Does he take any medications that may promote weight gain? These include antiepileptics such as phenytoin and valproate, antipsychotics such as olanzapine, systemic corticosteroids and hormonal contraceptives including the oral contraceptive pill.

Social conditions and habits
• Ask about his diet and specifically his daily calorie intake (if known).
• Is his lifestyle active or sedentary? Does he take regular exercise?
• Are there social or psychological issues that promote overeating, reduced physical activity and weight gain?

Family history
• Does obesity run in the family?
• Is there a family history of hypertension, diabetes mellitus, thyroid disease or coronary artery disease?

Motivation
• Is there willingness and motivation to change his lifestyle and diet?
• Is there an underlying cause for his obesity?

You call Mr Butcher into the consulting room. You introduce yourself and ask about his concerns. You concentrate on his weight. He tells you he has had difficulty with his weight for the last 10 or so years. He is now suffering from pain and stiffness in his knees and hips. He gets recurrent severe pain in his big toe on the right foot that usually resolves on taking ibuprofen for a few days. He asks you if you know the cause and can prescribe any medication for him.

Gastroenterology: Clinical Cases Uncovered, 1st edition.
© S. Keshav and E. Culver. Published 2011 by
Blackwell Publishing Ltd.

All his family members are 'big boned', and he is comfortable with his habitus, although he is aware that it may place him at risk of other illness. His work is physically demanding, and he also walks his dog for at least 20 min most days. He thinks he gets enough exercise from this. His diet is varied, although he likes his burger and chips on a Friday night, and a pint with the boys in the local pub.

Examination
What is the body mass index and how is it measured?

The BMI is a simple and widely used method for estimating body fat mass. It is calculated as weight in kilograms divided by the square of the height in metres:

$$BMI = [weight\ (kg)]/[height\ (m)^2]$$

Excess weight may, of course, not be necessarily due to excess fat. Therefore in athletes, with high muscle mass, the BMI may be high without indicating overweight or obesity. Table 22.1 shows BMI and the classification of body habitus.

There are also other methods to estimate body fat:
- *Skin-fold thickness*: measure using callipers, typically at the forearm.
- *Electrical impedance of the body*: this can be measured by passing a low electric current through the lower limbs. The greater the electrical impedance, the greater the proportion of body fat.
- *Distribution of fat*: truncal or central obesity indicates excess fat in the omentum. This is the greatest risk for cardiovascular and metabolic consequences.

Methods to estimate truncal obesity include measuring the waist circumference, with greater than 102 cm in men and 88 cm in women indicating obesity, and estimating the waist to hip circumference ratio, with greater than 0.9 in men and 0.85 in women indicating obesity.

Table 22.1 Body mass index and body habitus.

BMI (kg/m²)	Classification
<18	Underweight
18–25	Normal
25–30	Overweight
30–35	Obese
>35	Morbidly obese

General examination
- Vital signs, especially the pulse and blood pressure. Hypertension is associated with obesity and excessive alcohol consumption. Hypothyroidism, which may be associated with a low pulse rate, may present with excessive weight gain.
- The presence of fluid, such as peripheral oedema or ascites.
- Look for signs of thyroid or adrenal gland disease. Hypothyroidism may present with excessive weight gain. Cushing's syndrome, due to corticosteroid excess, may cause obesity.

Mr Butcher is a round-shaped man, his height is 1.6 m and his weight is 92 kg. His waist circumference is 108 cm. His blood pressure is 140 mmHg systolic, 95 mmHg diastolic. His pulse rate is 80 beats/min, and there are no sign of thyroid or other endocrine disease. There is no detectable peripheral oedema or ascites, and no signs of chronic liver disease. There is no detectable joint disease. Respiratory and cardiac examination is normal.

What investigations should be done?

Medical conditions that increase the risk of obesity include hypothyroidism, Cushing's syndrome, growth hormone deficiency and several rare genetic syndromes. Binge eating disorders also increase risk. Obesity is not regarded as a psychiatric disorder.

Obesity is associated with dyslipidaemia, impaired glucose metabolism, diabetes mellitus and fatty liver disease. It is reasonable, therefore, in an obese individual, to check the fasting lipid profile, fasting glucose level and liver tests. Thyroid dysfunction is common, particularly in women, and one could argue in favour of checking the TSH level to exclude hypothyroidism.

Other endocrine tests can be directed by history and examination findings.

What is the cause of his symptoms?

This man is morbidly obese. The pain and stiffness in his joints are probably due to osteoarthritis and his painful toe is likely to be caused by gout, which typically causes a recurrent monoarthritis. He is hypertensive, and therefore at increased risk of cerebrovascular and coronary artery disease. The risk is particularly high in those with an increased waist circumference, which he has.

Although he is comfortable with his physique, he is aware of the risks of obesity, and therefore may be receptive to ideas about how he could lose weight.

What diseases does obesity put him at a higher risk of?

Obesity reduces life expectancy. The metabolic syndrome is a constellation of medical disorders including diabetes mellitus type 2, hypertension, hypercholesterolaemia and hypertriglyceridaemia. It increases the risk of:

• Cerebrovascular disease such as stroke, vascular dementia and intracranial hypertension.

• Cardiovascular disease including coronary artery disease, myocardial infarction, congestive cardiac failure, hypertension and hypercholesterolaemia.

• Liver disease such as fatty liver and steatohepatitis.

• Gastrointestinal disease such as gastro-oesophageal reflux and cholelithiasis.

• Diabetes mellitus.

• Psychological distress from depression and social stigmatisation.

• Rheumatological complaints like gout, osteoarthritis, lower back pain and poor mobility.

• Dermatological problems such as stretch marks, cellulitis, acanthosis, hirsuitism and intertrigo.

• Respiratory conditions such as obstructive sleep apnoea and obesity hypoventilation syndrome.

• Sexual dysfunction and erectile problems.

• Malignant disease including breast and colon cancer.

He is concerned by this information and wants to try to lose weight. He has tried dieting before but put all the weight back on quickly.

What options are available?
Diet manipulation

A healthy diet, avoiding excessive calories and maintaining intake of micronutrients, is sensible. However, as most people can attest, following a modified diet to lose weight can be difficult and potentially unrewarding as initial loss of weight is frequently followed by reduced vigilance and eventual weight gain after a period of weeks or months. Numerous careful clinical trials demonstrate that weight loss is usually followed by weight gain, and measures to reduce this risk include concomitant counselling or coaching, increased physical exercise to raise the basal metabolic rate, and a gradual and sustained reduction in calories initially, to allow physiological adjustments and facilitate a longer term change in eating behaviour.

A realistic target weight should be agreed and a plan for steady weight loss made. Advice should be tailored to different individuals depending on their motivational factors and previous attempts. Regular supervision, a weight chart and a slimming group or organisation (as part of Weight Watchers) improves success. Restricting the size of portions served at mealtimes, and restricting or eliminating snacks between meals can help to reduce the overall number of calories consumed. Adequate hydration, especially with meals, helps to limit calorie intake by causing gastric distension, and probably by reducing craving for salty foods caused by dehydration.

Calorie-restricted diets allow gradual weight loss. However, very low calorie diets can result in malnutrition and metabolic complications. Low fat diets limit the fat content to between 20–30% of dietary intake, and as fats are the most energy-dense foods, these help to limit overall calorie intake.

Exercise

A change in lifestyle should accompany dietary interventions. Regular exercise increases the basal metabolic rate, suppresses appetite temporarily and consumes calories, contributing to the loss of weight. However, even vigorous exercise only consumes a modest number of calories compared to the amounts ingested. For example, cycling for 30 min may consume 250 calories, which is 5–10% of a typical total daily intake. Therefore it is not wise to recommend that people 'burn off' food that they should have avoided in the first place!

Medication

Pharmacological measures to limit weight generally target appetite and digestion. Only two antiobesity medications are approved by the Food and Drug Agency (FDA) of the United States of America. Both should be combined with dietary intervention.

• *Orlistat* (Xenical) is an intestinal lipase inhibitor, blocking fat absorption and digestion. Weight loss is associated with improved glucose tolerance, reduced complications of type 2 diabetes, lower cholesterol and low density lipoprotein. The main side effect is oily loose stool. In the UK, orlistat can be purchased without a prescription.

• *Sibutramine* (Meridia) is an appetite suppressant, inhibiting deactivation of the neurotransmitters norepinephrine, serotonin and dopamine. It has cardiotoxic side effects.

• *Metformin*, which is used to treat type 2 diabetes mellitus, polycystic ovary syndrome and fatty liver disease, may promote weight loss.

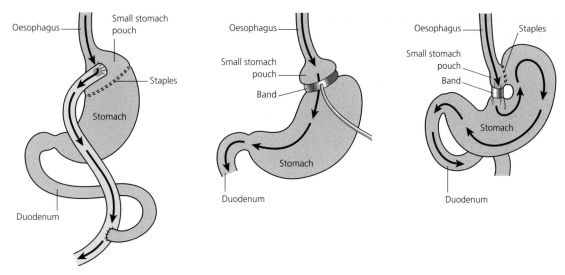

Fig. 22.1 Diagrams of (a) Roux-en-Y gastric bypass; (b) adjustable gastric bands; and (c) vertical banded gastroplasty (From Wikimedia Commons).

Trials of agonists and antagonists of peptide hormones that are involved in the control of appetite are being conducted.

Endoscopy

A relatively new endoscopic technique to reduce food intake involves the placement of a balloon within the stomach to reduce the size of the gastric reservoir. This is often used prior to gastric surgery for obesity.

Surgery

This aims to promote weight loss by restricting the size of the stomach, or by restricting intestinal absorption, and is termed bariatric surgery. Bariatric surgery (Fig. 22.1) is advocated in those with a BMI of greater than 35 with co-morbidity, although indications are increasing as surgical experience increases.

• *Laparoscopic gastric band surgery*: this causes early and prolonged satiety by creating a small gastric pouch and a small pouch outlet. Dietary compliance is needed, individuals eating small frequent meals. Postoperative symptoms include bloating, vomiting and diarrhoea.

• *Bypass operations*: operations such as the Roux-en-Y gastric bypass cause malabsorption and restriction of the gastric reservoir to achieve weight loss. Complications include anastamotic leakage, strictures, ulceration and hernias. Jejunal enteric bypass also causes malabsoprtion, but can result in malnutrition and steatohepatitis, so is not recommended.

• *Liposuction*: this removes adipose tissue but is mainly cosmetic with short-term benefits. Complications include scarring and infection.

He is determined to try and loose weight. You agree a plan of weight loss; firstly, to modify his diet by cutting out his daily high fat snacks and replacing them with more vegetables at dinner time; secondly, to increase his exercise to 30 min daily walking the dog; and thirdly, to reduce the calorie intake at the pub by reducing his alcohol consumption.

Unfortunately, he returns 2 months later and is the same weight. He tells you he managed to drop 2 kg in weight over the first month but then put it back on. He has also stopped smoking and this has lead to him eating to compensate.

You reinforce the positive step in stopping smoking but remind him about the need to manage his weight despite of this. He decides to try again, although he takes away some information about orlistat to consider additional help.

CASE REVIEW

Obesity is usually the consequence of a lifestyle of excessive calorie intake, which is very easy in modern Western societies, where carbohydrate and fat-rich foods are readily available, combined with sedentary work and leisure. It is not classified as a psychiatric illness.

Patients need education and support to help them loose weight and maintain weight loss. This will help to reduce obesity-associated morbidity and mortality. Knowing that there are multiple potential measures allows health care workers to introduce interventions and follow them depending on success or failure. The patient needs to understand both the process, chance of success and potential benefit to remain motivated and committed to a potentially arduous set of interventions.

KEY POINTS

- Obesity is the most prevalent health problem in the Western world, and is associated with increased risk of illness including heart disease, stroke, diabetes, liver disease and cancer.
- Overweight and obese patients should have their blood pressure monitored, and their serum glucose and lipids checked.
- The BMI is a guide to a healthy body weight.
- Other helpful measurements include the waist size and waist : hip ratio.
- Treating overweight and obesity requires attention to diet and exercise in the first instance.
- Medicines to help reduce weight include orlistat, which inhibits the digestion of fat, and sibutramine, which suppresses appetite.
- Endoscopic and surgical techniques to limit food intake and absorption are increasingly being refined and made available, particularly for those with a very high BMI and resulting co-morbidity.

Case 23 A 21-year-old student with chronic abdominal pain

Lisa Pike, a 21-year-old university student, came with her mother to your clinic. She tells you she has been suffering from lower abdominal pains on and off for the last year or so, and that they are getting gradually worse. This is associated with loose, sometimes offensive-smelling, bowel motions. She has tried paracetamol with little relief. Her mum wants to know what is causing the pain and what you can do to help her.

What features of the history will help you make a diagnosis and guide investigations?

Abdominal pain
• Character: dull ache, colicky spasms, deep or superficial.
• Location.
• Radiation: to back, loins, groin, chest, shoulder tip or other area of the abdomen.
• Onset: sudden or gradual.
• Progression: is it becoming more severe and intense or constant?
• Intensity: grading scale from 1 to 10, with 10 the worst pain imaginable.
• Frequency: this can be number of times in a day/week/month/year.
• Duration: when was it first noticed? This may be a prior episode.
• Aggravating and relieving factors: related to posture, eating meals, worsened by movement, inspiration or coughing, better after passing stool. Is it related to or aggravated by the menstrual cycle? Is it related to anxiety or stress?
• Associated symptoms.

Differentiate abdominal pain from cardiac, respiratory, musculoskeletal, renal, gynaecological and spinal pain.

Bowel habit
Describe her normal bowel habit and how this differs from her norm.
• Determine the duration of altered bowel habit. How chronic is the problem; has it affected her from childhood?
• Describe the stool frequency, consistency, colour and odour. Is there any blood in the stool (fresh or altered)? Is there any mucus?
• Does she describe stool urgency and is this at any particular time of the day? Are there nocturnal symptoms?
• Is there a sensation of incomplete rectal emptying after passage of a stool? Does she have obstructive symptoms?

Associated symptoms
• Has she noticed a change in appetite or unexplained weight loss? This may be associated with malabsorption or an inflammatory process.
• Does she suffer from bloating and abdominal distension? Ask about diurnal variation. This may occur in bacterial overgrowth or irritable bowel syndrome.
• Does she complain of excessive flatulence and belching? Consider malabsorption, bacterial overgrowth and functional disorders.
• Does she have persistent nausea or vomiting? Consider peptic ulceration or inflammation, gallstone disease and pancreatic inflammation.
• Does she have tiredness and lethargy? Think of thyroid disorders, inflammatory disorders and malabsorption. This symptom is very non-specific and may occur in many disorders.
• Does she have any urinary symptoms such as urgency, frequency or pain on urination? Consider urinary tract or kidney problems. Irritable bladder and bowel often coexist.

Gastroenterology: Clinical Cases Uncovered, 1st edition.
© S. Keshav and E. Culver. Published 2011 by Blackwell Publishing Ltd.

153

• Does she experience pain or discomfort during sexual intercourse (dysparenuria)? This may by gynaecological in origin, psychological or functional.

• Are there any problems with the menstrual cycle and does this influence her symptoms? Irritable bowel can be influenced by the menstrual cycle. Gynaecological problems such as cysts or fibroids can cause pain. The duration of symptoms exclude pregnancy as a cause, although it should always be tested for if there are concerns.

• Has she experienced recurrent mouth ulceration, new rashes, arthralgia or inflammation of the eyes? Consider inflammatory bowel or celiac disease.

Past medical history

• Does she have a history of anxiety or depressive illness?

• Does she have any gynaecological problems? She is young, but she may have children, if she does were there any obstetric problems? If she were older, has she had a hysterectomy?

• Does she have any known gastrointestinal disease?

Medications

• Is she taking any medications that may cause abdominal pain or loose bowel motions?

• Is she taking regular NSAIDs?

• Does she take any laxatives or has she used them excessively in the past?

Social history

• Is she intolerant of any specific food types? Are her symptoms intensified by any component of her diet? Has she changed her eating habits accordingly? Lactose intolerance, gluten and wheat sensitivity may be important.

• Does she drink alcohol or excessive caffeine? Does this affect her symptoms? Peptic ulceration, gallstone and pancreatic disease may all be affected by alcohol.

• Does she smoke or is she a recent ex-smoker?

• Does she describe a stressful life at home or work or social unrest? If so, does this intensify her symptoms? Irritable bowel may be intensified by stressful situations, as can other disease processes.

Family history

• Is there a history of inflammatory bowel disease or coeliac disease?

• Is there a family history of colorectal carcinoma at a young age?

Lisa explains that her symptoms started 2 years ago and were originally a background ache in the abdomen at the end of the day, associated with some bloating and distension. She noticed the stool frequency in the last year, with the stool loose, brown and without any blood. She opens her bowels up to three times per day with morning urgency but never gets up at night to pass a stool. The symptoms affect her most days. Her menstrual cycle has always been problematic with no fixed pattern and no new changes. She has no urinary symptoms.

She denies any previous medical problems and remembers taking citalopram prescribed a few years ago by her GP for low mood. She takes ibuprofen for headaches only. She has been very stressed since being at university; she is studying as a mechanical engineer and finds the balance between her studies, family commitments and financial problems difficult.

She smokes five cigarettes a day and is trying to quit. She drinks alcohol 'like everyone else at university' most nights and, if anything, it helps her symptoms. She has changed her diet considerably, trying to improve her symptoms. She thinks milk may intensify her problems. There is no family history of note.

What do you look for on examination?

This is done to exclude any evidence of organic pathology and will be directed by the history.

General examination

• Inspect for conjunctival pallor of anaemia and oral mouth ulceration of inflammatory bowel disease or coeliac disease.

• Palpate for cervical lymphadenopathy.

Abdominal examination

• Palpate for abdominal tenderness: is this deep or superficial and muscular in origin?

• Palpate for an abdominal or pelvic mass.

Rectal examination

Given the history of diarrhoea, a DRE should be done to look for perianal fissures and exclude a rectal mass.

Gynaecological examination

A gynaecological examination should be done if suggested by the history.

Examination demonstrats mild abdominal tenderness in the lower abdomen with no guarding, rebound or palpable masses. The rectal examination is normal.

What are your differential diagnoses?

The possible diagnoses for this young woman with a 2-year history of abdominal discomfort and loose stool are:

- Irritable bowel syndrome.
- Coeliac disease.
- Lactose intolerance.
- Crohn's disease.
- Small bowel bacterial overgrowth.
- Microscopic colitis associated with NSAID use and coeliac disease.

What indicators of organic disease must be excluded?

The indicators that suggest organic disease include:

- New onset of symptoms over the age of 50 years.
- Progressive or severe symptoms.
- Nocturnal symptoms.
- Rectal bleeding.
- Anorexia and unexplained weight loss.
- Persistent symptoms despite all therapy.
- Family history of carcinoma, inflammatory bowel disease and coeliac disease.
- Abnormal physical findings such as mouth ulcers or abdominal mass.
- Anaemia.
- Fever.
- Raised inflammatory markers.

What is the most likely cause of her symptoms?

Lisa has no indicators of organic disease. Her symptoms are suggestive of irritable bowel syndrome (IBS). The most common symptoms of irritable bowel are lower abdominal pain (which may ease after defecation), altered bowel habit (which may be diarrhoea, constipation or both), bloating and abdominal distension, urgency especially in the morning, and the passage of mucus with or without stool.

Additional symptoms include belching and excessive flatulence, loss of appetite, nausea and sometimes vomiting, tiredness, urgency and frequency of urination (irritable bladder), dysparenuria and an increased intensity of symptoms during menstruation.

The diagnosis of IBS is made by validated clinical criteria called the Rome III criteria. Abdominal bloating and the passage of mucus per rectum are supportive but not essential for diagnosis. The absence of alarm features increases specificity but not sensitivity.

There are four main subtypes of IBS:

- *Pain-predominant (IBS-P)*: central or iliac fossa pain or persistent ache which is poorly localised and is present on most days. It is usually related to defecation and worse during stressful periods or during menstruation.
- *Diarrhoea-predominant (IBS-D)*: morning frequency and urgency with or without abdominal pain, which is relieved by defecation.
- *Constipation-predominant (IBS-C)*: sensation of incomplete evacuation and associated with mucus production.
- *Alternating pattern (IBS-A)*: alternating hard stool, usually in the morning, followed by watery loose stool during the rest of the day.

IBS overlaps with other functional disorders such as non-ulcer dyspepsia and pelvic pain syndrome.

Box 23.1 Rome III criteria for IBS

A. Abdominal pain or discomfort >12 weeks in the last 6 months
B. Associated with two of the following:
   - Relieved by defecation
   - Associated change in stool frequency
   - Associated change in stool consistency

KEY POINTS

- It is important to search for and exclude indicators of organic disease.
- The Rome III criteria are validated in the diagnosis of irritable bowel syndrome.
- There are different subtypes of irritable bowel depending on which symptoms predominate. This will guide therapeutic strategies.

You explain the diagnosis of IBS to Lisa and her mother. Lisa asks 'what are the causes of IBS' and 'do I need any tests'?

Pathophysiology of irritable bowel syndrome

The cause of IBS is not known for certain, but it may occur after a gastrointestinal infection (in up to 20% of patients) or a stressful life event. There is no evidence it is linked to cancer.

Table 23.1 Pathology of different kinds of IBS.

Constipation-predominant IBS	Diarrhoea-predominant IBS	Pain-predominant IBS
Slow-transit constipation	Coeliac disease	Abdominal wall pain
Defecation disorder	Bile salt malabsorption	Gynaecological causes
Pseudo-obstruction	Bacterial overgrowth	Renal pain
Pelvic floor dysfunction	Inflammatory bowel disease	Spinal pain
	Lactulose intolerance	
	Microscopic colitis	

Some proposed mechanisms include visceral hypersensitivity, shown to be important by studies investigating the effects of ileal and anorectal balloon distension, altered intestinal motility and transit time, altered enteric and nervous system function, increased sensitivity to certain foods and food intolerance, altered bowel flora that may be influenced by probiotics, and psychological factors that influence pain perception and health-seeking behaviour.

The pathology to consider depends on the type of IBS (Table 23.1).

Investigations

Avoid over-investigation in patients with IBS, but exclude serious underlying pathology. There is no specific diagnostic test for functional disorders. Explain that the tests arranged are expected to be normal. Not all tests will be indicated in each patient, this will depend on the list of differential diagnoses based on history and examination findings.

• *Urine dipstick.* Look for blood or protein caused by renal tract disease and leucocytes/nitrites as evidence of urinary tract infection.

• *Blood tests:*
  • Full blood count for anaemia and thrombocytopenia of inflammatory disorders.
  • Urea and electrolytes and liver function tests.
  • C-reactive protein as a marker for inflammatory disease.
  • Coeliac serology.
  • Thyroid function and calcium in IBS-C and IBS-D.
  • Haematinics including ferritin, B_{12} and folate to look for malabsorption in IBS-D.

• *Stool sample.* Stool culture for IBS-D (to exclude bacterial infections)

• *Proctoscopy.* To exclude an anterior mucosal prolapse in IBS-C if there is a sensation of incomplete evacuation.

• *Sigmoidoscopy.* To look for inflammatory changes of colitis. If normal, a rectal and left-sided colonic biopsy is needed for microscopic colitis and Crohn's disease.

• *Colonoscopy.* Should be done if there are alarm features at any age or persistent symptoms refractory to all drugs and diet management.

• *Upper GI endoscopy.* This is advocated if there is evidence of iron deficiency (not in premenopausal women) or dyspepsia that is unresponsive to a 1-month trial of PPI and if the patient has had 'test and treat' for *Helicobacter pylori*.

• *Abdominal ultrasound.* This should only be done if the upper abdominal pain is episodic, endoscopy is normal and gallstone, pancreatic or liver disease is a possibility.

• *Pelvic ultrasound.* If lower abdominal pain is related to menstruation or there are other gynaecological symptoms.

• *Small bowel radiology.* Considered if weight loss, abdominal pain and diarrhoea are suggestive of Crohn's disease with a normal colonoscopy for jejunal diverticulosis and strictures causing bacterial overgrowth.

• *Breath tests:*
  • A hydrogen breath test after lactulose is non-invasive but has a low sensitivity and specificity for bacterial overgrowth. Breath test >20ppm in under 2h indicates overgrowth. A trial of antibiotic metronidazole twice daily is usually given for a week instead as a diagnostic test.
  • A lactose breath test is the most convenient method of confirming hypolactasia, but many document symptoms before and after stopping milk products for 1 week. Lactose intolerance can be temporary.

Lisa and her mum are happy with your explanation. Blood tests including full blood count, urea and electrolytes, liver function and C-reactive protein are normal. There is no indication for further investigation currently, so she is given some advice to manage her symptoms.

What advice do you give to manage her symptoms?

Management includes establishing a firm diagnosis of IBS using the Rome III criteria, excluding serious organic pathology, education and reassurance. Symptoms improve and disappear in about half of patients after 12 months.

Look at diet and lifestyle factors

Ensure her diet is well balanced, and that she is eating three regular meals daily with smaller portions containing less fat. Use fresh ingredients rather than ready-meals or take-aways. Have a dedicated time to sit down and eat. Drink plenty of fluids, at least eight cups per day. Avoid dietary substances (and alcohol in some) that aggravates symptoms. Take regular exercise.

Explore external stress

If stress is a trigger for IBS then take time to relax. Try relaxation, yoga, massage and aromatherapy sessions. Enlist the support of your family and friends.

Consult a dietician

If there is no improvement in symptoms despite diet intervention and lifestyle modification after 4–6 weeks consider dietician advice. Dieticians can help to identify food intolerance by exclusion diets and the reduction of resistant starches. Such foods can be reintroduced over a few months.

Medications

The placebo effect of tablets is high, with about 30–50% of patients responding in clinical trials. Pharmacological treatments are directed towards the predominant symptoms. Antispasmodics and smooth muscle relaxants are given to relieve pain from bloating and spasm. Antidiarrhoeal agents are chosen for loose stool. Laxatives and fibre supplements are useful for those with constipation. Probiotics such as Actimel may improve flatulence.

Pain-predominant IBS

• Antispasmodics: mebeverine, peppermint oil capsules, alverine citrate.
• Amitriptyline.

Diarrhoea-predominant IBS

• Loperamide, an opioid analogue (avoid codeine).
• Amitriptyline.

Constipation-predominant IBS

• Fibre supplements and increased fluid intake.
• Stool softener and osmotic laxative such as lactulose.

Complementary therapies

Consider these if conventional management fails or as an adjunct to treatment. This includes hypnotherapy, acupuncture and cognitive-behavioural therapy.

Lisa altered her diet and increased her consumption of fresh fruit and vegetables. She found rice and potatoes particularly problematic, causing bloating and abdominal aching so excluded these from her diet with success. There was no change to her symptoms on discontinuing milk products for a week-long trial.

She tried to deal with her stressful life by confiding in her mum about her problems. She moved out of university accommodation and back into her house, where she could be cooked healthy meals, see her family and had less financial problems. She tried peppermint oil and mebeverine for the abdominal discomfort with little effect.

When she returned to your clinic 3 months later, her symptoms were manageable and her quality of life had improved dramatically. She was reassured there was nothing wrong.

CASE REVIEW

Irritable bowel syndrome can be diagnosed using validated clinical criteria called the Rome III criteria. Organic disease should be excluded by looking for alarm features and investigating as appropriate. The patient should be told that these are likely to be normal. Education and reassurance that there is no significant organic pathology is important.

There are four different subtypes of irritable bowel depending on the symptoms that predominate. Each subtype requires different management strategies.

Management is aimed at lifestyle, diet and behavioural change. This is generally effective over a period of months. There is a placebo effect with medications although there is little evidence that most have more of an effect than this.

KEY POINTS

- IBS is a common condition, affecting around 1 in 5 people. Over three-quarters of these never seek medical advice.
- Women have a 2–4-fold increase in the prevalence of IBS and are more likely to seek medical advice.
- IBS is less common in those over the age of 65 years.
- IBS may manifest with a variety of symptoms, which vary between different individuals. These include abdominal discomfort and/or altered bowel habit.

- The Rome III criteria provide an objective method of diagnosis although there is no reliable diagnostic test for functional disorders.
- Symptoms of IBS can be distressing, but they do not predispose to serious illness or cancer so reassurance is appropriate and helpful.
- Symptoms often continue for months to years, and may be relieved but are not always cured.
- Although treatment remains unsatisfactory, combination treatment is often effective.
- In many cases symptoms resolve or abate spontaneously.

MCQs

1 Which one of the following statements is definitely true?

a. Elevated serum AST and ALT indicate hepatitis
b. Elevations in the serum bilirubin, together with ALP and γ-GT, indicate gallstones or biliary disease rather than viral hepatitis
c. The higher the AST and ALT, the more damaged the liver and the worse the liver function is
d. ALT and AST are enzymes found in muscles
e. An elevated bilirubin indicates good synthetic function and impaired excretory function

2 In a patient with dyspepsia, which one of the following is not regarded as an alarm feature?

a. Weight loss
b. Dysphagia
c. No response to proton pump inhibitors
d. Iron-deficiency anaemia
e. Previous gastric ulcer

3 Which one term best describes the following symptoms: central upper abdominal or retrosternal discomfort with heaviness, unease, post-prandial fullness and early satiety that may be related to eating, or hunger, or may be unrelated to food altogether?

a. Heartburn
b. Indigestion
c. Biliousness
d. Dyspepsia
e. Gastro-oesophageal reflux

4 Dysphagia may occasionally be associated with which one of the following haematological abnormalities?

a. Thrombocytopenia
b. Iron deficiency
c. Macrocytosis
d. Thrombocytosis
e. Neutropenia

5 Which one of the following is not a recognised complication of vomiting?

a. Haematemesis
b. Hypokalaemia
c. Aspiration
d. Acid damage to teeth
e. Papilloedema

6 Metoclopramide, domperidone and prochlorperazine as antiemetics act on which one of the following receptors?

a. Acetylcholine
b. Serotonin (5-HT)
c. Dopamine
d. Purine
e. Histamine

7 Which one of the following is unlikely to be the cause of rectal bleeding when the blood is mixed with stool?

a. Fissure in ano
b. Colorectal cancer
c. Bacterial dysentery
d. Ulcerative colitis
e. Diverticular disease

8 Which one of the following is unlikely to be helpful in someone with rectal bleeding?

a. Colonoscopy
b. CT scan of the abdomen
c. Abdominal ultrasound scan
d. Rigid sigmoidoscopy
e. Upper endoscopy

Gastroenterology: Clinical Cases Uncovered, 1st edition.
© S. Keshav and E. Culver. Published 2011 by
Blackwell Publishing Ltd.

9 Which one factor from the following list is strongly associated with death after upper gastrointestinal haemorrhage?

a. Low haemoglobin
b. Coexisting renal or liver disease or cancer
c. Low blood pressure
d. Mallory–Weiss tear
e. Being 60 years old

10 Which one of the following clinical signs suggests intestinal blood loss as cause of iron-deficiency anaemia?

a. Dupuytren's contracture
b. Freckles around the mouth
c. High blood pressure
d. Frontal balding
e. Tremor

11 Which one of these criteria make a positive diagnosis of IBS?

a. Abdominal pain and change in bowel habit for over 12 weeks in the preceding 6 months, accompanied by anxiety and depression, with normal blood tests
b. Abdominal pain and change in bowel habit for over 12 weeks in the preceding 6 months, accompanied by bloating, mucus and rectal bleeding
c. Abdominal pain or discomfort for over 12 weeks in the preceding 6 months, relieved by defecation, or associated with a change in stool frequency or consistency
d. Abdominal pain or discomfort for over 12 weeks in the preceding 6 months, with bloating and dyspepsia; the patient is known to have a normal endoscopy
e. Abdominal pain or discomfort for over 12 weeks in the preceding 6 months that is aggravated by eating wheat, tomatoes and mushrooms; the patient is a menstruating female who is mildly anaemic

12 Which one of the following is true of coeliac disease?

a. It is strongly associated with a particular HLA type: DQ2
b. It is not familial, but rather is related to diet
c. It mainly affects Africans
d. Iron deficiency occurs because of the high risk of lymphoma and other cancers
e. Duodenal biopsy is necessary because there is no reliable blood test

13 Which one of the following drugs is most likely to cause constipation?

a. Metformin
b. Codeine phosphate
c. Digoxin
d. Tramadol
e. Movicol

14 Which one of the following is most likely to cause travellers' diarrhoea?

a. *Echinococcus*
b. *Campylobacter*
c. *Entamoeba*
d. *Schistosoma*
e. Rotavirus

15 Which one of the following organisms is most likely to cause bloody diarrhoea?

a. Norovirus
b. Dengue
c. *Giardia*
d. *Campylobacter*
e. Rotavirus

16 Which one of the following is unlikely to be a manifestation of inflammatory bowel disease?

a. Arthralgia
b. Anaemia
c. Arthritis
d. Skin ulcer
e. Wheezing

17 Which one of the following is more likely to feature in Crohn's disease and not in ulcerative colitis?

a. Arthralgia
b. Anaemia
c. Diarrhoea
d. Rectal bleeding
e. Perianal abscess

18 Which one of the following is not a recognised cause of pancreatitis?

a. Gallstones
b. Anaemia
c. Hypertriglyceridaemia

d. Hypercalcaemia

e. Alcohol

19 Which one of the following is not a recognised complication of gallstones?

a. Pancreatitis

b. Cholangitis

c. Intestinal obstruction

d. Hypercalcaemia

e. Cancer of the gallbladder

20 Which one of the following is least likely to be helpful in determining the cause of jaundice?

a. Ultrasound scan

b. Hepatitis serology

c. Abdominal X-ray

d. Full blood count

e. Urine dipstix

21 Which one of the following is typical of chronic liver disease rather than acute liver disease?

a. Jaundice

b. Malaise

c. Ascites

d. Spider naevi

e. Coagulation disorders

22 Which one of the following typically causes a transudate?

a. Tuberculosis

b. Budd–Chiari syndrome

c. Cirrhosis

d. Ovarian cancer

e. Pancreatitis

23 Which one of the following questions is not part of the CAGE questionnaire for alcohol misuse?

a. Have you ever had a drink first thing in the morning (eye-opener) to steady your nerves or to get rid of a hangover?

b. Have people annoyed you by criticising your drinking?

c. Has anyone ever felt you should cut down on your drinking?

d. Have you ever felt guilty about your drinking?

e. Do you regularly crave alcohol?

24 Which one of the following is not a typical feature of the clinical picture of colon cancer?

a. Rectal bleeding

b. Altered bowel habit

c. Anaemia

d. Dyspepsia

e. No symptoms

25 Which one of the following is a fat-soluble vitamin?

a. Hydroxocobalamin

b. Cholecalciferol

c. Pyridoxine

d. Selenium

e. Cholesterol

26 Obesity is not associated with which one of the following adverse events?

a. Colon cancer

b. Obstructive sleep apnoea

c. Crohn's disease

d. Diabetes mellitus

e. Poor wound healing

27 *Helicobacter pylori* is a major cause of intestinal disease. Which one of the following statement about it is true?

a. *H. pylori* is a normal commensal in the colon

b. *H. pylori* used to be considered a *Campylobacter*-like organism

c. *H. pylori* is the only *Helicobacter* found in humans

d. Acute *H. pylori* infection is characterised by a transient hepatitis

e. *H. pylori* can only survive at pH 4 or lower

EMQs

1 Liver disease

a. Liver biopsy

b. MRI of the liver

c. MRCP

d. Corticosteroids

e. ERCP

f. Abstinence from alcohol and recheck progress and liver chemistry

g. Liver screen by blood and urine tests

h. Weight reduction and exercise and then repeat liver biochemistry in 3–6 months

i. Abdominal ultrasound

For each of the statements below, choose the most likely answer from the list above. Each answer may be chosen once, more than once or not at all.

1. The first line investigation for gallstone disease is …

2. Acute onset of jaundice with a bilirubin of 155 μmol/L (elevated), ALP of 360 U/L (elevated) and γ-GT of 200 IU/L (elevated) should be initially investigated by …

3. Chronic alcohol excess causing a γ-GT of over 200 IU/L with otherwise normal liver function should be treated by …

4. Right upper quadrant intermittent colicky pain, in the absence of gallstones on ultrasound scan, should be investigated by …

5. Non-alcoholic fatty liver disease with an ALT of 60 U/L should be treated by …

6. A woman with known primary sclerosing cholangitis develops malaise and arthralgia, and has a change in the pattern of her liver tests with an ALT elevated to over 100 U/L; she should have …

7. A man with persistently abnormal liver tests for 6 months with an ALP of 350 U/L and γ-GT of 120 IU/L should have …

8. Autoimmune liver disease confirmed on liver biopsy should be treated with …

2 Gastro-oesophageal disease

a. Prokinetic medications, such as metoclopramide or domperidone

b. Barium swallow

c. Upper endoscopy

d. *H. pylori* breath test followed by eradication if positive

e. 24 h pH monitoring

f. Empirical proton pump inhibitor therapy trial for 4–6 weeks

g. Oesophageal manometry

h. Gastric emptying scan

i. Distal duodenal biopsies

For each of the statements below, choose the most likely answer from the list above. Each answer may be chosen once, more than once or not at all.

1. In a 35-year-old man with a 6-week history of dyspepsia, the optimum initial management options is …

2. Progressive dysphagia to solids and then liquids should be investigated by …

3. A diabetic woman with early satiety and abdominal bloating had a trial of omeprazole and a normal endoscopy; the next lines of investigation and management are …

4. The gold standard investigation for achalasia is …

5. A young man with persistent gastro-oesophageal reflux every time he leans over or shortly after he has a meal should have …

6. The gold standard test to diagnose coeliac disease is …

Gastroenterology: Clinical Cases Uncovered, 1st edition.
© S. Keshav and E. Culver. Published 2011 by Blackwell Publishing Ltd.

7. The ideal first line investigation for oesophageal dysmotility disorders is …
8. The most likely gastroenterological test to yield a diagnosis of Whipple's disease is …

---

3 Colorectal disease
a. Prostatomegaly
b. Diverticulosis
c. Anal fissure
d. Haemorrhoids
e. Ulcerative colitis
f. Crohn's disease
g. Rectal cancer
h. Irritable bowel syndrome
i. Abdominal tuberculosis

For each of the statements below, choose the most likely answer/s from the list above. Each question may have more than one answer. Each answer may be chosen once, more than once or not at all.
1. On performing a digital rectal examination for rectal bleeding, you may find …
2. Diarrhoea may be caused by …
3. The Rome III criteria are used to diagnose …
4. Complete colonoscopy and biopsies are particularly helpful in …
5. Dietary advice forms an essential part of the management strategy in …
6. Surgery is frequently an option in some patients with …
7. Granulomas may be seen in biopsy samples in …
8. Fever and abdominal pain may be a feature of …

---

4 Gastrointestinal bleeding
a. Administer intravenous pamidronate
b. Take blood tests to check the blood count and cross-match
c. Insert a large bore cannula
d. Perform upper endoscopy
e. Administer 4 units of O-negative blood immediately
f. Administer recombinant activated factor VIIa
g. Give an injection of vitamin K, and order fresh frozen plasma
h. Make a 'do not resuscitate decision' as the patient has a terminal illness
i. Perform colonoscopy

For each of the statements below, choose the most appropriate answer/s from the list above. Each question may have more than one answer. Each answer may be chosen once, more than once or not at all.
1. An 80-year-old man with multiple myeloma comes into the emergency room after haematemesis and melaena, with a blood pressure of 90/50 mmHg. He should be managed by …
2. In a patient with advanced liver cirrhosis with massive haematemesis, immediate management should be …
3. In patients with a bleeding diathesis and melaena, their coagulopathy should be reversed by …
4. In an elderly woman with one episode of coffee-ground vomit, appropriate management includes …
5. Persistent melaena in a middle-aged man with a normal initial upper endoscopy should be further investigated by …
6. The most appropriate initial investigation(s) for an 88-year-old woman with iron-deficiency anaemia is/are …
7. Profuse bright red rectal bleeding in a 60-year-old man should prompt …
8. In a gastrointestinal bleed, the following is/are not appropriate …

---

5 Anaemia
a. Dietary iron insufficiency
b. Menstrual bleeding
c. Peptic ulceration
d. Smoking
e. Coeliac disease
f. Colon cancer
g. Crohn's disease
h. Dyspepsia
i. Iron supplements

For each of the statements below, choose the most appropriate answer/s from the list above. Each question may have more than one answer. Each answer may be chosen once, more than once or not at all.
1. In a woman of child-bearing age, the following are potential causes of anaemia …
2. A combination of folate and iron deficiency in a young woman is most likely caused by …
3. Altered bowel habit is often associated with anaemia in …

4. The most common causes of an iron-deficiency anaemia in females under the age of 45 years are …
5. Endoscopic examination is important in diagnosis of …
6. Black stool may be described in association with …
7. Epigastric discomfort and bloating may occur in …
8. The following are associated with an increased risk of gastrointestinal malignancy …

---

6 Coeliac disease
a. Abnormal liver chemistry
b. Lymphoma
c. Cerebellar ataxia
d. Dermatitis herpetiformis
e. Anaemia
f. DEXA bone scan
g. Strict gluten-free diet
h. Non compliance with gluten-free diet
i. Duodenal biopsies

For each of the statements below, choose the most appropriate answer/s from the list above. Each question may have more than one answer. Each answer may be chosen once, more than once or not at all.
1. … may be attributed to the disease, and may regress on a gluten-free diet
2. The diagnosis of coeliac disease is made by …
3. Management of patients with this disease includes …
4. Persistent symptoms of bloating and diarrhoea may suggest …
5. Monitoring of blood tests in coeliac patients may detect …
6. … would be useful to detect osteopenia or osteoporosis.
7. Itch may be attributed to …
8. Further imaging may be required for …

---

7 Gastrointestinal pathology
a. Fever
b. Abdominal pain
c. Loose stool
d. Difficulty passing stool
e. Rectal bleeding
f. Weight loss
g. Needing to strain when defecating
h. Infrequent defecation
i. Flushing

For each of the statements below, choose the most appropriate answer/s from the list above. Each question may have more than one answer. Each answer may be chosen once, more than once or not at all.
1. The following symptoms may be reported by a patient with idiopathic constipation …
2. The following symptoms may occur in a patient with coeliac disease …
3. In a severe flare of ulcerative colitis, symptoms may include …
4. Proton pump inhibitors can cause …
5. Chronic pancreatitis may result in …
6. Insufficient relaxation of the puborectalis muscle can lead to …
7. A rectal adenocarcinoma can cause …
8. Anal fissures may result in …

---

8 Inflammatory bowel disease
a. Fever
b. Weight loss
c. Small bowel enema
d. Rectal bleeding
e. Arthralgia
f. Mouth ulcers
g. Ileocolonoscopy
h. Upper endoscopy
i. Loose stools

For each of the statements below, choose the most likely answer/s from the list above. Each question may have more than one answer. Each answer may be chosen once, more than once or not at all.
1. The following symptoms may be reported by a patient with ulcerative colitis …
2. Crohn's disease may be diagnosed by the following investigations …
3. Coeliac disease and inflammatory bowel disease may both cause …
4. Colorectal cancer and inflammatory bowel disease may both have …
5. Isolated terminal ileal Crohn's disease is diagnosed by …
6. Microscopic colitis may cause …
7. Behcet's disease and colonic Crohn's disease share the following features …
8. Extraintestinal manifestations of inflammatory bowel disease include …

9 Abnormal liver function

a. Gilbert's syndrome
b. Viral hepatitis
c. Congestive cardiac failure
d. Peptic ulcer
e. Haemolysis
f. Alcohol-associated liver disease
g. Gentamicin
h. Flucloxacillin
i. Azathioprine

For each of the statements below, choose the most likely answer/s from the list above. Each question may have more than one answer. Each answer may be chosen once, more than once or not at all.

1. The following are associated with jaundice …
2. A cholestatic pattern of liver injury may be the result of …
3. Elevated serum transaminase may be the result of …
4. An abdominal ultrasound shows hepatomegaly; the most likely causes are …
5. Fever and mylagia can be seen with …
6. Liver function is not typically affected by …
7. Cirrhosis may occur in patients with/taking …
8. Upper endoscopy may be diagnostic in patients with/taking …

10 Chronic liver disease

a. Hypoalbuminaemia
b. Variceal haemorrhage
c. Splenomegaly
d. Hyperammonaemia
e. Haemolysis
f. Obesity
g. Thrombocythaemia
h. Gynaecomastia
i. Spironolactone

For each of the statements below, choose the most likely answer/s from the list above. Each question may have more than one answer. Each answer may be chosen once, more than once or not at all.

1. The following occur typically in patients with chronic liver disease …
2. Portal hypertension may result in …
3. Inflammatory disorders may cause …
4. Terlipressin may be useful in …
5. Peripheral pitting oedema may be the result of …
6. Hepatic encephalopathy in a patient with chronic liver disease may be triggered by …
7. In the absence of cirrhosis, alcohol may cause …
8. The following may occur in portal vein thrombosis …

1 What medical term is used to denote central upper abdominal or retrosternal discomfort with heaviness, unease, post-prandial fullness and early satiety that may be related to eating, or hunger, or may be unrelated to food altogether?

2 A young girl with asthma develops increasing difficulty swallowing food, because she says it gets stuck. Her parents are certain that she does not have an eating disorder, although it has been suggested by some medical people. At endoscopy, apart from some white plaques, the oesophagus appears normal. What is the likely diagnosis?

3 An 80-year-old patient with multiple myeloma comes to the emergency room following an episode of haematemesis and melaena. His blood pressure is 90/50 mmHg. What is the pre-endoscopy Rockall score?

4 A 24-year-old man with iron deficiency, weight loss and diarrhoea comes to the clinic complaining of an itchy vesicular rash on his elbows. What diagnosis springs to mind?

5 What is the cause of coeliac disease?

6 What is the mainstay of managing acute diarrhoea and vomiting caused by an infection?

7 What treatments are available for IBD?

8 What features indicate severe acute pancreatitis?

9 What is the difference between cholelithiasis, cholecystitis and cholangitis?

10 What are the complications of ascites?

Gastroenterology: Clinical Cases Uncovered, 1st edition.
© S. Keshav and E. Culver. Published 2011 by
Blackwell Publishing Ltd.

1. d: Elevations in AST and ALT typically indicate hepatocellular injury, while elevations in ALP and γ-GT indicate biliary disease. However, there is major overlap in these patterns, and typically they coexist. A common misconception is that AST and ALT are only found in the liver. Another major source particularly of AST is skeletal muscle. Bilirubin levels rise when deconjugation (detoxification) or biliary excretion are impaired. Hepatic synthetic function is reflected in reduced serum albumin, or prolonged prothrombin time.

2. c: Dyspepsia is extremely common in the general population, and may be caused by hyperacidity, or not. Rarely, it indicates serious illness, such as peptic ulcer or cancer, therefore alarm features such as weight loss, dysphagia, iron deficiency or a previous gastric ulcer highlight the need to investigate further. However, non-response to proton pump inhibitors by itself is not an alarm feature, and may indicate rather that the dyspepsia is not related to hyperacidity at all.

3. d: Biliousness and indigestion are not medical terms and are best avoided. Gastro-oesophageal reflux is what may be occurring in a patient with heartburn. Symptoms alone rarely indicate that this is happening. The complex of symptoms is related to dysfunction of the foregut – oesophagus, stomach and duodenum – and the term dyspepsia is used to capture it as a medical entity. The causes of dyspepsia vary, and include gastritis, peptic ulcer, gastro-oesophageal reflux, biliary disease, etc.

4. b: Iron deficiency may occur with many intestinal diseases, including reflux oesophagitis, which can itself lead to stricturing of the oesophagus and dysphagia. A more esoteric link is between idiopathic oesophageal stricture and iron deficiency in the so-called Plummer–Vinson or Paterson–Kelly syndrome.

5. e: Haematemesis can occur from a superficial tear in the oesophageal mucosa (Mallory–Weiss tear); loss of gastric and intestinal fluid can cause hypokalaemia, hyponatraemia, metabolic alkalosis or acidosis. Recurrent vomiting, particularly if consciousness is impaired, can lead to aspiration and pneumonia, and stomach acid can damage the teeth and gums. Papilloedema is a sign of raised intracranial pressure, which can cause vomiting.

6. c: Metoclopramide, domperidone and prochlorperazine act on dopamine D_2 receptors, blocking their function. Other receptors involved in vomiting are acetylcholine, serotonin and histamine.

7. a: Fissure in ano and haemorrhoids typically cause bleeding that is bright red and seen on the surface of faeces, or is noticed when wiping after defecation. Therefore, in the appropriate clinical setting, and after careful local examination, patients can often be reassured that such bleeding does not indicate serious illness in the colon, necessitating colonoscopy or other investigation.

8. c: Brisk upper GI bleeding sometimes causes fresh blood to be present in the stool, when there has not been sufficient time in the intestine to digest the blood, therefore upper endoscopy may be helpful. Sigmoidoscopy and colonoscopy can clearly help to identify a source of bleeding, while an abdominal CT scan can delineate the colon and blood vessels. Abdominal ultrasound is mainly used to examine the solid organs and large blood vessels such as the aorta, vena cava and portal vein. It is a poor test for air-filled organs.

9. b: Upper GI haemorrhage is life-threatening. However, some causes typically are self-limiting and

Gastroenterology: Clinical Cases Uncovered, 1st edition.
© S. Keshav and E. Culver. Published 2011 by
Blackwell Publishing Ltd.

usually non-serious, such as a Mallory–Weiss tear following prolonged retching or vomiting. The Rockall score is used to measure risk prospectively, and having coexisting renal or liver disease or cancer has been shown to confer the greatest risk of death. Other poor prognostic factors are age over 80 years, systolic blood pressure less than 100 mmHg, and continued or recent bleeding at the time of endoscopy.

10. b: Perioral freckles occur in Peutz–Jeghers syndrome, which is associated with intestinal polyposis that can cause bleeding. Dupuytren's contracture is associated with alcohol misuse and liver disease.

11. c: The Rome III consensus conference on functional bowel disorders has revised clinical criteria that allow one to make a firm positive diagnosis of IBS in patients with typical symptoms lasting over 6 months. Patients must still fulfil the *sine qua non* criterion of having no other clearly defined cause for these symptoms, and clinical or laboratory evidence of a lack of organic pathology. Anxiety and depression are associated with IBS, although the causal relationship remains unknown. Chronic symptoms could plausibly exacerbate or induce anxiety and depression. Rectal bleeding may signify inflammation or neoplasia, and the cause must be determined before a diagnosis of IBS is entertained. Anaemia, even in a menstruating female must raise the suspicion of significant organic illness such as coeliac disease, inflammatory bowel disease or peptic ulcer and gastritis. Functional bowel disorders, including non-ulcer dyspepsia may be related to IBS. However, IBS is now a specific diagnosis that must include defecatory disturbance associated with abdominal pain.

12. a: Coeliac disease is an abnormal reaction to gliadin peptides found in cereals such as wheat, rye, and barley. It is almost always associated with carriage of the HLA-DQ2 allele, which is quite common. The disease tends to run in families and family members of affected individuals should probably be screened. There is an excellent serological test for screening – the anti-TTG antibody or endomysial antibody test. Duodenal biopsy, which shows increased intraepithelial lymphocytes and may show damage to the villus epithelium, supports the diagnosis, and allows one to recommend, with confidence, the appropriate dietary restriction. For

some reason, the disease is very common in Southern and Western Europe, and is often seen in Asians, although it seems not to affect Africans. Iron deficiency is one of the earliest signs, because immune damage to the duodenum profoundly affects the ability to absorb iron.

13. b: Opiates such as morphine, codeine, fentanyl and tramadol may all cause constipation, although tramadol is least likely to do so. Metformin frequently causes diarrhoea, digoxin may cause nausea and vomiting, and Movicol is an osmotic laxative.

14. b: Bacteria such as *Escherichia coli*, *Salmonella* and *Campylobacter* species are common causes of travellers' diarrhoea. *Entamoeba coli* is a rarer, although important, cause. *Schistosoma* causes urinary and colonic infection and bleeding. *Echinococcus* is the cause of hydatid cyst disease. Rotavirus is an important cause of gastroenteritis in infants and children.

15. d: Bacteria such as *E. coli*, *Shigella* and *Campylobacter* species are common causes of bacterial dysentery that is characterised by diarrhoea and rectal bleeding. Rotavirus is an important cause of gastroenteritis in infants and children. Norovirus typically causes vomiting and diarrhoea, *Giardia* causes non-bloody diarrhoea often associated with bloating and excess wind, and dengue can cause haemorrhagic fever.

16. e: Arthralgia and arthritis occur in approximately 15% of patients with IBD. Cutaneous manifestations such as erythema nodosum, pyoderma gangrenosum and Sweet's syndrome are also relatively common. Anaemia is often found particularly in Crohn's disease. Lung disease associated with IBD is extremely rare, and does not typically cause wheezing.

17. e: Ulcerative colitis and Crohn's disease both typically cause diarrhoea, and ulcerative colitis usually causes rectal bleeding, which is not universal in Crohn's disease. Extraintestinal manifestations such as arthralgia and anaemia do not distinguish the two diseases; however, perianal abscesses and fissures are much more likely to occur as part of Crohn's disease.

18. b: There are many causes of acute pancreatitis, of which gallstones and alcohol use are the most common. Anaemia may occur in severe pancreatitis, and is not a cause.

19. d: Gallstones can obstruct the gallbladder and biliary tract, or the common duct to the pancreas, causing pancreatitis. Rarely, they may pass into the intestine and cause obstruction. Longstanding stones in the gallbladder increase the risk of cancer.

20. c: Gallstones, which are an important cause of jaundice, are readily detected on ultrasound scan, and poorly detected by X-ray. Other causes of jaundice include hepatitis and haemolysis, for which a full blood count is helpful. Dipstix may detect bilirubinuria in jaundice.

21. d: Acute and chronic liver disease can share many features, because acute liver disease can progress very rapidly in some cases. However, some features such as gynaecomastia, reduced body hair, testicular atrophy and spider naevi are more frequently found in chronic liver disease.

22. c: Ascites associated with cirrhosis is typically a transudate, with a low albumin concentration. Most other causes are exudates, although nephritic syndrome and congestive cardiac failure may also cause a transudate.

23. e: The CAGE questions are: c (cut down), b (annoyed), d (guilty) and a (eye-opener).

24. d: Colon cancer is the second commonest cause of cancer-related death, and may be completely asymptomatic. Typical symptoms include altered bowel habit, rectal bleeding and abdominal pain or discomfort. Microcytic anaemia with no apparent cause should also alert one to the possibility of a colonic tumour, while dyspepsia points to the stomach and upper intestinal tract.

25. b: The fat-soluble vitamins are A (retinoic acid), D (cholecalciferol), E (tocopherol) and K (phytomenadione). Hydroxocobalamin is vitamin B_{12}, and pyridoxine is vitamin B_6. Selenium is a metallic element, and cholesterol is a minor lipid macronutrient.

26. c: Crohn's disease typically causes weight loss and, when it affects young children, it retards growth. There is no evidence that obesity predisposes to Crohn's disease, although it does to all of the other options.

27. b: Before its classification as a *Helicobacter*, *H. pylori* was often termed a *Campylobacter*-like organism, based on its morphology. Hence the term CLO test for the commonly used urease-based colorimetric assay for *H. pylori* in gastric biopsies. The urease of *H. pylori* neutralises stomach acid locally in the stomach by producing alkaline ammonia and carbon dioxide from urea, hence its ability to survive in harsh stomach acid. Non-human *Helicobacter* species from cats, for instance, may rarely be found in the stomach, and may even cause disease. Acute infection is usually asymptomatic, and no clear syndrome has been described except experimentally when gastritis is the main feature. Drs Marshall and Warren, who shared the Nobel Prize for discovering the link with peptic ulcers, induced gastritis in themselves to demonstrate the pathogenicity of *H. pylori*.

EMQs answers

1
1. i
2. i
3. f
4. c
5. h
6. i
7. i
8. d

2
1. d
2. b
3. h
4. g
5. f
6. i
7. g
8. i

3
1. a, c, d, f, g
2. b, e, f, g, h, i
3. h
4. e, f, g, i
5. b, c, d, h
6. b, c, d, e, f, g
7. f, i
8. b, e, f, g, i

4
1. b, c, d
2. b, c, d, g

3. g
4. b, c, d
5. b, d, i
6. d, i
7. b, c, i
8. a

5
1. a, b, c, e, f, g
2. a, e
3. e, f, g
4. a, b
5. c, e, f, g
6. c, i
7. c, e, f, g, h
8. d, e, f, g

6
1. a, c, d, e
2. i
3. f, g
4. b, h
5. a, e, h
6. f
7. d, e
8. a, b, c, e

7
1. b, c, d, e, g, h
2. a, b, c, f
3. a, b, c, e, f
4. c
5. b, c, f

6. b, d, g, h
7. a, b, c, d, e, f, g, h
8. d, e, h

8
1. a, b, d, e, f, i
2. c, g, h
3. b, f, i
4. a, b, d, i
5. c, g
6. b, i
7. a, b, d, e, f, i
8. e, f

9
1. a, b, e, f, h
2. c, f, h
3. b, c, f, h, i
4. b, c, f
5. b, i
6. d, e, g
7. b, c, f, h
8. d

10
1. a, b, c, h
2. b, c, d
3. a, c, e, g
4. b
5. a
6. b, d, i
7. f, h
8. b, c

Gastroenterology: Clinical Cases Uncovered, 1st edition.
© S. Keshav and E. Culver. Published 2011 by
Blackwell Publishing Ltd.

1 Dyspepsia.

2 Eosinophilic oesophagitis. This is a well-recognised cause of dysphagia and food bolus obstruction, especially in young atopic individuals with eczema, asthma, etc. White plaques in the oesophagus may represent candidal infection, which when severe can cause odynophagia (painful swallowing) and even dysphagia. However, the plaques of candidiasis are typically surrounded by an area of inflamed mucosa where the *Candida* adheres.

3 The Rockall score for this patient is 7. The Rockall score is calculated as follows:

Rockall score (max. score 11)				
	0	**1**	**2**	**3**
Age	<60 years	60–79 years	>80 years	
Shock	None	Pulse >100 mmHg (and systolic BP >100 mmHg)	Systolic BP <100 mmHg	
Co-morbidity	None		Cardiac failure Ischaemic heart disease Major co-morbidity	Renal failure Liver failure Disseminated malignancy
Endoscopic diagnosis	Mallory–Weiss tear or no lesion *and* no sign of bleeding	All other diagnoses	Malignancy of upper GI tract	
Major stigmata of recent haemorrhage	None or dark spot only		Blood in upper GI tract Adherent clot Visible or spurting vessel	

Gastroenterology: Clinical Cases Uncovered, 1st edition.
© S. Keshav and E. Culver. Published 2011 by
Blackwell Publishing Ltd.

PART 3: SELF-ASSESSMENT

A score of 7 is the highest score before endoscopy is performed and other prognostic markers can be evaluated. It predicts a mortality risk of 50%.

4 Coeliac disease with dermatitis herpetiformis. Some patients with coeliac disease develop a characteristic vesicular rash that responds to a gluten-free diet, and is associated with the dermal deposition of anti-TTG antibodies.

5 Coeliac disease is an abnormal reactivity to gliadin peptides found in cereals such as wheat, rye and barley. It is almost always associated with carriage of the HLA-DQ2 allele, which is quite common. The disease tends to run in families and family members of affected individuals should probably be screened. Gliadin peptides from the diet interact with antigen presenting cells bearing the HLA-DQ2 protein, and stimulate T cells, which produce inflammatory mediators that damage the intestinal epithelium, causing malabsorption.

6 The great majority of cases of viral and bacterial gastroenteritis are self-limiting. The mainstay of management is supportive and in particular maintaining hydration in the acute phase. Especially in children and those who are frail, dehydration and loss of electrolytes is the greatest immediate danger.

7 IBD may be treated medically or surgically. Medical treatments include 5-aminosalicylates and immunosuppressants such as corticosteroids, thiopurines, methotrexate and anti-TNF antibodies. Antibiotics are generally ineffective unless there are particular infective complications such as abscess or perforation.

8 The Glasgow score specifies a number of features including hypoxia, hypocalcaemia, hypoglycaemia, low serum albumin, leukocytosis and raised urea and LDH concentrations.

9 Cholelithiasis refers to the presence of gallstones, which are quite common in older people; they are mainly asymptomatic and harmless. They may be associated with inflammation of the gallbladder, termed cholecystitis, or they may pass into the biliary tract, cause obstruction and infection, which is termed cholangitis.

10 Ascites due to cirrhosis is a sign of decompensated liver disease, and may precede other complications of the compromised hepatic function, such as variceal haemorrhage and encephalopathy. There is a high risk of spontaneous bacterial peritonitis in patients with ascites associated with cirrhosis. Tense ascites may also be associated with renal dysfunction and the hepatorenal syndrome.

Further reading

Allum AW, Griffin SM, Watson A, Colin-Jones D (2002) *Guidelines for the Management of Oesophageal and Gastric Cancer*. British Society of Gastroenterology, London. www.bsg.org.uk/pdf_word_docs/ogcancer.pdf.

Boon NA, Colledge NR, Davidson S, Walker BR (2006) *Davidson's Principles and Practice of Internal Medicine*, 20th edn. Churchill Livingstone, Edinburgh. Cash WJ, McConville P, McDermott E, McCormick PA, Callender ME, McDougall NI (2010) Current concepts in the assessment and treatment of hepatic encephalopathy. *Q J Med* **103**(1): 9–16.

Cerulli MA, Iqbal S (2009) Upper gastrointestinal bleeding. *Emedicine: Gastroenterology*, November.

Chey WD, Wong BY and the Practice Parameters Committee of the American College of Gastroenterology (2007) Guideline on the management of *Helicobacter pylori* infection. *Am J Gastroenterol* **102**: 1801–25.

Coeliac UK. www.coeliac.org.uk.

Day CP (2002) Non-alcoholic steatohepatitis (NASH): where are we now and where are we going? *Gut* **50**: 585–8.

Delaney BC, Qume M, Moayyedi P, *et al*. (2008) *Helicobacter pylori* test and treat versus protein pump inhibitor in the initial management of dyspepsia in primary care: multicentre randomised controlled trial (MRC-CUBE trial). *Br Med J* **336**(7645): 651–4.

Dunlop MG (2002) Guidance on large bowel surveillance for people with two first degree relatives with colorectal cancer or one first degree relative diagnosed with colorectal cancer under 45 years old. *Gut* **51** (Suppl. V): v17–20.

Fauci AS, Braunwald E, Kasper DL, *et al*. (2008) *Harrison's Principles of Internal Medicine*, 17th edn. McGraw-Hill Medical Publishing Division, USA.

Feldman M, Friedman LS, Brandt LJ (2006) *Sleisinger and Fordtran's Gastrointestinal and Liver Disease: Pathophysiology, Diagnosis, Management*, 8th edn. WB Saunders, Edinburgh.

Forrest EH, Morris AJ, Stewart S, *et al*. (2007) The Glasgow alcoholic hepatitis score identifies patients who may benefit from corticosteroids. *Gut* **56**(12): 1743–6.

Garden OJ, Rees M, Poston GJ, *et al*. (2006) Guidelines for resection of colorectal cancer liver metastases. *Gut* **55** (Suppl. III): iii1–8.

Goddard AF, James MW, McIntyre AS, Scott BB (2005) *Guidelines for the Management of Iron Deficiency Anaemia*. British Society of Gastroenterology, London. (Due to be updated 2010.)

Keshav S (2005) *The Gastrointestinal System at a Glance*, 2nd edn. Blackwell Publishing, Oxford.

Kumar P, Clark ML (2009) *Clinical Medicine*, 7th edn. WB Saunders, Edinburgh.

Leggett BA, Halliday JW, Brown NN, Bryant S, Powell LW (1990) Prevalence of haemochromatosis amongst asymptomatic Australians. *Br J Haematol* **74**: 525–30.

Lewis NN, Scott BB (2007) *BSG Guidelines for Osteoporosis in Inflammatory Bowel Disease and Coeliac Disease*. British Society of Gastroenterology, London.

Longmore M, Wilkinson I, Davidson E, Foulkes A, Mafi A (2010) *Oxford Handbook of Clinical Medicine*, 8th edn. Oxford Handbook Series. Oxford University Press, Oxford.

Malfertheiner P, Megraud F, O'Morain C, *et al*. and the European Helicobacter Study Group (EHSG) (2007) *Helicobacter pylori*: current concepts in the management of *Helicobacter pylori* infection – the Maastricht III Consensus Report. *Gut* **56**: 772–81.

Mathurin P, Louvet A, Dharancy S (2008) Treatment of severe forms of alcoholic hepatitis: where are we going? *J Gastroenterol Hepatol* **23** (Suppl. 1): S60–2.

Moore KP, Aithal GP (2006) Guidelines to the management of ascites in cirrhosis. *Gut* **55**: 1–12.

National Institute for Health and Clinical Excellence (NICE) (2004) *NICE Guidelines: Dyspepsia*. NICE, London.

National Institute for Health and Clinical Excellence (NICE) (2004) *NICE Guidelines: Eating Disorders. Core Interventions in the Treatment and Management of Anorexia Nervosa, Bulimia Nervosa and Related Eating Disorders*. Clinical Guideline No. 9. NICE, London.

National Institute for Health and Clinical Excellence (NICE) (2006) *NICE Guidelines: Obesity. Guidance on the Prevention, Identification, Assessment and Management of Overweight and Obesity in Adults and Children*. Clinical Guideline No. 43. NICE, London.

National Institute for Health and Clinical Excellence (NICE) (2007) *Palliative Photodynamic Therapy for Advanced Oesophageal Cancer.* NICE, London. www.nice.org.uk/nicemedia/live/11278/31659/31659.pdf

National Institute for Health and Clinical Excellence (NICE) (2009) *NICE Guidelines: Coeliac Disease.* NICE, London.

National Institute for Health and Clinical Excellence (NICE) (2010) *NICE Guidelines: Alcohol Use Disorders. Diagnosis and Clinical Management of Alcohol Related Physical Complications in Adults and Children (over the Age of 10 yrs).* NICE, London.

National Institute for Health and Clinical Excellence (NICE) (2011) *NICE Guidelines: Alcohol Use Disorders. Diagnosis, Assessment and Management of Harmful Drinking and Alcohol Dependence.* NICE, London. (In progress.)

National Institute for Health and Clinical Excellence (NICE) (2011) *NICE Guidelines: Colorectal Cancer.* NICE, London. (In progress.)

National Institute for Health and Clinical Excellence (NICE) (2012) *Gastrointestinal Bleeding: Management of Upper Gastrointestinal Bleeding.* NICE, London. (In progress.)

Owens MD, Warren DA (2010) *Salmonella* infection. *Emedicine: Emergency Medicine,* May.

Robinson MK (2009) Surgical treatment of obesity – weighing the facts (Editorial). *N Engl J Med* **361**: 520–1.

Royal College of Psychiatrists (RCP) (2005) *Guidelines for the Nutritional Management of Anorexia Nervosa.* Council Report CR130. RCP, London.

Scottish Intercollegiate Guidelines Network (SIGN) (2003) *Guideline 74: The management of harmful drinking and alcohol dependence in primary care. A national clinical guideline.* Scottish Intercollegiate Guidelines Network, Edinburgh. http://www.sign.ac.uk/pdf/sign74.pdf

Scottish Intercollegiate Guidelines Network (SIGN) (2006) *Management of Oesophageal and Gastric Cancer.* www.sign.ac.uk/pdf/sign87.pdf.

Scottish Intercollegiate Guidelines Network (SIGN) (2008) *Guideline 105: Management of Acute Upper and Lower Gastrointestinal Bleeding.* Scottish Intercollegiate Guidelines Network, Edinburgh. www.sign.ac.uk/pdf/qrg105.pdf

Skelly MM, James PD, Ryder SD (2001) Findings on liver biopsy to investigate abnormal liver function tests in the absence of diagnostic serology. *J Hepatol* **35**: 195–9.

Spiller R, Aziz Q, Creed F, *et al.* (2007) Guidelines on the irritable bowel syndrome: mechanisms and management. *Gut* **56**: 1770–98.

Swain S, Krause T, Laramee P, *et al.* (2010) Diagnosis and clinical management of alcohol related physical complications: summery of NICE guidance. *Br Med J* **340**: 1412–13.

Travis SPL, Ahmed T, Collier J, Steinhart AH (2005) *Pocket Consultant: Gastroenterology,* 3rd edn. Blackwell Publishing, Oxford.

UK Working Party on Acute Pancreatitis (2005) UK guidelines for the management of acute pancreatitis. *Gut* **54**: 1–9.

Williams EJ, Green J, Beckingham I, Parks R, Martin D, Lombard M (2008) *BSG Guidelines on the Management of Common Bile Duct Stones (CBDS).* British Society of Gastroenterology, London.

Index of cases by diagnosis

Upper gastrointestinal

Case 1 Dysphagia due to oesophageal carcinoma, 29

Case 2 Gastro-oesophageal reflux disease, 34

Case 3 Non-ulcer dyspepsia, 40

Case 4 *Helicobacter pylori* infection, 45

Case 5 Nausea and vomiting due to hypercalcaemia, 51

Case 6 Gastrointestinal bleeding from small bowel angiodysplasia, 56

Case 7 Coeliac disease, 63

Lower gastrointestinal

Case 8 Obstructive defecation disorder and diverticular disease, 69

Case 9 Chronic diarrhoea due to inflammatory bowel disease, 74

Case 10 *Salmonella* gastroenteritis, 80

Case 11 Colorectal carcinoma, 85

Case 12 Rectal bleeding from an anal fissure and haemorrhoids, 90

Case 13 Iron deficiency anaemia, 95

Liver disease

Case 14 Abnormal liver function tests secondary to fatty liver disease, 100

Case 15 Acute jaundice from alcoholic hepatitis, 109

Case 16 Chronic liver disease with decompensation, 115

Case 17 Ascites from cardiac failure, 120

Case 18 Alcohol dependence and withdrawal, 125

Biliary and pancreatic disease

Case 19 Gallstone disease, 131

Case 20 Acute pancreatitis and complications, 136

Nutrition

Case 21 Anorexia nervosa, 143

Case 22 Obesity and the metabolic syndrome, 148

Functional disorders

Case 23 Irritable bowel syndrome, 153

Gastroenterology: Clinical Cases Uncovered, 1st edition.

© S. Keshav and E. Culver. Published 2011 by
Blackwell Publishing Ltd.

Index

Note: page numbers in *italics* refer to figures,
those in **bold** refer to tables and boxes

abdomen
   distension 15, 18
   examination 23–4
abdominal discomfort 23
abdominal discomfort, upper 40–4, 159
   altered bowel habit 85
   causes 40, 45, 46–7
   coeliac disease 47
   colicky 131–5
   dyspepsia 47
   endoscopy 47
   examination 41–2, 46
   gallstone disease 47
   gastro-oesophageal reflux disease 47
      with heartburn 45–50
   Helicobacter pylori 46, 47–50
   history 40–1, 45, 131, 132
   peptic ulceration 46
   tests 47
abdominal pain 14, 17–18
   abdominal ultrasound 138, 139
   abdominal X-ray 138
   acute 136–42
   associated symptoms 153–4
   blood tests 138
   bowel habit 153
   causes 18, 40, 155
   chronic 153–8
   chronic diarrhoea 74
   constipation 69
   diagnosis 139
   differential diagnosis 138, 155
   examination 137, 154
   haematemesis 57
   history 17–18, 80, 120, 136–7, 153–4
   investigations 138–9
   organic disease indicators 155
abdominal quadrants *24*
abdominal swelling 120–4
   causes 120
   diagnosis 122–3
   examination 121
   history 120
   investigations 122
abdominal ultrasound 26–7
   abdominal pain 138, 139
   abnormal liver function 103
   alcohol use/abuse 129

altered bowel habit 66
ascites 122
   chronic diarrhoea 77
   dyspepsia 43
   gallstone disease 132
   jaundice 112, 113, 117
   nausea and vomiting 53
abdominal X-ray
   abdominal pain 138
   chronic diarrhoea 77
   constipation 72
   gallstone disease 132
   nausea and vomiting 82
acetaminophen *see* paracetamol
acute liver disease 161
   causes 113
acute liver failure, paracetamol-induced 12
Addison's disease 106
adrenal insufficiency 106
alanine aminotransferase (ALT) 102, 159
   abnormal levels 103–6
albumin, serum levels 102
alcohol detoxification 127, 129
alcohol use/abuse 10, 22, 125–30
   abdominal ultrasound 129
   abnormal liver function 106–7
   acute pancreatitis 139
   addiction 128
   blood tests 129
   CAGE questionnaire **125,** 161
   chest X-ray 129
   dependence 128
   ECG 129
   endoscopy 129
   examination 127
   gastritis 46
   history 125, 126–7
   investigations 129
   jaundice 110
   liver disease 113
   management 127
   neurological signs 127, **128**
   physical harm **128**
   psychological harm **128–9**
   social harm **128–9**
   withdrawal seizures 125, 127, 128, 129
alcohol withdrawal syndrome 128
alcoholic hepatitis 113, 114
alcoholism 128
5-aminosalicylate (5-ASA) 77–8
amoebal infections 9, 22

ampulla of Vater 4, 28
anaemia 95–9, 163–4
   barium contrast 97
   blood transfusions 98
   causes **96**
   coeliac disease 12, 66–7
   colonoscopy 97
   correction 98
   diet 22
   differential diagnosis 96
   endoscopy 97
   examination 96
   follow-up 98
   Helicobacter pylori infection 97
   history 95
      retaking 98
   investigations 96–7
   iron-deficiency 96, 97, 98–9, 160
   symptoms 98
   urinalysis 97
angiography, CT 61
anorectal physiology, constipation 72
anorexia 20
anorexia nervosa 106, 143–7
   complications 146
   examination 144–5
   history 143–4
   investigations 145
   management 145–6
   psychological/psychiatric treatment 146
anti-TNF-α antibodies 78, 79
antibiotics 83
anticoagulants 58, 60
antiemetics 54, 82, 159
antiendomysial antibody 76, 97
antimitochondrial antibody (AMA) test 12
antiplatelet drugs
   haematemesis 58, 60
   upper gastrointestinal bleeding 60
antispasmodics 93
α₁-antitrypsin deficiency 106
anus 4
anxiety management 73
approach to patient 14–28
arterial blood supply 1
ascites 121–4
   abdominal ultrasound 122
   autoimmune hepatitis 115
   blood tests 122
   cardiac failure 121, 123

Gastroenterology: Clinical Cases Uncovered, 1st edition. © S. Keshav and E. Culver. Published 2011 by Blackwell Publishing Ltd.

ascites (continued)
    causes **122, 123**
    chest X-ray 122
    diagnosis 122–3
    examination 121
    investigations 122
    risk factors 120–1
    treatment 123–4
ascitic tap 117, 122
    complications 123
aspartate aminotransferase (AST) 102, 159
    abnormal levels 103–6
aspirin
    erosive gastritis 97
    haematemesis 58
autoimmune hepatitis (AIH) 105, 113, 115–19
autoimmune liver disease 67, 68
autoimmunity *11*, 12
autonomic nervous system 1, *3*
azathioprine 78

bacterial infections 9, 22
    see also Helicobacter pylori
bacterial overgrowth, small bowel 26
bariatric surgery 151
barium contrast 27
    anaemia 97
    chronic diarrhoea 77
barium swallow
    dyspepsia 43
    dysphagia 31, *32*
Barrett's oesophagus **37**
belching 15, 18
benzodiazepines 127, 129
bile 4
bile duct carcinoma **134**
biliary fistula **134**
biliary obstruction 113
biliary tract disease, acute pancreatitis 139
bilirubin
    conjugated **21**
    unconjugated **21**
    urinalysis 103, 112
biofeedback for constipation 73
biological agents, Crohn's disease 78
biopsy 28
    altered bowel habit 65–6
    Crohn's disease 77
    see also liver biopsy
bisphosphonates 58
bloating 15, 18, 22
blood tests 25–6
    abdominal pain 138
    alcohol use/abuse 129
    altered bowel habit 65
    ascites 122
    chronic diarrhoea 76–7
    constipation 71
    dyspepsia 43
    gallstone disease 132
    haematemesis 56
    jaundice 112
    nausea and vomiting 82
    rectal bleeding 92
blood transfusions, anaemia 98

body mass index (BMI)
    anorexia nervosa 144
    calculation 149
    increased 148–52
botulinum toxin 73
bowel habit, altered 15, 18, 63–8
    abdominal pain 153
    abdominal ultrasound 66
    biopsy 65–6
    blood tests 65
    colonoscopy 66, 87
    diarrhoea 80
    differential diagnosis 65, 86
    endoscopy 65–6
    examination 64–5, 86
    gastroscopy 66, Plate 7.1
    histology 65–6
    history taking 64
    investigations 65–6, 85–7
    management 88
    mass lesions 87, Plate 11.1
    risk factors 86
    staging CT 87, *88*
    with weight loss 85–9
breath tests 26
Bristol stool chart *76*, 80
Budd–Chiari syndrome 113
buscopan 83

caecum 4
caffeine intake 22
CAGE questionnaire **125**, 161
cancer 12–13
    ascites risk 120–1
    familial syndromes 13
    prevention 13
    risk with coeliac disease 67
capsule endoscopy 28
    upper gastrointestinal bleeding 61
cardia adenocarcinoma 32
cardiac failure
    ascites 123
        risk 121
    treatment 124
cardiovascular examination 121
ceruloplasmin 106
chest pain 34–9
    associated symptoms 34
    endoscopy 36, **37**
    examination 35
    history taking 35
    investigations 35
    medications 35, 36
    presentation 34
    re-presentation 36
    treatment 35–6
chest X-ray
    alcohol use/abuse 129
    ascites 122
    haematemesis 56
cholangitis 133, **134**
    bacterial 134
cholecystitis **134**
cholera 8
cholestasis, medication-induced 12

cholestatic jaundice **21**, 112
chronic liver disease 161, 165
chronic obstructive pulmonary disease
        (COPD) 123
chylomicrons 6
cirrhosis 10
    ascites risk 120
    causes 116, **118**
    decompensated 116
    diagnosis 116
    hereditary haemochromatosis risk 104
    investigations 116–17
    liver disease 107
    primary biliary cirrhosis 12
    risk factors 107
    symptom palliation 117
    treatment 117–18, 119
clopidogrel, haematemesis 58
Clostridium difficile 82, 83
co-morbidity 21–2
coeliac disease *11*, 12, 22, 66–8, 160, 164
    aminotransferase elevation 106
    anaemia 66–7
    duodenal histology 66, Plate 7.1
    endomysial antibody 97
    genetic susceptibility 66
    gluten-free diet 66
    liver function 67
    malignancy risk 67
    presentation 66
    tests 65
    treatment 66–7
    upper abdominal discomfort 47
colon, blood supply 5
colon cancer 12, 13, 161
    smoking 22
colon transit studies 27, 72, *73*
colonocytes 5
colonoscopy 13, 28
    altered bowel habit 66, 87
    anaemia 97
    chronic diarrhoea 77
    constipation 72
    upper gastrointestinal bleeding 60
colorectal cancer 13, 23
colorectal disease 163
common bile duct (CBD) stones 132, 134–5
computed tomography (CT) 27
    angiography 61
    chronic diarrhoea 77
    high-resolution 28
    jaundice 117
    pancreatitis 140, *142*
    staging in altered bowel habit 87, *88*
    triple-phase 28
constipation 15, 19–20, 22, 69–73
    abdominal X-ray 72
    advice to patient 71
    aetiology 20
    anorectal physiology 72
    biopsy 72
    blood tests 71
    causes **20, 71**, 160
    colon transit studies 72, *73*
    colonoscopy 72

defecating proctogram 72
definition 85
differential diagnosis 70–1
  examination 70
  flexible sigmoidoscopy 72
  histology 72
  history 19, 69–70
  investigations 71–2
  slow transit 72–3
  spinal MRI 72
  treatment 71, 72–3
  with weight loss 85
corticosteroids
  alcoholic hepatitis 113, 114
  Crohn's disease 78, 79
Crohn's disease 12, 160
  biopsy 77
  chronic diarrhoea 76, 77–9
  diagnosis 77
  outcome 79
  relapse 79
  remission 79
  smoking 22, 77
  surgery 78
  treatment 77–9
crypts, intestinal 4
cytomegalovirus (CMV)
  abnormal ALT/AST levels 103
  hepatitis 113

dairy product intolerance 22
defecating proctogram, constipation 72
defecation 5
  difficulty 15, 20
defecation disorder 73
delirium tremens 127, 129
diarrhoea 8, 9, 15, 19
  bloody 160
  caffeine intake 22
  causes 19
  chronic 74–9
    abdominal ultrasound 77
    associated symptoms 74
    barium contrast 77
    blood tests 76–7
    colonoscopy 77
    CT 77
    differential diagnosis 75
    endoscopy 77
    examination 75
    history 74, 75
    investigations 76–7
    management 75–6
    MRI 77
    plain abdominal radiographs 77
    presentation 74
    risk factors 74
  dietary causes 22
  history 19
  with nausea and vomiting 80–4
  osmotic 8
  risk factors 19
  stool examination 26
  symptoms 19
  see also traveller's diarrhoea

diazepam 127
diet
  coeliac disease 66
  gastrointestinal pathology 22
  manipulation in obesity 150
Dieulafoy lesion 60
digestion 6–8
digestive enzymes 6, 7
diverticular disease 92–4
  management 93
diverticulitis 93
diverticulosis 93
domperidone 82, 159
  dyspepsia 42
duodenum
  anatomy 3–4
  coeliac disease 66, Plate 7.1
  function 4, 7
dysentery 9, 22
dyspepsia 42–4, 159
  causes 45
  investigations 42, 43
  management 42
  non-ulcer 47
  organic causes 42
dysphagia 14, 15, 23, 159
  abdominal examination 30
  causes 30–1
  complications 29
  differential diagnosis 30
  examination 30
  history taking 29
  investigations 31, 32
  malignancy 32–3
  management 32
  oesophageal stents 32
  predisposing factors 29–30
  progressive 29–33

eating disorders see anorexia nervosa
elastase, faecal 65
electrical impedance of body 149
electrocardiogram (ECG)
  alcohol use/abuse 129
  haematemesis 56
encephalopathy, West Haven criteria for
    grading 111
endomysial antibody 76
  coeliac disease 97
endoscope 27, 28
endoscopic retrograde
    cholangiopancreatography (ERCP) 28, 112
  cholangitis 134
  gallstone disease 133, 134
endoscopy 28
  alcohol use/abuse 129
  altered bowel habit 65–6
  anaemia 97
  chest pain 36, 37
  chronic diarrhoea 77
  dyspepsia 43
  dysphagia 31, 32
  nausea and vomiting 53
  obesity 151
  portal hypertension 117

rectal bleeding 92
  upper abdominal discomfort 47
  upper gastrointestinal bleeding 60, 61
  see also capsule endoscopy
enterocytes 4
enteroscopy 28
  upper gastrointestinal bleeding 61
Epstein–Barr virus (EBV)
  abnormal ALT/AST levels 103
  hepatitis 113
erythema nodosum 80
examination of patient 23–5
exercise 150

faecal elastase 65
faecal incontinence 15, 19
familial syndromes 23
  cancers 13
family history 23
fat, body
  distribution 149
  estimation 144, 149
fatty acids 6–7
fibre intake 22, 93
flatulence 15, 18
flexible sigmoidoscopy
  constipation 72
  nausea and vomiting 82
  rectal bleeding 92
fluorography 28
food poisoning 8
fundoplication, gastro-oesophageal reflux 37–8

gallbladder carcinoma 134
gallbladder empyema 134
gallstone disease 132–5
  abdominal ultrasound 132
  abdominal X-ray 132
  blood tests 132
  common bile duct stones 132, 134–5
  complications 133, 161
  consequences 134
  ERCP 133
  examination 132
  history 132
  investigations 132–3, 134
  jaundice 112, 113, 133
  MRCP 133
  obstructive 133, 134
  pain 131
  surgery 134, 135
  treatment 133, 134–5
  types 132
  upper abdominal discomfort 47
gastric acid reflux 13
gastric band surgery, laparoscopic 151
gastric cancer 12
gastritis
  alcohol excess 46
  erosive 97
  NSAIDs 46
gastro-oesophageal reflux 14, 17, 35, 36, 47,
    162–3
  alcohol consumption 127
  fundoplication 37–8

gastro-oesophageal reflux (continued)
  investigations prior to surgery 38
  surgery 37–8
gastroenteritis 8, 9–10, 22
  dietary causes 22
gastrointestinal bleeding 163
gastrointestinal bleeding, upper 160
  assessment 61
  cause 60
  colonoscopy 60
  differential diagnosis 59
  endoscopy 60
  investigations 61
  medications 60
  Rockall score 59
  treatment 61
gastrointestinal pathology 8–10, *11*, 12–13, 164
  diet 22
  medication-induced 22
gastrointestinal symptoms 14–21
gastroscopy, altered bowel habit 66, Plate 7.1
genitalia, examination 24
giardiasis 22
Glasgow alcoholic hepatitis score (GAHS) 113,
  114
Glasgow scoring system for pancreatitis 140
gliadin peptides 12
  antibodies 76
glucose, blood level in anorexia 143
glucose, oral rehydration solutions 8
gluten 12, 22
  sensitivity 67
gluten-free diet
  coeliac disease 66
  compliance 67
  osteoporosis 67
goblet cells 4, 5
Guillain–Barré syndrome 80–1
gums 23

H_2-receptor antagonists, dyspepsia 42
habits 22
haematemesis
  antiplatelet drugs 58
  associated symptoms 57
  blood tests 56
  cause 60
  chest X-ray 56
  confounding factors in shock 58
  differential diagnosis 60
  ECG 56
  examination 57–8
  history 57–8
  interventions 59
  medications 57–8, 60
  with melaena 56–62
  NSAIDs 57, 60
  resuscitation 56
haemochromatosis 23
haemoglobin 98
haemolysis, screening in jaundice 112
haemolytic uremic syndrome (HUS) 80
haemorrhoids, rectal bleeding 93
heartburn 14, 17
  alcohol consumption 127
  causes 45
  with upper abdominal discomfort 45–50

Helicobacter pylori 10, 161
  anaemia 97
  cancer development 13
  culture 48
  diagnosis 47–8
  eradication 13, 48–9
  histology 48
  lifestyle modifications 49
  peptic ulceration 46
  retesting 49
  serology 48
  stool antigen enzyme immunoassay 48
  tests 47–8
  treatment 49
  upper abdominal discomfort 46, 47–50
  urease breath test 26
  urease test 48
hemolytic uraemic syndrome (HUS) 82
hepatic steatosis 106–7
hepatitis
  alcoholic 113, 114
  causes 113
  see also autoimmune hepatitis (AIH);
    non-alcoholic steatohepatitis
    (NASH)
hepatitis, viral 10, 113
  abnormal ALT/AST levels 103–4
  intravenous drug use 22
hepatitis A virus 10, 113
hepatitis B virus 10, 22, 113
  abnormal ALT/AST levels 103–4
  liver cancer 12, 13
  prevention 13
  treatment 13
hepatitis C virus 10, 22, 113
  abnormal ALT/AST levels 104
hepatitis E virus 10, 113
hepatobiliary system 5–6
hepatocellular carcinoma 113
  hereditary haemochromatosis risk 104
hepatocellular jaundice **21**, 112
hepatocytes 6
hepatomegaly 111, 112, 113
hereditary haemochromatosis 104
hernial orifices 24
hiatus hernia 37
histology 28
history taking 14–21
HIV infection 22
hookworms 9
hypercalcaemia, nausea and vomiting 54
hypermotility 8
hyperparathyroidism 54–5
hypersecretion 8

ileoscopy 28
ileum 4
  function 7
imaging 26–8
immune system 1–2, *11*, 12
immunosuppressive therapy
  Crohn's disease 78
  inflammatory bowel disease 12
incomplete evacuation 15, 18, 20
incontinence *see* faecal incontinence
infections 8–10
  see also named organisms and conditions

inflammatory bowel disease 12, 160, 164
  smoking 22
  see also Crohn's disease; ulcerative colitis
infliximab, Crohn's disease 78
international normalized ratio (INR) 58
intestinal tract
  absorption 6–8
  anatomy 2–5
  blood supply 1, 4, 5
  embryology 1
  function 2–5
  immune-mediated damage 12
  inflammation 8
  lymphatic drainage 4
  nerve supply 1
  pathology 8–10, *11,* 12–13
  physiological measurements 26
  structure 1
  toxic damage 10, 12
  see also immune system
intravenous fluids, nausea and vomiting 82,
  83
investigations 25–8
iron supplementation 98
irritable bowel syndrome (IBS) 23, 155–8
  alternating pattern 155
  constipation-predominant 155, 157
  diagnosis 160
  diarrhoea-predominant 155, 157
  investigations 156
  management 156–7
  pain-predominant 155, 157
  pathophysiology 155–6
  subtypes 155, 157
  symptom management 156–7

jaundice 15, 21
  abdominal ultrasound 112, 113, 117
  with abnormal liver tests 115–19
  acute 109–14
  alcohol excess consumption 110
  blood tests 112
  causes **21**, 109–10, 161
  cholestatic **21**, 112
  CT 117
  examination 111, 115–16
  gallstone disease 112, 113, 133
  haemolysis screening 112
  hepatocellular **21**, 112
  history 21, 109–10
  investigations 112–13, 116–17
  liver biopsy 117
  management 113
  obstructive 112
  pre-hepatic **21**
  types 109, 112
jejunum 4

Kayser–Fleischer rings 106
Korsakoff's psychosis 111, 127
Kupffer cells 6

lactose breath test 26
lactose insufficiency 22
lactose intolerance 26
lactulose breath test 26
lansoprazole 42

laparotomy, surgical for upper gastrointestinal
  bleeding 61
large intestine
  anatomy 4–5
  blood supply 5
  function 5
  nerve supply 5
laxatives 71, **72**
  osmotic 93
  slow-transit constipation 72–3
LeVeen shunt 124
lifestyle changes in obesity 150
liposuction 151
lips 23
liver
  anatomy 5
  chemistry 102
  imaging 28
  specialised cells 6
  vascular damage 113
liver biopsy 28, 105
  abnormal liver function 107, 117
liver cancer 10, 12
  hepatitis B virus 12, 13
liver disease 161, 162
  acute 113, 161
  alcohol use/abuse 113
  alcoholic 10, 22
  autoimmune 67, 68
  causes 113
  chronic 161, 165
  decompensated 21, 115–19
    investigations 116–17
  diagnosis 28
  familial 23
  hepatitis viruses 10
  inherited **105**
  medication-induced 12
  necrosis 12
  see also autoimmune hepatitis (AIH);
      non-alcoholic fatty liver disease
liver failure
  acute paracetamol-induced 12
  treatment 124
liver fibrosis 116
  risk factors 107
liver function 5–6, 7
  abnormal 100–8, 165
    diagnosis 106–7
    differential diagnosis 102
    examination 101–2
    history 100–1
    investigations 102–3
    with jaundice 115–19
    malnutrition 147
  coeliac disease 67
liver function tests (LFTs) 102
liver transplantation 124
lorazepam 127

Maddrey's discriminant function 113, 114
magnetic resonance cholangiopancreatography
    (MRCP) 28, 112
  gallstone disease 133
magnetic resonance imaging (MRI) 26, 27, 28
  chronic diarrhoea 77
  spinal in constipation 72

malabsorption 7
  blood tests 65
  chronic pancreatitis 141
  coeliac disease 12
  stool examination 26
malignancy see cancer
Mallory bodies 113
malnutrition 143, 147
mass lesions
  altered bowel habit 87, Plate 11.1
  management 88
mebeverine 93
medications
  abnormal liver function 100
  acute liver failure 113
  chest pain 35, 36
  gastrointestinal disease induction 22
  haematemesis 57–8, 60
  liver damage 12
  obesity 150–1
melaena 116
  assessment 61
  with haematemesis 56–62
  investigations 61
Mental Health Act (1983) 146
mercaptopurine 78
metabolic syndrome 150
metastases, liver 113
metformin 150
metoclopramide 82, 159
micronutrient transport 6–7
milk intolerance 22
mineral deficiencies 143, **144**
Mirizzi's syndrome **134**
mouth
  anatomy 2–3
  examination 23
  function 2–3
  painful 14, 15
muscle disorders 106

Na⁺/glucose transporter 8
nausea and vomiting 14, 16–17,
    51–5
  abdominal ultrasound 53
  abdominal X-ray 82
  associated symptoms 51
  blood tests 53, 82
  causes **16–17, 53**
  complications 80–1
  with diarrhoea 80–4
  differential diagnosis 52, 82
  endoscopy 53
  examination 52–3, 81–2
  flexible sigmoidoscopy 82
  history 52, 80, 81
  hypercalcaemia 54
  investigations 53, 82
  management 53–4
  oral rehydration 54
  potassium replacement 83
  presentation 51
  rehydration 82, 83
  risk factors 81
  treatment 82–3
  urine tests 53
  see also vomiting

neoplasia 12–13
  see also cancer
neuroendocrine cells 4
non-alcoholic fatty liver disease 100–8
  causes **104–5**
  management 106
  raised ALT/AST 104
non-alcoholic steatohepatitis (NASH) 104–5,
    106–7
non-steroidal anti-inflammatory drugs
    (NSAIDs)
  abnormal liver function 100
  gastritis 46
  haematemesis 57, 60
  peptic ulceration 46
notifiable diseases, Salmonella 83
nutritional deficiency 22

obesity 148–52
  adverse events 161
  associated symptoms 149
  endoscopy 151
  estimation 149
  examination 149
  history 148
  investigations 149
  management 150–1
  medications 150–1
  risk of other diseases 150
  surgery 151
  truncal 149
odynophagia 14, 15
oesophageal cancer 13
oesophageal stents, dysphagia 32
oesophageal strictures, endoscopic dilatation 32
oesophageal varices 117
oesophagitis 13
  reflux **37**
oesophagus
  anatomy/function 2–3
  see also gastro-oesophageal reflux
oesphageal manometry 38
omeprazole 36, 37
  dyspepsia 42
  nausea and vomiting 53
oral rehydration solutions 8
  nausea and vomiting 54, 82
orlistat 150
osteoporosis, gluten-free diet 67

p53 gene mutation 13
pain
  gallstone disease 131
  swallowing 15
  see also abdominal pain
pancreas 6
  abscess **141**
  anatomy 6
  function 6, 7
  imaging 28
  necrosis **141**
  secretions 4, 6
pancreatic carcinoma, risk 142
pancreatic enzymes 4, 6
pancreatic pseudocyst 141, 142
pancreatitis 133, **134**
  acute 139–42

pancreatitis (continued)
    causes 139
    complications 141
    investigations 139–40, 141
    recurrent idiopathic 141
    severity markers 140
    treatment 140–1
  alcoholic 22
  ascites risk 121
  causes 160–1
  chronic 141
  CT imaging 140, *142*
  Glasgow scoring system 140
  hereditary 142
Paneth cells 4
paracetamol 83
  abnormal liver function 100
  acute liver failure 12, 113
parasitic infections 9, 22
parathyroid adenoma 54–5
penis, examination 24
peptic ulceration 46
percutaneous transhepatic cholangiography 134
peripheral oedema 120
peristalsis 4
  increased 8
pH studies, gastro-oesophageal reflux 38
pharynx, anatomy/function 2–3
physiological measurements 26
picolax 72
plain abdominal X-ray 27
portal hypertension 115
  endoscopy 117
potassium levels 82
potassium replacement, nausea and vomiting 83
presenting complaint 14
primary biliary cirrhosis (PBC) 12
prochlorperazine 159
proctoscopy 25
  rectal bleeding 91
prothrombin time (PT) 102
proton pump 3
proton pump inhibitors (PPIs) 36, 37
  dyspepsia 42
  haematemesis 58
  upper gastrointestinal bleeding 60
pyruvate dehydrogenase (PDH) 12

radio-isotope scanning 26
radionucleotide scanning 28
ranitidine 42
reabsorption 7–8
recreational drugs 22
rectal bleeding 15, 20, 90–4, 159
  blood tests 92
  causes 20, 92, *93*
  differential diagnosis 91
  endoscopy 92
  examination 91, **92**
  flexible sigmoidoscopy 92
  haemorrhoids 93
  history 90–1
  investigations 92
  proctoscopy 91
  rigid sigmoidoscopy 91
  symptoms 90

rectal examination 24–5
red blood cells (RBCs) 98
refeeding syndrome 127, 146
  treatment 146–7
reflux oesophagitis **37**
rehydration, nausea and vomiting 82, 83
Reiter's syndrome 80
rigid sigmoidoscopy, rectal bleeding 91
Rockall score for upper gastrointestinal
    bleeding 59
Rome III criteria for irritable bowel
    syndrome 155, 156, 157
roundworms 9
Roux-en-Y gastric bypass 151

salivary glands 2
salivation
  excess **38**
  increased 17
Salmonella enteritidis 83
Salmonella enteritis **83–4**
scrotum, examination 24
seizures, alcohol withdrawal 125, 127, 128,
    129
sepsis 81
sexual activity 22
shock
  confounding factors 58
  upper gastrointestinal bleeding 58, 60
sibutramine 150
sigmoidoscopy 25, 28
  rigid 91
  see also flexible sigmoidoscopy
skin-fold thickness 144, 149
small intestine
  anatomy 4
  angiodysplastic lesions 61, Plate 6.2
  bacterial overgrowth 26
  blood loss investigations 61
  blood supply 4
  function 4
  lymphatic drainage 4
  organisation *3*
smell sense 2
smoking 22
  Crohn's disease 77
  peptic ulceration 46
sodium ions 8
stem cells 4
steroids
  alcoholic hepatitis 113, 114
  Crohn's disease 78, 79
stomach, anatomy/function 3
stool(s)
  abnormal colour **18**
  blood mixed with 159
  examination 26, 82
  incomplete evacuation 18, 20
  loose 63, 64
  melaena 57, 116
  samples 65
  tests 26
stool chart 76, 80
swallowing, examination 23
swallowing difficulty *see* dysphagia
systemic inflammatory response syndrome 81

tapeworms 9
taste sense 2
  altered 17, **38**
teeth 2
  examination 23
tenesmus 15, 18
testes, examination 24
thiamine 127
thiopurines, Crohn's disease 78
throat examination 23
thrombocytopenia 147
thyroid disorders 106
thyroid tests 65
tiredness with altered bowel habit 63–8
tongue 2, 23
toxic damage 10, 12
tranexamic acid 61
transjugular intrahepatic portal-systemic shunt
    (TIPSS) 124
transporter proteins 6
transudates 161
travel 22–3
traveller's diarrhoea 23, 160
tuberculosis, ascites risk 121

ulcerative colitis 12, 160
  smoking 22
ultrasound 26–7
  see also abdominal ultrasound
urease breath test 26, 48
urease test 48
urinalysis, bilirubin 103, 112
urine tests 26
urobilinogen 112

veno-occlusive disease, hepatic 113
venous drainage 1
villi, intestinal 4
viral infections 9, 10
vitamin(s)
  deficiencies 143, **144**
  fat-soluble 161
vitamin K deficiency 147
vomiting
  complications 159
  melaena 56–9
  recurrent 54
  see also nausea and vomiting
von Willebrand factor (vWF), anaemia 97

waist to hip circumference ratio 149
water, intestinal absorption 8
waterbrash 17, **38**
weight gain, constipation 69
weight loss 15, 20
  with altered bowel habit 63–8, 85–9
  amount 85
  causes **20–1**
  diet 22
  obesity management 151
Wernicke's encephalopathy 111, 127, **128**
West Haven criteria for grading
    encephalopathy **111**
Wilson's disease 23, 105–6

X-rays 26, 27